Volume 33, Supplement 1,
September 2006

Transfusion Medicine and Hemotherapy

Founded in 1973 as «Die Infusionstherapie» by H. Reissigl, H. Grobecker, U. Henneberg, K.H. Bäßler
Continued by: H.-D. Viering (1973–1977), A. Grünert (1982–1992), G. Kleinberger (1982–1988), K. Widhalm (1988–1992), G. Wolfram (1990–1992), J. Eckart (1992–1997), H. Forst (1992–1997), K. Meßmer (1992–1997), K. Peter (1992–1997), K.H. Usadel (1992–1997), B. Zwißler (1995–1997), K. Gutensohn (1998–2001), V. Kretschmer (1990–2002) , W. Stangel (1992–2005), W. Dzik (1998–2005), H.G. Klein (1998–2005)

Official Organ of
German Society of Transfusion Medicine and Immunohematology

Deutsche Gesellschaft für
Transfusionsmedizin und
Immunhämatologie

DGTI

KARGER
Basel · Freiburg · Paris · London · New York ·
Bangalore · Bangkok · Singapore · Tokyo · Sydney

Impressum

Die Zeitschrift erscheint zweimonatlich; pro Jahr erscheint 1 Band zu je 6 Heften. DGTI-Mitglieder erhalten die Zeitschrift im Rahmen ihrer Mitgliedschaft. Der Bezug ist im Rahmen des Mitgliedsbeitrags abgegolten. Für den Jahrgang 33, 2006, gelten folgende Bezugspreise: Print-Abonnement EUR 157,–, Online-Abonnement EUR 157,–, Kombi-Abonnement Print/Online EUR 194,–, einschließlich MWSt., zuzüglich Postgebühren. Der Abonnementpreis ist im voraus zahlbar. Das Abonnement der Zeitschrift läuft weiter, wenn es nicht spätestens 4 Wochen vor Abschluss eines Bandes abbestellt wird. Abonnementbestellungen können bei jeder Buchhandlung oder direkt beim Verlag aufgegeben werden:

Deutschland:
S. Karger Verlag für Medizin und Naturwissenschaften GmbH
Lörracher Str. 16a
D-79115 Freiburg
Tel. +49 761 45 20 70
Fax +49 761 4 52 07 14
E-mail Information@Karger.de

Übrige Länder:
S. Karger AG
Allschwilerstr. 10
Postfach
CH-4009 Basel
Tel. +41 61 3 06 11 11
Fax +41 61 3 06 12 34
E-mail Karger@Karger.ch

Anzeigen:
S. Karger Verlag für Medizin und Naturwissenschaften GmbH
Lörracher Str. 16a
D-79115 Freiburg,
Tel. +49 761 45 20 70
Gültig ist die Preisliste Nr. 20 vom 1. Januar 2006.

Supplement 1 zu Band 33, September 2006
ISBN 10: 3-8055-8196-3
ISBN 13: 978-3-8055-8196-7

Verlagsleitung und presserechtlich verantwortlich: Sibylle Hopf
Produktionsleitung: Georg Brunner
Anzeigenleitung: Susanne Meister

Gesamtherstellung:
KONKORDIA GmbH, Bühl
Das Medienunternehmen

Bibliographische Dienste
Biological Abstracts
Current Contents/Clinical Medicine
Excerpta Medica/EMBASE
Medical Documentation Service
Reference Update
Research Alert
Science Citation Index
SCISEARCH Database

Transfusion Medicine and Hemotherapy

Transfus Med Hemother 2006;33 (suppl 1)

Supplement 1,
Vol. 33,
September 2006

39th Annual Congress of the German Society for Transfusion Medicine and Immunohematology (DGTI)

in Collaboration with the
International Society for Cellular Therapy (ISCT-Europe)

Frankfurt, September 19–22, 2006

ABSTRACTS

Editor
Erhard Seifried, Frankfurt/M.

KARGER
Basel · Freiburg · Paris · London · New York ·
Bangalore · Bangkok · Singapore · Tokyo · Sydney

Transfusion Medicine and Hemotherapy

Contents · Inhalt

Vol. 33, Supplement 1, September 2006

Continued on p. VI

KARGER

Fax +49 761 4 52 07 14
E-mail Information@Karger.de
www.karger.com

Accessible online at:
www.karger.com/tmh

Transfusion Medicine and Hemotherapy

Contents · Inhalt

Vol. 33, Supplement 1, September 2006

Transfusion Medicine and Hemotherapy

Abstracts

Transfus Med Hemother 2006;33(suppl 1):1–82

Oral Sessions

OS1: Stem Cells

OS1.1

German Registry for Stem Cell Transplantation (DRST): A National Transplant Registry as Basis for Quality Assurance and Scientific Studies

H. Schrezenmeier[1], *C. Müller*[2], *D.W. Beelen*[3], *H. Ottinger*[3]
[1]Institut für Klinische Transfusionsmedizin und Immungenetik, Ulm, D; [2]Zentrales Knochenmarkspender-Register für die Bundesrepublik Deutschland, Ulm, D; [3]Klinik für Knochenmarktransplantation, Essen, D

The German Registry for Stem Cell Transplantation ("Deutsches Register für Stammzelltransplantationen e.V.;" DRST) collects data on all hematopoietic stem cell transplantations (SCT) in Germany since 1998 in close cooperation with all German centers currently performing SCT. The DRST provides valuable early information on trends in SCT. The number of allogeneic SCT (allo SCT) in Germany increased from 1118 in the year 1998 to 1889 SCT in 2005 (first SCT only). Main indications for allo SCT in the year 2005 were acute myeloid leukemia (AML) (36% of all allo SCT), acute lymphoblastic leukemia (15.8%) and myelodysplastic syndrome (10.4%). The number of SCT for chronic myeloid leukemia declined (from 30% of all allo SCT in 1998 to only 5.6% in 2005). From 1998 to 2000 the majority of allo SCT were performed from related donors. In 2001 for the first time the number of unrelated donor SCT exceeded the related donor SCT. The unrelated transplants further increased to 1157 in 2005 (61% of all allo SCT). Peripheral blood stem cells (PBSC) are now the preferred stem cell source over bone marrow (BM). Eighty-four percent of all allo SCT performed in Germany in the year 2005 used PBSC. After a transient decrease the number of autologous SCT (auto SCT) is again continuously increasing since 2002 and reached a total number of 2615 in 2005 (first transplants only). This reflects the transplant activity for the main indications of auto SCT, i.e. multiple myeloma and Non-Hodgkins-Lymphoma, whereas number of auto SCT for solid tumors has now almost disappeared. In the period from 1998 to April 2006 the DRST has collected information on 10575 allo SCT. Among these are e.g. 3120 transplants for AML; but also number of registered SCT for rare diseases like aplastic anemia (n = 247) or immunodeficiencies (n = 104) are now noteworthy. The overall number of registered auto SCT is now 19973. The DRST has been successfully established as National Registry for SCT in Germany. Given the large number of registered transplants it provides the basis for national multi-center studies. We will give an overview on the currently registered data on SCT. This should encourage studies on a national basis to analyze the impact of e.g. conditioning regimens, donor compatibility, graft source or graft manipulation on outcome of SCT.

OS1.2

The Mitochondrial ATP Dependent K+ Channel Regulates Growth and Differentiation of Hematopoietic Cells

S. Körper, G. Baur, H. Schrezenmeier
Institut für klinische Transfusionsmedizin und Immungenetik Ulm, D

Despite the abundance of mitochondria in the cytosol of myeloid cells little is known about their physiological function in hematopoiesis. To get more insight in the role of mitochondria in myeloid cells we examined the effect of gating modifiers of the mitochondrial ATP dependent K+ channel (mitoKATP) on proliferation and differentiation on different CD34+ cells. Diazoxide is a highly selective opener of mitoKATP and depolarises the mitochondrial membrane without apoptosis induction. 5-HD blocks this channel. Depolarised mitochondria have been linked to higher clonogenity of hemoatopoietic stem cells in mouse transplantation models. Proliferation was measured in the CD34+ cell line KG-1a, the c-kit+/CD34+ cell line CS-1, and in CD34+ selected bone marrow progenitor cells (BMC). Proliferation was determined either by a cell counter or by flow cytometry with the membrane dye PKH67. Intracellular Ca2+ and mitochondrial membrane potential (MP) was measured by confocal laser scanning microscopy. Differentiation was determined by assessment of CD11c expression and morphology. Diazoxide inhibited the proliferation of the CD34+ cell lines KG-1a and CS-1. In ex-vivo expansion assays of BMC the proliferation was also inhibited (20.1 ± 4.9 fold expansion in the control vs. 12.9 ± 3.0). Cytokine depletion induced also a lower MP and growth inhibition in BMC. The growth inhibiting effect was more pronounced if CS-1 cells were stimulated by SCF. 5-HD promoted the proliferation of KG-1a and CS-1 cell lines. Diazoxide inhibited capacitive Ca2+ entry into CS-1 cells. Depletion of extracellular Ca2+ by addition of EGTA in the culture medium resulted in marked growth inhibition. 5-HD induced up-regulation of the differentiation marker CD11c in promyelocytic cell line NB-4 and in CD34+ cell line KG-1 but not in KG-1a cells, that are less mature subclones of KG-1 cells. The differentiation induction was confirmed by assessment of cell morphology. Here we provided pharmacological evidence that alteration of MP by opening or closing of mitoKATP contribute to the regulation of growth of CD34+ hematopoietic cells by the control of store operated Ca2+ entry. Such a mechanism can also be postulated for cytokine depletion in BMC. Stabilisation of MP by maintained closure of mitoKATP promoted the differentiation of hematopoietic cells.

OS1.3

Differentiation Potential of Human Lipoaspirate Derived Mesenchymal Stem Cells into Retinal Pigment Epithelium

S. Kühl, U. Vossmerbäumer, S. Kern, H. Klüter, J.B. Jonas, K. Bieback
Institut für Transfusionsmedizin und Immunologie, Mannheim, D

Purpose: Age related macular degeneration (ARMD) counts among the most frequent causes for legal blindness in the senescent population in industrialized countries. In dry ARMD retinal pigment epithelium (RPE) cells slowly perish resulting in the gradual disintegration of the retinal tissue architecture. This paves the way for an cell therapeutic approach to replace the vanishing RPE by stem or progenitor cells. We investigated the potential of lipoaspirate derived Mesenchymal Stem cells (MSC) to differentiate towards the neuroectodermal lineage into cells expressing RPE characteristics. **Methods:** MSC from human lipoaspirate were cultured in MSC medium as undifferentiated condition. Differentiation towards the RPE lineage was induced by exposure to conditioned media from porcine RPE cells, and/or Vasoactive Intestinal Peptide (VIP). The expression of RPE lineage markers like RPE 65, Bestrophin and Cytokeratin 8 and 18 was verified by immunocytochemistry. A hint for functional activity towards RPE characteristics was the formation of granula after melanocyte stimulating hormone (MSH) exposure. **Results:** Following culture of undifferentiated MSC with preconditioned medium and/or VIP, expression of the MSC marker CD90 remained nearly unaltered. In contrast, the expression of all three differentiation markers, was induced in 80.9 ± 6.3% (Bestrophin), 61.3 ± 19.6% (RPE 65) and 52.6 ± 14.4% (Cytokeratin 8/18) of the MSC. All three conditions trigger the expression of RPE specific markers with significant changes compared to primary MSC medium, neither a single one nor the combination of both factors being superior. Production of brown granules after MSH treatment further supported the notion of RPE specific transdifferentiation of MSC. **Conclusions:** We found expression of RPE specific markers in MSC derived cells upon induction with RPE conditioned medium, VIP and a combination of both. Despite the stimulated expression of RPE markers, the constant staining for CD90 seems to indicate that cells do not undergo a complete transdifferentiation but retain certain properties of their origin. Nevertheless, the attained level of differentiation seems to be sufficient to enable the formation of brown granulas stimulated by á-MSH. Further refinement of analysis could eventually point to novel

Accessible online at:
www.karger.com/tmh

options for a tissue regeneration therapy in degenerative macular disease, where perishing RPE causes severe visual impairment.

OS1.4

Two Steps to Clinical MSC without Animal Serum

C. Malischnik, K. Schallmoser, E. Rohde, W. Linkesch, G. Lanzer, D. Strunk

Medical University of Graz, A

Ex vivo expansion of multipotent mesenchymal stromal cells (MSC) is a prerequisite for evaluating their therapeutic potential in ongoing clinical trials. However, even large volumes of starting material and extended culture periods do not assure to obtain >2 × 10E6 MSC/kg/adult patient. Further limitation results from using animal serum for MSC expansion in most established protocols. We introduce a new two-step procedure to propagate >1.5 × 10E8 MSC from <5 mL bone marrow within less than 4 weeks without animal serum. We analyzed the influence of log-fold decreased MSC seeding (2,500–250–25–2.5/cm^2) on clinical scale expansion, MSC phenotype and immunomodulatory function combined with multiplex cytokine display. Maintenance of MSC characteristics was tested in CFU-F and differentiation assays. Reduced seeding density boosted MSC propagation. Low density expanded MSC were CD13+/29+/73+/90+/105+/146+/34−/45−/133−/HLA−AB+, retained their differentiation potential, and inhibited lymphocyte proliferation accompanied by deregulated cytokine production. Seeding 0.7–1 × 10E6 MSC derived from a 10 day primary culture at low density permitted propagation of 1.5–10 × 10E8 MSC within a unique 11–15 day secondary expansion step. Clinical scale expansions were even more effective with human platelet lysate substituting for bovine serum as growth factor supplement under good manufacturing practice conditions. This two-step procedure for clinical scale MSC propagation without animal serum should largely facilitate rational clinical testing of MSC based therapies.

OS1.5

Aptamer Based Isolation of Mesenchymal Stem Cells in Comparison to Plastic Adherence Method

R. Schäfer, G. Ke-Tai, A. Paul, A. Gerber, H. Northoff, G. Ziemer, H.P. Wendel

Universitätsklinikum Tübingen, D

Purpose: Adult mesenchymal stem cells (MSC) are a heterogeneous population of progenitor cells with mesenchymal differentiation potential which can be isolated by density gradient and plastic adherence and expanded in culture. Although in the focus of stem cell research for several years, there still is a lack of a distinct surface epitope pattern to characterize and isolate these progenitor cells sufficiently by antibodies in contrast to hematopoietic stem cells (CD34+, AC 133+). Here we established a new neither antibody- nor plastic adherence- based method for the isolation and enrichment of MSC. **Methods:** Aptamers are specific binding nucleic acids emerging from an in vitro selection procedure called systematic evolution of exponential enrichment (SELEX). Targeting porcine MSC we identified an aptamer that binds to porcine MSC with high affinity and specificity. **Results:** Using this specific molecule we isolated MSC from porcine bone marrow. The isolated cells were expanded and characterized in vitro evaluating their differentiation and proliferation capacity. Compared to the conventional plastic adherence method the yield of MSC (CD29+, CD44+, CD90+, CD45−) was considerabily higher (no detection of MSC after seeding 500 cells isolated by density gradient and plastic adherence vs. confluent colonies of MSC after seeding 500 cells isolated by aptamer technique) and the cells showed adaequate differentiation and proliferation capacity. **Conclusions:** This new application of aptamers can facilitate MSC isolation and enrichment greatly, thereby enhancing the rate of MSC-derived cells after in vitro differentiation for various applications in regenerative medicine.

OS1.6

Feasibility and Efficacy of Peripheral Blood Progenitor Cell Mobilisation with Pegfilgrastim for Allogeneic Stem Cell Transplantation

F. Kroschinsky[1], K. Hölig[1], R. Ordemann[1], A. Haack[1], K. Poppe-Thiede[1], M. Blechschmidt[1], G. Rall[2], M. Bornhäuser[1], C. Rutt[1], G. Ehninger[1]

[1]Universitätsklinikum Carl Gustav Carus an der TU Dresden, D; [2]DKMS Deutsche Knochenmarkspenderdatei, Tübingen, D

Short-term administration of rhG-CSF is a safe and effective procedure for mobilization of allogeneic PBPC in healthy related and unrelated donors. Pegfilgrastim (Neulasta™, Amgen Inc., Thousand Oaks, USA) is a covalent conjugate of filgrastim and polyethylene glycol with an increased elimination half-life due to decreased serum clearance. We report on 25 allogeneic PBPC donors (15 related, 10 unrelated, 16 male, 9 female), who have undergone a mobilization treatment with pegfilgrastim. The median age was 43 (range 28–74) years. Donors received a single subcutaneous injection of 2 vials (12 mg) pegfilgrastim resulting in a median dose of 161 μg/kg body weight (range 126–203). Monitoring included complete blood cell counts, number of CD34+ cells in peripheral blood (PB-CD34) and cytokine related side effects. PBPC were collected by large-volume leukaphereses (4 × blood volume) using Cobe Spectra 7.0 (Gambro BCT Inc.). Within 24 hours after pegfilgrastim administration an increase in all peripheral leukocyte subsets was observed. The maximum WBC counts were in median 7fold (range 4–14fold) higher than the baseline values and occurred in 13 donors (52%) on day 4. The maximum number of circulating CD34+ cells was found on day 5 (median 67/μL, range 10–385/μL). CD34+ cell counts on day 4 (median 61/μL, range 4–135/μL) ranged below the values of day 5 but were higher than on day 6 (median 30/μL, range 9–180/μL). All aphereses started on day 5. In 20 out of 25 donors (80%) sufficient PBPC yields were achieved by a single apheresis. The median apheresis yield was 7.50 × 10^6 CD34+ cells/kg donor weight (range 2.37–29.32), corresponding to a median of 9.30 × 10^6 CD34+ cells/kg recipient (range 3.22–39.71). Apheresis products contained in median 3.9 × 10^8 CD3+ T-cells. Bone pain and headaches were the main adverse events of mobilization, occurring in 76% and 44% of donors, respectively. Engraftment data are available from 23 patients. Stable engraftment of neutrophils occurred in 20 patients, whereas platelet reconstitution and independency from transfusions was achieved in 19 cases. Pegfilgrastim is able to mobilize a sufficient number of CD34+ PBPC for stem cell collection in allogeneic donors. Schedule for mobilization and apheresis is very similar to conventional, non-pegylated rhG-CSFs. However, the PB-CD34+ cells were found to be higher on day 4 than on day 6. Pegfilgrastim is well tolerated and side effects are similar to Filgrastim. The most important benefit for the donor is the simplified once-per-mobilization dosing. Further evaluation with respect to graft function and incidence of graft-versus-host-disease is ongoing.

OS1.7

Immunomodulatory Properties of Human Stem Cells Isolated from Adipose Tissue and Amniotic Membrane

M. Fahrner[1], S. Wolbank[1], A. Peterbauer[2], S. Hennerbichler[1], M. van Griensven[2], H. Redl[2], C. Gabriel[1]

[1]Blood Transfusion Service for Upper Austria, Linz, A; [2]Ludwig Boltzmann Institute for Experimental and Clinical Traumatology, Linz, A

Purpose: The immunomodulatory properties of mesenchymal stem cells from bone marrow have already been characterised by multiple studies. There is a body of evidence that adult stem cells can also be isolated from alternative tissue sources like adipose tissue and amniotic membrane. The immunosuppressive effect of these cells is still under investigation. In this study we present the in vitro comparison of the immunomodulatory potency of human stem cells (SC) derived from adipose tissue and amniotic membrane. **Methods:** The influence of stem cells on the stimulation of peripheral blood mononuclear cells (PBMC) by either a mitogen or an allogeneic mixed lymphocyte reaction (MLR) was examined. PBMC proliferation was assessed by BrdU incorporation. **Results:** A cell contact- and dose-dependent inhibition of PBMC responses in MLR (66 to 93% inhibition at equal amounts of SC and PBMC) and mitogen activation assays (67 to 96% inhibition at equal amounts of SC and PBMC) was demonstrated. A SC to PBMC ratio of 1 to 8 was able to significantly inhibit PBMC proliferation. While subcultivation (from passage 2 to 6) did not alter the immunoinhibitory properties cryopreservation significantly reduced the immunomodulatory potential. Additionally we observed no or at most mild alloreactions when SC were cocultured with allogeneic PBMC. **Conclusions:** In this study we could demonstrate a contact- and dose-dependent immunomodulation of human amniotic mesenchymal and epithelial cells as well as adipose derived stem cells. These cells may therefore be promising candidates for regenerative medicine and cell therapy. This work was partially supported by the European STRP project Hippocrates (NMP3-CT-2003-505758) and the Lorenz Boehler Fonds and it was carried out under the scope of the European NoE Expertissues (NMP3-CT-2004-500283).

OS1.8

High-Grade Depletion of CD45/Glycophorin-A Positive Cells Decreases the Yield of Mesenchymal Stem Cells from Human Umbilical Cord Blood

A. Dada, B. Schneider, S. Barlage, M. Marx-Müller, M. Weiss-Penzel, G. Schmitz

Klinikum der Universität Regensburg, D

Objective: Cord blood has been successfully used for hematopoetic stem cell transplantation. Mesenchymal stem cells (MSCs) are multipotent precursors for various lineages of mesenchymal tissues. The aim of this study was to inquire into umbilical cord blood as an alternative source for mesenchymal stem cells and to optimize isolation and culture conditions. Therefore we investigated wether a very efficient depletion of CD 45/glycophorin-A positive cells has an effect on yield of MSCs. **Methods:** Mononuclear cells (MNCs) were separated by negative immunodepletion of CD45+ and glycophorin-A+ cells. We used a magnetic-activated cell sorting (autoMACS) programme of very high compared to one of lower efficiency for the depletion of CD45/glycophorin-A positive cells. Isolated MNCs cells were equally cultivated under selective culture conditions. Differentiation was inducted by treatment with chondrogenic and osteogenic conditioned media. Cell differentiation was characterized by morphology, histology and immunhistochemistry. **Results:** After 6–8 weeks in culture cultured MNCs gave rise to a population which exhibited a characteristic fibroblast-like morphology and were CD105+, CD90+, CD29+, CD13+ and CD14−, CD34−, CD45−. Moreover this population could be expanded extensively. Surprisingly, when compared with the standard autoMACS programme we obtained a very poor yield of mesenchymal stem cells with no growth of the cultures separated by the high-grade depletion programme. Chondrogenesis was demonstrated by alcian blue staining and the presence of collagen II, osteogenesis by alizarin red staining and measurement of alkaline phosphatase activity. **Conclusion:** MSCs from human cord blood have capacities for chondrogenic and osteogenic differentiation and may be an ideal source for clinical application. However, a high-grade depletion of CD45/glycophorin-A positive cells using the autoMacs system dramatically decreases the yield of MSCs. Further investigations are needed to assess the role of residual CD45/glycophorinA positive cells in highly CD45/glycophorin-A depleted stem cells from human cord blood.

OS2: Immunohematology – Red Cells, Granulocytes, Platelets

OS2.1

Multi-Variant Genotyped Donor Panels in Usage for Performance Comparison of Three Commercially Available RHD/ABO Serotyping Methods

C. Gassner[1], G.F. Körmöczi[2], C. Jungbauer[3], D. Wessin[4], P. Schwind[5], H. Schennach[1], D. Schönitzer[1]

[1]Central Institute for Blood Transfusion and Immunological Department, Innsbruck, A; [2]Department of Blood Group Serology and Transfusion Medicine, Vienna, A; [3]Austrian Red Cross Blood Donation Center, Vienna, A; [4]Medical Central Laboratory, Feldkirch, A; [5]Medion Diagnostics AG, Düdingen, CH

Background: Performance evaluations of routine serological methods – usually requiring large numbers of samples – could be improved and still be simplified using predefined donor test panels. Using local blood group DNA-typing records of the last 12 years and considering knowledge about Caucasian RHD and ABO alleles and their frequencies, a Caucasian-specific donor panel was compiled. This donor panel was used for a performance comparison of three commercially available serological methods MDmulticard (Medion Diagnostics), ID-System (DiaMed) and ScanGel (BioRad). **Methods:** Samples were investigated with the methods mentioned above and retyped on DNA level. Samples consisted of standard and variant RHD and ABO phenotypes and included the following (numbers): all C/c/D/E/e permutations (20), partial Ds DNB(3), DFR(4), Rh33(1), D categories IV type IV(2), VI type I(5) VI type II(2), VII(4), weak D types 1(4), 2(5), 3(4), 4.0 or 4.1(3), 4.2(1), 5(3), 15(3), 26(2), DELs RHD(M295I)(4), RHD(IVS3 + 1G > A)(1), D neg RHD-CE(2–9)-D hybrid (8), and D neg ccDCesee (1) resulting in a 81 sample panel for D serology. For ABO, genetically defined O1O2(8), O1A2(3) and O1A"3"(3) samples were collected to interpret weak serological reactivity for blood group

A specificity. **Results:** The 81 sample panel for D serology included all regular phenotypes and all "representative" rare variants and hence reflected a much larger sample collective, than just chosen by chance. Focusing on specific results of performance for variant phenotypes, pronounced differences in reaction strengths could be observed. Exemplary results were: MDmulticard and ScanGel defined D category VII and DNB samples as weakly D+, ID-System showed regular D+. Weak D type 5 was reliably detected as D+ by MDmulticard, but only very weakly by the ID-System and ScanGel. **Conclusion:** Predefined multi-variant test panels allow for more significant performance evaluation of new serological test procedures compared to such based on sample numbers only.

OS2.2

RHD Gene Carriers among Serologically D Negative Donors: Alleles and Population Frequency in Southwest Germany

I. von Zabern[1], F.F. Wagner[2], W.A. Flegel[1]
[1]Institut für Klinische Transfusionsmedizin und Immungenetik Ulm, D;
[2]DRK Blutspendedienst NSTOB, Springe, D

Introduction: The D negative phenotype in Europeans is predominantly due to the absence of the RHD gene. Less frequently the lack of D antigen expression is associated with the presence of the RHD gene. Some serologically D neg. donors may harbor weak D types, DEL types (D positive by adsorption/ elution only) or D chimeras. Such red blood cells (RBC) units are a potential risk for anti-D immunization in D negative recipients. Materials and **Methods:** From Jan 2002 until Dec 2005 first time donors in Southwest Germany typing D negative by serological methods including the indirect antiglobulin test were tested for the presence of the RHD gene. Pools of 20 donor samples were tested for RHD intron 4 by PCR-SSP. RHD gene positive samples were further investigated by PCR-SSP and nucleotide sequencing. The DEL phenotype was determined by adsorption/elution. **Results:** Among 29,823 first time donors, 61 were RHD gene carriers. New D neg. alleles were: RHcE(1–3)–D(4–10) (n = 4), RHD(343delC) (n = 2), RHD(IVS3 + 2T > A) (n = 2), RHD (660delG) (n = 1), RHD(712delG) (n = 1), RHD(785delA) (n = 1), RHD(Y269X) (n = 1) and RHD(R318X) (n = 1). New DEL alleles were: RHD(147delA;IVS1 + 6delA) (n = 2), RHD(93–94insT) (n = 1) and RHD(L153P) (n = 1). RHD(V56M, W90X) (n = 1) was a new allele not tested for DEL. 7 alleles were known: RHD(IVS3 + 1G > A) (n = 11), RHD-CE(8–9)–D (n = 11), RHDΨ (n = 8), RHD(M295I) (n = 7), RHD(K409K) (n = 2), RHD(W16X) (n = 2) and RHD(1252–53insT) (n = 1). The molecular evaluation of 1 sample is pending. D negative types comprised 11 different alleles, DEL types 7 different alleles. No chimera was detected. **Discussion:** Among serologically D negative donors the prevalence of RHD gene carriers was 1:489, of whom 43% were DEL. DEL RBC units are potentially immunogenic and at least the transfusion to D negative girls or women of childbearing age should be avoided. Many different serologically D negative RHD alleles are encountered in Europe: 19 alleles were observed in this study and further are known. In Asians the serologically D negative phenotype is often associated with the DEL allele RHD(K409K), while the prevalent African RHDΨ and Ccdes alleles do not express D antigen: To investigate D negative carriers for the RHD gene, different diagnostic approaches may be required depending on the ethnic background of the population.

OS2.3

Prokaryotic versus Eukaryotic Recombinant Lutheran Blood Group Protein for Antibody Identification

A. Seltsam, D. Grüger, R. Blasczyk
Hannover Medical School, Hanover, D

Background: At present, identification of antibodies against high frequency antigens is reserved for reference laboratories having blood cell specimens from individuals with rare blood group phenotypes. The resulting delay in antibody detection usually prolongates the blood supply of immunized patients. Antibodies against Lub, an high frequency antigen of the Lutheran blood group system, are among the most frequent, clinically relevant antibody specificities directed against high frequency antigens. **Methods:** Soluble recombinant fusion proteins were generated consisting of the three N-terminal extracellular immunoglobulin superfamily domains of the Lutheran glycoprotein and a C-terminal V5/His-Tag. Secreted eukaryotic recombinant fusion protein was produced in stably transfected HEK293 cells and isolated and purified using Anti-V5 sepharose. The prokaryotic fusion protein was expressed in E. coli, purified by Ni-NTA and refolded by chromatographic procedures. Eight sera from anti-Lub immunized individuals, 10 anti-Lua sera, 20 sera from individuals immunized against various other blood group antigens and 100 sera from randomly selected blood donors were used for antibody screening. **Results:** The recombinant Lutheran proteins could be immunoblotted with anti-Lu monoclonal antibodies. Both eukaryotic and prokaryotic recombinant proteins specifically inhibited hemagglutination of Lub-positive red blood cells by human anti-Lub antisera, whereas the reaction of antisera directed against other blood group antigens was not inhibited. In solid phase ELISA, the antibody specificity of all anti-Lub sera tested was successfully identified with both types of proteins. While for the human anti-Lub antisera titres in the range from 1 to 16 were detectable in gel agglutination tests, antibody titres of up to 1024 could be determined by the ELISA technique. **Conclusion:** Antibody detection systems based on soluble eukaryotic or refolded prokaryotic recombinant blood group proteins have the potential to replace the current use of red blood cells for identification of alloantibodies against high or low frequency antigens. This approach brings specialized antibody diagnostics closer to routine laboratories, improving the blood supply of patients with hard to identify alloantibodies.

OS2.4

The Neutrophil Specific Antigen NB1 Is a Counterreceptor for PECAM-1 on Endothelial Cells

S. Santoso[1], U. Sachs[1], C. Andrei-Selmer[1], A. Maniar[1], T. Weis[1], T. Chavakis[2]
[1]Clinical Immunology and Transfusion Medicine, Giessen, D;
[2]Experimental Immunology Branch, Bethesda, USA

Human neutrophil specific NB1 is involved in different syndromes such as immune neutropenia, transfusion related acute lung injury (TRALI). Recent evidence indicated that NB1 transcript is strongly upregulated in bacterial infection and sepsis. However, little is known about the role of NB1. To study the function of NB1, we sought to determine the ligand of NB1 by the use of soluble recombinant NB1-Fc fusion protein. Screening with different extracellular matrix proteins failed to elicit any ligand of NB1-Fc. In contrast, flow cytometry analysis showed specific binding of NB1 to human endothelial cells (HUVEC). Immunoprecipitation of surface labelled HUVEC with soluble NB1 yielded a specific band of ~120 kDa. This band could be identified as platelet endothelial cell adhesion molecule-1 (PECAM-1) when analyzed with a panel of mabs in immunoblotting. Real-time protein-protein analysis confirmed this result. Purified PECAM-1 bound to NB1 with a Kd of 8.15×10^{-7}M. Adhesion of U937 stably expressing NB1 showed a specific binding to immobilized PECAM-1, which could be inhibited with by mab MEM 166 against NB1 as well as mabs specific for PECAM-1 (clones PECAM 1.1 and 1.2). No inhibition was observed with mabs PECAM 1.3, Gi18 and Gi34 against PECAM-1. These results indicate that NB1 interacts with domains 5 and 6 of PECAM-1.In transmigration assay, NB1 transfected cells migrated faster through HUVEC monolayer towards MCP and significant inhibition was observed in the presence of purified NB1 protein. In summary, we identified endothelial PECAM-1 as the counter receptor of neutrophil specific antigen NB1. This novel heterophilic binding opens a new concept of multistep interaction between neutrophils and endothelium; an important process of neutrophil transmigration during inflammation.

OS2.5

Further Analysis of the Molecular Structure of the Antigen in Heparin-Induced Thrombocytopenia Indicates Formation of the Antigen by Approximation of Two PF4 Molecules

A. Greinacher[1], M. Gopinadhan[1], J. Guenther[1], M. Omer-Adam[1], U. Strobel[1], T. Warkentin[2], G. Papastavrou[3], W. Weitschies[1], C. Helm[1]
[1]Ernst-Moritz-Arndt-Universität Greifswald, D; [2]McMaster University, Hamilton, CA; [3]University of Geneva, Genf, CH

Background: Heparin-induced thrombocytopenia (HIT) is induced by antibodies against platelet factor 4 (PF4) and heparin. We recently characterized the structural characteristics of these complexes by atomic force microscopy (AFM) and photon correlation spectroscopy (PCS). We now investigated why the anticoagulant fondaparinux, a pentasaccharide, induces antibodies serologically indistinguishable from those generated in patients with (HIT), as formation of the antigens in HIT on platelet factor 4 (PF4) is believed to require heparin molecules of at least 10–12 saccharide units in length. **Methods:** PF4 was purified from human platelets, the interactions of fondaparinux, low-molecular-weight and unfractionated heparin with PF4 were compared using photon correlation spectroscopy and atomic force microscopy. **Results:** PF4 alone had a height of 4 nm and a width of 26 nm. The single PF4 molecules kept a distinct distance of 10–20 nm from each other, most likely due to their strong positive charge. In the presence of UFH, LMWH and fondaparinux PF4 formed complexes of up to 200 nm hydrodynamic radius (PCS). AFM visualized polysaccharide-induced reorganization of single PF4 tetramers into linear structures of up to 150–200 nm length, with slightly reduced height compared to PF4 alone. In these complexes PF4 molecules lost their distance and showed continues surfaces. This is most likely the structural change leading to antigen formation. We then visualized binding of single IgG molecules to these neo epitopes showing for the first time a single molecule ELISA approach. **Conclusion:** The antigen in HIT is formed by charge neutralization of PF4 which allows close approximation of two PF4. HIT could be an important model for the pathomechanism of other auto-immune diseases.

OS2.6

Anti-Inflammatory Protection of the Endothelium via Heme Oxygenase-1 Gene Induction: A Novel Therapeutic Target for the Treatment of Autoimmune Hemolytic Anemia

S. Immenschuh, L.C. Andrei-Selmer, G. Bein, S. Santoso
Justus-Liebig Universität, Giessen, D

Hemolysis has fatal consequences in clinical conditions such as autoimmune hemolytic anemia (AIHA) or transfusion reactions due to the toxicity of the prooxidant heme. This heme-dependent toxicity is reflected by a local inflammation of the vascular endothelium. Heme oxygenase-1 (HO-1) as the inducible isoform of the rate-limiting enzyme of heme degradation is not only highly up-regulated by heme, but also protects against the toxic effects of this compound as well as the detrimental effects of other pro-inflammatory stimuli such as lipopolysaccharide in endothelial cells (EC). Accordingly, genetic deficiency of HO-1 in humans as well as knock out mice cause chronic damage of the endothelium. To further evaluate the protective potential of endothelial HO-1 we investigated the regulation of HO-1 gene expression via the major endothelial receptor platelet endothelial cell adhesion molecule-1 (PECAM-1, CD31). PECAM-1 is an important transducer of intracellular signaling pathways and for the present study stable cell lines expressing PECAM-1 were established. In comparison to non-transfected cell lines, PECAM-1 transfectants showed significantly higher endogenous HO-1 gene expression and HO-1 promoter activity. When PECAM-1 transfectants were exposed to the proinflammatory mediator LPS, no effect on HO-1 gene expression was detected. A marked up-regulation of HO-1, however, was observed in non-transfected cells. Vice versa, LPS induced cyclooxygenase-2 (COX-2) gene expression in PECAM-1 transfectants, but had no effect in non-transfected cells. Finally, we compared the LPS-dependent regulation of the HO-1 gene in human umbilical vein endothelial cells (HUVEC) expressing high surface PECAM-density (~800.000 molecules/cell) with monocytic cells carrying low density of PECAM-1 (~50.000 molecules/cell). While LPS did not affect HO-1 gene expression in HUVEC cells, significant up-regulation of HO-1 was detected in monocytes. Thus, comparable LPS-dependent gene regulation patterns of HO-1 were observed in HUVEC (high PECAM-1 expression) and in PECAM-1 overexpressing cells. Since AIHA is associated with endothelial inflammation the present data may suggest that HO-1 gene regulation is a novel therapeutic target for the treatment of AIHA.

OS2.7

Human Platelets Recruit Dendritic Cells via JAM-C/Mac-1 Interaction

S. Santoso[1], H. Langer[2], Kissel[1], M. Gawaz[2]
[1]Clinical Immunology and Transfusion Medicine, Giessen, D; [2]Medizinische Klinik III, Tübingen, D

Human platelets represent an important linkage among inflammation, thrombosis, and atherogenesis. Moreover, there is growing evidence regarding the importance of dendritic cells (DCs) in the pathogenesis of atherosclerosis and vulnerable coronary plaque. However, the mechanisms involved in the recruitment of circulating DCs towards vascular lesions are poorly understood. Recently, we described that platelets can recruit neutrophils by interaction via junctional adhesion molecule-C (JAM-C) on platelets and Mac-1 integrin (alphaMbeta1) on neutrophils. In this study, we investigated the molecular interaction of platelets with DCs. To test whether DCs bind to adherent platelet, adhesion assay was performed under static conditions. Isolated platelets were allowed to adhere to microtiterwell coated with collagen. Subsequently, monocyte derived DCs were added to the wells and adhesion of DCs was evaluated. Under this condition, DCs substantially adhered to immobilized platelets but not to immobilised collagen. Adhesion of DCs to platelets was dependent on the maturation status, as DCs cultivated in the presence of CD40L showed enhanced adhesion onto platelets compared to immature DCs generated in the absence of CD40L. Analysis of potential adhesive receptors on DCs showed that Mac-1 integrin is highly expressed on DCs, and this expression was enhanced in mature DCs. Moreover, alpha4beta1 integrin and PSGL-1 were substantially surface expressed on DCs. When DCs were preincubated with blocking Mac-1 antibody, adhesion of DCs to immobilized platelets was reduced significantly. Contrary, inhibition of alpha4beta1 had no effect on adhesion of DC to immobilized platelets. In order to identify the exact adhesion mechanism, we generated soluble recombinant JAM-C protein, which is known as counterreceptor of Mac-1. When soluble JAM-C was immobilized on microtiterwells specific adhesion of DCs was observed. Furthermore, preincubation of DCs with soluble JAM-C reduced DC-platelet interaction significantly. In the control experiment, soluble recombinant JAM-A showed no effect. In addition, analysis of DC-platelet interaction under arterial flow conditions showed that the rolling of mature DCs was significantly enhanced on platelets compared to the collagen as control. Preincubation with a blocking mab against PSGL significantly reduced the rolling of DCs on adherent platelets. These data indicate that PSGL-1 mediates an initial contact between DCs and platelets under arterial flow conditions. Subsequently, firm adhesion of DCs onto platelets occurs under dynamic flow conditions mediated through Mac-1 integrin binding to platelets JAM-C.

OS2.8

A New Platelet Alloantigen, Swi(a), Located on Glycoprotein Ia (Alpha2 Integrin Subunit) Identified in a Family with Fetal and Neonatal Alloimmune Thrombocytopenia

H. Kroll[1], K. Köhl[2], C. Zwingel[2], J. Hoch[3], R. Bald[4], S. Santoso[2]
[1]DRK Blutspendedienst NSTOB, Dessau, D; [2]Clinical Immunology and Transfusion Medicine, Giessen, D; [3]Institute for Transfusion Medicine and Experimental Haemostaseology, Bonn, D; [4]Clinics for Gynecology and Obstetrics, Leverkusen, D

We describe a new low frequency alloantigen, Swi(a), which was identified in a family with fetal and neonatal alloimmune thrombocytopenia. The first pregnancy was uneventful and the child born with normal platelet count. The second child was lost due to prenatal intracranial hemorrhage. During the third pregnancy, the fetus was treated with repeated intraumbilical platelet transfusions. The newborn required one further transfusion and recovered completely. Analysis of maternal serum in MAIPA assay with paternal platelets showed reactivity with integrins alphaIIbbeta3 and alpha2beta1, but not with alpha5beta1 and alpha6beta1, indicating anti-HPA-1a and an additional alloantibody against alpha2 (anti-Swi(a)). Extended family and population studies showed that 4 of 10 members of the paternal family but none of 500 unrelated blood donors were Swi(a) carriers. By immunochemical studies, the localization of the Swi(a) antigen on alpha2beta1 could be confirmed. Analysis of paternal alpha2 cDNA showed a C3389T bp substitution in exon 28 resulting in a Thr-Met amino acid substitution. Reanalysis of family members by

RFLP using Msl I endonuclease showed perfect correlation with phenotyping. There was no relation of the Swi(a) antigen to HPA-5 or -13. A Swi(a) allele-specific cDNA construct in the mammalian expression vector pMPSV was generated by site-directed mutagenesis and transfected into CHO cells. Expression of the recombinant Swi(a) antigen on CHO cells was confirmed by immunoprecipitation and MAIPA assay. Swi(a) platelets showed a normal aggregation response to collagen and other standard agonists. Adhesion of CHO cells expressing recombinant Swi(a) to immobilized collagen was not impaired compared to wild type controls. Furthermore, anti-Swi(a) did not influence the adhesion onto collagen. B-cells from a Swi(a) individual were immortalized by EBV transfection. In summary, we report the third alloantigen on alpha2, Swi(a). Inclusion into the HPA-nomenclature is proposed.

OS3: Best of Abstracts

OS3.1

Pharmacogenetics of Oral Anticoagulation – VKORC1-Haplotypes Determine the Inter-Individual and Inter-Ethnical Variability

C. Geisen[1], M. Watzka[2], K. Sittinger[1], B. Luxembourg[3], M. Steffens[4], C.R. Müller[5], T.F Wienker[2], E. Lindhoff-Last[3], E. Seifried[1], J. Oldenburg[2]

[1]DRK Blutspendedienst BW-Hessen, Frankfurt, D; [2]Institut für Exp. Hämatologie und Transfusionsmedizin, Bonn, D; [3]Medizinische Klinik III, Frankfurt am Main, D; [4]Institut für Medizinische Biometrie, Bonn, D; [5]Institut für Humangenetik, Würzburg, D

Purpose: Coumarins are known for their high inter-individual and inter-ethnical variability of the dose-response association (i.e. significant higher maintenance dose in Africans and lower dose in Chinese). Recently, common SNPs of the VKORC1 gene (encoding the molecular target of coumarins, vitamin K epoxide reductase) were shown to be associated with lower warfarin dose requirement (c.−1639G > A [rs17878363], c.173 + 1000C > T [rs9934438]). In order to clarify whether these SNPs are part of more extended haplotypes, we established a comprehensive haplotype map of the entire VKORC1 gene locus. VKORC1-haplotype association with coumarin dose requirement was analysed in different ethnical populations and patient cohorts. **Methods:** In 200 german blood donors the VKORC1 gene locus was analysed by direct sequencing. VKORC1 genotype data in 7 additional populations from Africa, Asia and Europe were retrieved from internet databases. Haplotype frequencies were inferred using EHplus and FAMHAP. Unselected patients receiving phenprocoumon (n = 61) and patient cohorts of European origin with either increased coumarin sensitivity (n = 14, weekly phenprocoumon dose <6 mg) or partial coumarin resistance (n = 36, weekly phenprocoumon/warfarin dose >42/>70 mg) were typed for VKORC1 haplotypes. **Results:** In 200 controls we identified 28 SNPs within the VKORC1 gene. 6 SNPs formed 3 main haplotypes covering more than 99% of the genetic variability of VKORC1 (VKORC1*2: 42%, VKORC1*3: 38%, and VKORC1*4: 20%). SNPs associated with low warfarin dose (rs17878363, rs9934438) were in complete linkage disequilibrium with the VKORC1*2 haplotype. Haplotype frequency in Africans and Chinese differed significantly from the European sample (for VKORC1*2: Europeans 42%, Chinese 95%, Africans 14%). In 61 unselected patients receiving phenprocoumon c.−1639AA genotype patients (homozygous VKORC1*2) required less phenprocoumon (1.40 mg/d) than AG (2.12 mg/d) and GG patients (3.02 mg/d). 13 of 14 patients (93%) with increased coumarin sensitivity but none of the patients with partial coumarin resistance were c.−1639AA. Vice versa, the c.−1639G allele (present in the non VKORC1*2 haplotypes) was found homozygous in 31 patients (86%) with partial coumarin resistance but in none of the patients with increased coumarin sensitivity. **Conclusions:** Three main haplotypes represent more than 99% of VKORC1's genetic variability in Europeans. VKORC1 haplotypes are strongly associated with the inter-individual and inter-ethnical variability of oral anticoagulation. In future studies, VKORC1-haplotype testing may provide a clinically relevant predictor of coumarin dosing and bleeding risk in oral anticoagulation.

OS3.2

The Novel Immunophilin-Binding Agent Sanglifehrin A Blocks Key Dendritic Cell Functions in vivo and Exhibits Synergy with Cyclosporine A

H. Hackstein, C. Steinschulte, S. Fiedel, V. Rathke, H. Hölschermann, G. Bein

Justus Liebig Universität Giessen, D

The immunophilin-ligands cyclosporine A (CsA), FK506 and rapamycin have revolutionized clinical immunosuppressive therapy. Sanglifehrin A (SFA) is a novel compound with unsurpassed cyclophilin-binding affinity but relatively low direct activity against lymphocytes. Here, we report for the first time on the capacity of SFA to impact on key DC functions in vivo and to inhibit acute and chronic heart allograft rejection. By using independent in vivo models, we provide evidence that SFA profoundly decreases DC receptor-mediated endocytosis, DC macropinocytosis and targets DC-T cell allostimulatory activity. Furthermore, SFA abrogates >90% of IL-12p70 production in vivo while having no effect on IL-10 and TNF-á. In a rat heart transplant model, animals rejected within 23 days after low-dose CsA, whereas addition of SFA promoted long-term (mean graft survival 82 days; p = 0.0007) graft survival. With respect to chronic rejection, SFA + CsA almost completely prevented graft arteriosclerosis compared to animals treated with CsA alone and controls. These results are the first to reveal the immunosuppressive activity of SFA in vivo. We propose that SFA represents a novel class of immunophilin-binding immunosuppressants with high activity against DCs and profound synergy with CsA.

OS3.3

Nonhuman Primate (Callithrix jacchus) Hematopoietic and Embryonic Stem Cells are Efficiently Transduced Using Foamyvirus Vectors

P.A. Horn[1], M. Wurm[2], K. Tani[3], D. Lindemann[4], E. Sasaki[5], R. Blasczyk[1], H. Hanenberg[2]

[1]Medizinische Hochschule Hannover, D; [2]Heinrich Heine University, Düsseldorf, D; [3]Medical Institute of Bioregulation, Fukuoka, JP; [4]University Hospital Dresden, D; [5]Central Institute for Experimental Animals, Kawasaki, JP

Purpose: Genetic modification of adult and embryonic stem cells will advance the use of stem cell based regenerative treatments. Preclinical large animal models are important tools for evaluating the safety and therapeutic efficacy of such new therapeutic modalities. Currently, no data on the transduction efficiency of foamyviral vectors for the transduction of nonhuman primate stem cells exists. **Methods:** We performed a direct comparison using gammaretroviral, lentiviral and foamyviral vector constructs on hematopoietic (HSC) and embryonic stem cells (ESC) from the common marmoset (Callithrix jacchus). All vectors were pseudotyped with a modified prototype foamy virus (PFV) Env and the lentiviral vector additionally with VSV-G. **Results:** Foamyviral vectors typed with the foamyviral envelope were the most efficient gene transfer tool for marmoset hematopoietic CD34-positive cells with stable transduction rates of over 80% as assessed in cells from liquid cultures by flow cytometry at 2 and 7 days after transduction and on average 88% transduction efficiency into colony forming cells (CFU-C). Transduction of CFU-C with the other vectors was always below 60%. In ESC, initial gene transfer rates of over 80% were achieved with the VSV-G pseudotype lentiviral vector, however, expression decreased to 13% after 7 days. In contrast, the foamyviral vector decreased only from 49% to 24% after 7 days. **Conclusions:** We achieved stable viral gene transfer and expression in ESC as well as highly efficient gene transfer into common marmoset hematopoietic CD34 positive cells using foamyviral vectors. These results suggest that foamyviral vectors may be highly feasible vectors for stem cell gene transfer and thus set the stage for a more detailed analysis of this vector system in transplantation studies in this nonhuman primate model.

OS3.4

Clinical HIT and HIT-Antibody Seroconversion in Trauma Patients Receiving Unfractionated Heparin vs. Certoparin: A Randomised, Double-Blind Study

N. Lubenow, P. Hinz, T. Lietz, A. Ladwig, M. Jünger, A. Ekkernkamp, A. Greinacher
Universität Greifswald, D

Introduction: Heparin-induced thrombocytopenia (HIT) is a severe adverse effect of heparin treatment. We prospectively assessed the frequency of HIT in trauma surgery patients receiving low-molecular-weight-heparin (LMWH) or unfractionated heparin (UFH). **Methods:** In this double-blind study, trauma patients were randomised to receive the LMWH certoparin (Mono-Embolex, Novartis) or UFH for thrombosis prophylaxis. Primary endpoint was HIT-antibody seroconversion after day 5 of heparin medication. A functional test (HIPA) and an ELISA were used for HIT-antibody detection. Secondary endpoints were the frequency of clinical HIT and the occurence of thromboses related to the two heparins used. Daily platelet counts and a lower limb ultrasound examination on discharge were performed. Patients were followed up for 3 months. **Results:** 295 (48.4%) LMWH and 314 (51.6%) UFH-treated patients were evaluable per protocol. Seroconversion occurred in 5 (1.7%) of the patients treated with LMWH and 21 (6.7%) of the patients treated with UFH (p = 0.002). Clinical HIT occurred in 1 (0.3%, LMWH) and 4 (1.3%, UFH) patients, respectively. Neither clinically relevant thromboembolic complications (TEC) nor all TECs differed (11 (3.7%) vs 9 (2.9%), p = 0.551; 23 (7.8%) vs 21 (6.7%, p = 0.597). Outcome after 3 months regarding TECs was also no different between the two groups. **Discussion:** In trauma patients HIT-antibodies are induced less frequently using LMWH for thrombosis prophylaxis as compared to UFH, and numerically less clinical HIT (1 (0.3%) vs 4 (1.3%) cases) occurred with LMWH. Symptomatic and proximal deep vein thromboses occurred at the same frequencies. Certoparin is safer than UFH in trauma surgery as it induces HIT less frequently.

OS3.5

Mechanism of Immunosuppression by Mesenchymal Stem Cells of Normal Adults and Aplastic Anemia Patients

V. Mailänder, E. Hennel, M. Rojewski, M. Wiesneth, H. Schrezenmeier
Universität Ulm – Institut für klinische Transfusionsmedizin und Immunogenetik, Ulm, D

Purpose: Mesenchymal stem cells (MSC) are increasingly used for therapy of GvHD or immunosuppression in autoimmune diseases. It was hypothesized that MSC from aplastic anemia patients are less immunosuppressive thus allowing immunoreaction against autologous hematopoesis. While the immunosuppressive effect of healthy MSC can be demonstrated in vitro and in vivo models as well as in clinical studies there is uncertainty about the mechanism. **Methods and Results:** MSC from bone marrow were characterized by FACS (CD9+, CD44+, CD105+, CD34−, CD45−) and differentiation assays. In a standard mixed lymphocyte reaction (MLR) MSC in a ratio of 1:1 to the responder cells clearly suppressed the MLR reaction (80–100% reduction of proliferation). A 1:10 ratio of MSC:responders was not effective in most experiments and at a 1:100 ratio we never observed a suppressive effect. MSC from patients with aplastic anemia were studied for their immosuppressive potential. In all experiments (n = 5) suppression of proliferation was observed contrary to the results of other groups (Bacigalupo A et al. Exp Hematol. 2005;33:819). In experiments with MSC supernatant we did not find any suppressive effect. In contrast there was some effect when we put the MSC in a transwell system (roughly 50% suppression of proliferation). Data in the literature on the mechanism are very controversial. Among others it was proposed that prostaglandin mediates the effect. However by inhibition of prostaglandin synthesis with indomethacin and NS398 we could not reduce the MLR-suppressive effect of MSC. Currently we are investigating whether depletion of tryptophan plays an important role. **Conclusions:** Immunosuppression by MSC of normal adults and aplastic anemia patients can be detected in direct cell-cell contact and in transwell experiments while no effect of MSC supernatant was seen. The mechanism of immunosuppression is not fully understood and further investigations are needed.

OS3.6

Granulocyte Apheresis Donors: The Impact of Hydroxyethyl Starch on Blood Coagulation

G. Stiegler, V. Kolovratova, G. Leitner, P. Höcker
Medizinische Universität Wien, A

Purpose: High molecular weight Hydroxyethyl Starch (HES) is used as sedimentation agent in granulocyte apheresis for achieving satisfying granulocyte yields due to its ability to coat red blood cells (RBC) leading to improved separation of RBCs and granulocytes. HES is known to impair blood coagulation and platelet function. Our primary aim was to investigate the effect of HES on donors thrombelastography and plasma coagulation. Secondary, the impact of granulocyte apheresis on donors blood counts, calcium, and fibrinogen was studied. **Methods:** 44 healthy donors (f/m = 7/37) underwent granulocyte collection (processed blood volume 6557 mL, ±430) with the Cobe Spectra (Gambro). Instead of ACD-A, 500 ml HES 6% (450 kd, Plasmasteril) and 30 mL 46.7% Natrium citrate were used as anticoagulant. Blood samples were taken before and after apheresis (blood count, natrium, potassium, calcium, PTT, fibrinogen). Whole blood clot formation profiles were measured with the Thrombelostograph Rotem (Pentapharm). The Mann-Whitney-U-Test was applied. **Results:** We observed decreased clot strength after apheresis (before 59 mm, ±4; after 53 mm, ±6; p = 1.3–5) and a compromised prothrombin time (before 95%, ±16; after 79%, ±15; p = 1.9–5). The other coagulation parameters remained unchanged. The number of red and white blood cells, and platelets was significantly decreased after apheresis. Levels of calcium (before 1.17 mmol/L, ±0.05; after 0.95 mmol/L, ±0.09; p = 3.9–10) and fibrinogen (before 315 mg/dL, ±64; after 249 mg/dL, ±59; p = 7.0–4) were reduced. **Conclusions:** HES induces transient hypocoagulation as reflected by impaired clot firmness and decreased prothrombin time after granulocyte collection. However, our donors did not report any bleeding events after apheresis. Nevertheless, this observation has to be taken into consideration for donors safety issues. Repeatedly granulocyte collections may lead to clinical significant impaired blood coagulation due to the coagulation-compromising effect of HES. Consecutive apheresis procedures of patients' relatives may aggravate this effect because of the loss of platelets, fibrinogen, and calcium.

OS3.7

Topical Use of Autologous Platelets in Maxillofacial Surgery Does Not Improve Bone Formation. Results of a Prospective Controlled Trail

K. Heidinger
Institute of Clinical Immunology and Transfusion Medicine, Giessen, D

Purpose: In order to enhance wound healing and formation of new bone, attempts were made to release peptide growth factors by the use of topically administered autologous platelets. We conducted a clinical, bicenter, randomized, prospective and controlled trial to prove the effect of platelets on wound healing and bone grafting in patients undergoing maxillofacial procedures. **Methods:** The trial has been set up as a two-center-study in Giessen and Erlangen. 53 patients were included who needed osteoplastic bone graft for sinusfloor augmentation prior to implant placement. Autologous platelet concentrate (APC) was obtained from platelet rich plasma (PRP) derived from 450 ml of CPD anticoagulated blood. After storage for 24 hours, PRP was concentrated and adjusted to 1010 platelets per ml. Platelet gel was generated intraoperatively from 3 ml platelet suspension by the use of 0.5 ml 10% calcium gluconat and 0.5 ml autologous native blood. This mixture was added to approximately 3 cm^3 autologous bone graft. Operation procedure was performed in every patient group by standardized protocol. The intervention group was additionally treated intraoperatively with local application of APC. Panoramic radiographics, computerized tomography and bone biopsy were taken 4 months later. **Results:** Histological evaluation of biopsy revealed numerous areas of osteoid and bone formation without evidence of inflammatory cell infiltrate. The bone volume reached 31% in the group with APC and 35% in the group without APC. Osteoid volume showed 6.1% in the APC group versus 6.5% in the group without APC. Results of CT-scans revealed −115 Houndsfield-Units (HU) in the group with APC (−105 HU in the control group) showing remarkably dense bone in sufficient quantity without any difference between both groups. **Conclusions:** Final data of the prospective controlled trial show that topical use of APC does not significantly improve osteoid bone formation in the maxilla compared to conventional treated patients.

OS3.8

CMV DNA and Detection of Infectious Virus: Loss of Infectivity during Storage at −30°C

H. Hennig[1], S. Hartz[1], K. Hamprecht[2], A. Unmack[1], M. Ziemann[1], S. Görg[1], H. Kirchner[1]

[1]Universität zu Lübeck, D; [2]Universität Tübingen, D

Purpose: The detection of Human Cytomegalovirus (CMV) DNA in human plasma is associated with an active CMV infection, but it is not evidence for the presence of infectious virus particles. We found a high prevalence of CMV-DNA at low levels in plasma of regular blood donors in connection with sero-conversion. The aim of this study was to correlate CMV DNA concentration and quantification of infectious CMV. Furthermore, the stability of CMV under laboratory and blood bank conditions was investigated. **Methods:** CMV strain AD169 was multiplied in human foreskin fibroblasts (HFF). Infectivity of virus lysate was tested by semilogarythmic titration and immunoperoxidase staining for CMV pp72 immediate-early antigen expression in HFF on day 7 after infection. CMV DNA was quantified using a newly developed TaqMan PCR. **Results:** A virus lysate containing 7.9 × 10e6 genome equivalents (geq) CMV DNA per ml showed an infectivity of 1.9 × 10e3 × ID-50 in our culture system. This suggested that at least 4 × 10e3 geq CMV DNA per ml would be necessary to infect every second culture. Fresh-frozen plasma (FFP, n = 4) which contained 130–600 (mean 360) geq CMV DNA per ml were tested negative for infectious virus in more than 2,300 HFF cultures. Further experiments on storage of virus lysate showed a reduction of infectivity after storage for 6 hours at room temperature as well as after storage for 7 days at −30°C. **Conclusions:** In comparison to CMV DNA levels which we normally found in FFP, higher concentrations seem to be necessary to infect HFF cultures in our system. Quarantine storage of CMV-containing FFP at −30°C probably leads to a significant loss of infectivity.

OS4: Plasmapheresis

OS4.1

The Second Vaccination in a Hyperimmunization Program for the Production of Plasma for Special Purposes with High Anti-Hbs-Antibody Levels

E. Ulrich[1], M. Lefmann[2], K. Krause[3]

[1]Haema AG, Dresden, D; [2]Haema AG, Berlin, D; [3]Haema AG, Leipzig, D

We perform a hyperimmunization program since 2004 in order to produce plasma for special purposes with high anti-Hbs-levels. 102 donors (80 male/22 female) were included. 51 (37 male/14 female) donors received a second vaccination with a combined hepatitis A (HAV) and B (HBV) vaccine (Twinrix® for adults) in conformity to the vote of the local ethic committee. All participants gave informed consent.Target was the investigation of the antibody levels before and after second vaccination and the analysis of drop outs. The anti-Hbs-antibody-levels were measured with the Abbott Axsym Anti-Hbs-EIA. **Results:** 96% of the 51 donors developed necessary anti-Hbs-levels of more than 50 IU/ml during the second vaccination. 9.8% of them had not enough anti-HBs after the first vaccination but developed necessary levels during the second one. 3.9% showed no response to the second vaccination. No side effects were observed during the program.

Table 1. Development of anti-Hbs-levels due to second vaccination

Anti-Hbs-level before 2. vaccination	Anti-Hbs-level after second vaccination
(MW ± SD) [IU/ml]	(MW ± SD) [IU/ml]
72.29207 ± 80.9841	105.88376 ± 84.0253
Median: 40.441	Median: 86.541

Table 2. Analysis of drop out reasons

Drop out reasons (number of donors n = 51 out of 102*)				
> 6 month not present/no donation	Other reasons	Incompliance	Own wish of the donor	Non responder
n = 12	n = 4	n = 4	n = 6	n = 1

*n = 24 gave no information up to now

During the second vaccination we found a higher response (96%) than in the first vaccination (60%) [1]. Between 2004 und 2006 we had a loss of 50% of participants mostly because of social-cultural reasons. The hyperimmunization program with the combined HBV/HAV-vaccine is successful and can be considered as safe.

1 Ulrich E, Mehl M, Krause K: Production of plasma for special purposes with high level of anti-Hbs-antibodies. Transfusion Medicine and Haemotherapy 32(suppl 1):26, 2005.

OS4.2

Comparison of Side Effects during Plasmapheresis with and without Saline Substitution.

K. Wolter[1], P. Prusa[2], S. Schmid[2]

[1]Baxter Healthcare SA, Wallisellen (Schweiz); [2]Baxter AG, Wien

Purpose: The substitution of plasma volume by sodium-chloride solution is a common and widespread practice in automated plasmapheresis. However, scientific evidence for its beneficial impact on donor safety is lacking. Some facilities refrain from using the common substitution protocol of saline solution after plasma donation and have not reported any increase in the occurrence of side effects. We investigated the influence of a modified plasmapheresis protocol and the resulting effects in regards to circulatory side effects ("mild" with dizziness, vertigo, anaemic pallor, nausea, blood pressure systolic >80 mmHg, "medium" with dizziness, vertigo, anaemic pallor, nausea, blood pressure systolic >70 mmHg, tachycardia 90–110 HR, bradykardia 40–50 HR, "severe" with vomitus, unconsciousness, hypoxia, blood pressure systolic <70 mmHg, tachycardia >110 HR, bradykardia <40 HR.) **Methods:** Over a period of 11 month (10/04–09/05) the influence of volume substitution by sodium-chloride solution (0.9% Sodium Chloride, 500 ml, Baxter) after automated plasmapheresis (collection volume 600–850 ml including anti coagulant) with Baxter Autopheresis-C APC 6.0, Model A-200 was observed in a plasmapheresis facility in Austria. During a period of 6 month 23492 donations were collected without saline substitution. The most occurring side effect circulatory collapse (including dizziness, vertigo, anaemic pallor, nausea) was compared to the occurrence of the same side effects during a 3 month control period (11264 donations) with saline substitution. The study was conducted under the supervision of the facility Head Physician and in accordance with EU and Austrian regulations. All donors volunteered and signed an informed consent. The non-saline protocol is a licensed procedure in Europe. **Results:** During the study period 11264 donations from 1436 donors (56% male, age ranging between 18–65 years) were collected using saline substitution and compared with 23492 donations from 1939 donors (55% male, age ranging between 18–65 years) collected under the saline substitution procedure. The total incidence of documented circulatory side effects was 1.18% (278) without, and 0.99% (111) with saline substitution after plasma donation. However, analysis of variances and frequencies resulted in no significant differences (Table 1.) for total and medium side effects. Due to the low incidence of severe side effects a valid statistical analyses could not be conducted. Graph 1: Boxplot of frequencies of occurance of vaso-vagal side effects in regards to saline substitution vs. no substitution (with • = mean). **Conclusion:** Although the volume substitution after automated plasmapheresis is not mandatory [1] saline substitution reflects the most common practice. Circulatory collapse represents the most frequent side effect during automated plasmapheresis. However, scientific evidence for the beneficial impact on donor safety and well being of saline substitution is not sufficient [2]. Data are available for therapeutic LDL-apheresis [3]. During our investigation no statistically significant differences in regards to variances and frequencies of total circulatory side effects could be demonstrated.

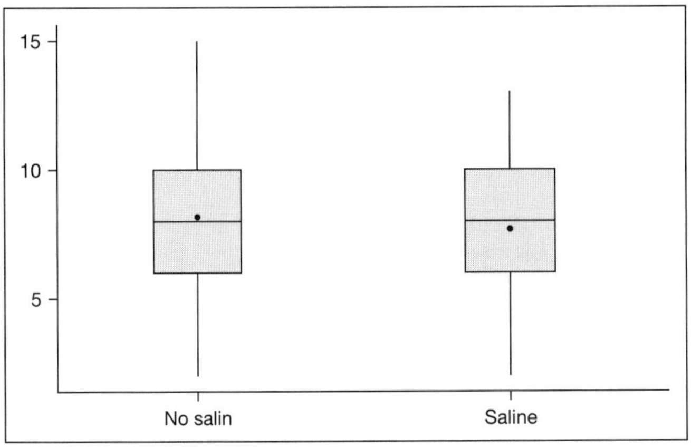

1 Baxter Healthcare Corp., Fenwal DivisionSRD-Operating Menus FE932-SRD-1505–2.0
2 Transfusion and apheresis science: official journal of the World Apheresis Association: official journal of the European Society for Haemapheresis, Vol. 32 (3), p: 283–6, 2005. Haemapheresis activities in Germany. Moog R.
3 Therapeutic apheresis and dialysis: official peer-reviewed journal of the International Society for Apheresis, the Japanese Society for Apheresis, the Japanese Society for Dialysis Therapy, Vol. 7 (4), p: 382–90, 2003. Low-density lipoprotein apheresis: an overview. Bambauer R; Schiel R; Latza R.

OS4.3

Berufliche Fremdblutexposition (FBE) in Plasmapheresezentren: Infektionsrisiko & Management

U. Diekamp
Humanplasma Deutschland GmbH, Bremen, D

FBE von Mitarbeitern durch Nadelstichverletzung (NSV) und Schleimhautkontamination (SHK) bedürfen eines Maßnahmeplans zur Infektionsrisikominimierung. Wichtige Infektionsrisiken nach Sarrazin treffen für diese Mitarbeiter oft zu: tiefe Stichverletzung, sichtbares Blut an verletzender Nadel, Kanüle zuvor in Vene der Indexperson (Sarrazin et al. Dtsch Ärztebl 2005; 102: A2234–9). Wir zeigen Daten zu NSV und SHK in 6 Plasmazentren von 2001 bis 2005 und empfehlen Maßnahmen. **Methoden:** Bei FBE unterscheiden wir NSV von SHK, vorgetestete oder nicht vorgetestete identifizierte von nicht identifizierter Indexperson. FBE-Daten entnehmen wir dem berufsgenossenschaftlichen Verbandsbuch und der Datei "besondere Vorkommnisse". Die EDV ermittelt die Anzahl der Punktionen (Spenden, Laborprobenentnahmen und Umpunktionen). Aus Mitarbeiterzahl und -beschäftigungsdauer errechnen wir Expositions-inzidenz pro Spenden, pro Mitarbeiterjahre und pro Punktionen. **Ergebnisse:** Wir finden 77 FBE, 54 NSV und 23 SHK und identifizieren 63 (82%) der Indexpersonen; bei 14 NSV-Fällen (26%) verletzt man sich an einer nicht zuordnungsfähigen Nadel (z.B. im Entsorgungsbereich). FBE betreffen 57 von 168 Mitarbeitern (34%), zu 51% nicht punktierendes Personal. Bei insgesamt 259 Jahren Beschäftigungsdauer registrieren wir 0,30 NSV/SHK pro Mitarbeiterjahr (bei nicht punktierendem Personal 1 NSV/SHK in 0,54 Mitarbeiterjahren). Bei 738.720 Punktionen kommt 1 NSV/SHK auf 9.595 Punktionen. 5,2% der Punktionen betreffen ungetestete Spendewillige. 4,8% der NSV betreffen ungetestete Indexpersonen. Gleichzeitig finden wir 33 HBV-, 15 HCV- bzw. 3 HIV-bestätigt reaktive unter ungetesteten Spendewilligen und 3 Serokonversionen, entsprechend 1 auf 760 Punktionen bei zuvor Ungetesteten und 1 auf 246.000 Punktionen bei Vorgetesteten. **Diskussion:** NSV/SHK sind meldepflichtige Arbeitsunfälle. 2002 arbeiten in Plasmapheresestationen 735 Ärzte und Entnahmepersonal (0,33% der im Gesundheitswesen mit NSV-/SHK-gefährdeten Aktivitäten Befassten). Infektions- & Erkrankungsrisiken sind am größten bei den ca. 5% zuvor ungetesteten Spendewilligen. Alle Mitarbeiter sind HBV-geimpft. Wir empfehlen postexpositionelle Prophylaxe nach Exposition ungeschützter Mitarbeiter zu Blut/Plasma von bekannt HIV- oder HBV-Infizierten. Bei HCV ist Prophylaxe erst bei symptomatischer Infektion angezeigt.

OS4.4

Haemodynamics of Vasovagal Reactions – Case Report of a Plasmapheresis Donor

R. Karger, M. Halbe, V. Kretschmer
Philipps-Universität Marburg, D

Background: Although vasovagal reactions are common in blood donors, the pathophysiological mechanisms leading to such reactions are only incompletely understood. **Methods:** In a prospective study, parameters of BV regulation were recorded in plasmapheresis (PP) donors undergoing PP using Haemonetics PCS2® machines. Haemodynamic parameters were determined non-invasively employing thoracic bioimpedance (GE Medical). In a control investigation, donors were kept in reclined donation position for the duration of a PP session without actually donating. We report on a male 34-year-old study participant who developed a cardiovascular reaction during his 15th PP. **Results:** During the first half of the donation, i.e. in the first 15 minutes, heart rate (HR), stroke volume (SV), cardiac output (CO) and cardiac index (CI) remained stable. Then, these parameters became much more variable, leading to a slow decrease of SV and CO whereas HR continuously increased from around 75/min to 95/min. Suddenly, approximately 25 min after beginning of donation, the donor collapsed. This reaction was followed by a sudden, steep fall of HR from 95/min to 51/min and a concomitant increase of SV from 70 mL/beat to 121 mL/beat. This, however, was insufficient to maintain CO which decreased from 6.8 L/min to 5.6 L/min. CI decreased from 3.3 L/min/m^2 to 2.7 L/min/m^2 during the reaction, i. e. by 18%, within 2 min. It is important to note, though, that the collapse of the donor preceded the drop of HR by more than 60 seconds. Systolic blood pressure dropped from 120 mm Hg to 85 mm Hg. The donor recovered within 10 minutes. Recovery was accomplished by an increase of HR to 67/min while SV still remained above 100 mL/beat leading to restoration of CO and CI. Thoracic fluid content did not change prior to the reaction; in addition, the extracorporeal blood volume at the time of the reaction was only approximately 11%, both indicating that a hypovolaemic origin of the reaction was highly unlikely. During the control investigation, the donor did not show any significant changes of haemodynamic parameters. **Conclusion:** This case report suggests that vasovagal reactions are preceded by haemodynamic disturbances that are neither recognized by the donors nor recognizable by the nurses. Our findings also provide direct evidence that the currently held belief that the parasympathetic cardiac response (bradycardia) in the course of a vasovagal reaction is of minor importance for the development of fainting might actually be true.

OS4.5

Prospective Study of Circulatory Reactions in Plasmapheresis Donors – Incidence, Pathophysiology and Risk Factors

R. Karger, V. Kretschmer
Philipps-Universität Marburg, D

Background: Circulatory reactions in plasmapheresis donors are rare and are usually considered to be vasovagal. However, because of the high extracorporeal blood volume developing during donation, it is possible that some of those reactions might be owing to hypovolaemia. This issue has never been addressed in a prospective study. **Methods:** During a one-year-period symptoms suggestive of cardiovascular origin were prospectively recorded in our plasmapheresis donors using a standardized questionnaire. In particular, parameters supposed to distinguish between vasovagal and hypovolaemic reactions were documented. Logistic regression was used to identify risk factors for circulatory reactions in plasmapheresis donors. Target donation volume per session was 650 mL including anticoagulant. **Results:** 6533 plasmapheresis procedures were performed during the study period. 43 systemic reactions with cardiovascular symptoms, involving 39 plasmapheresis donors, occurred. The incidence was 0.66%; 95% confidence interval (95%-CI) 0.46–0.85%. The most often observed symptoms were dizziness (in 63% of reactions), pallor (47%) and discomfort (44%). Severe symptoms only occasionally occurred: unconsciousness (4.7%), a fit (4.7%), and vomiting (2.3%). Based on our predefined criteria, only two reactions were considered to be possibly of hypovolaemic origin. However, the extracorporeal blood volume of the two donors at the time of the reaction was only 10.2 and 12.4%, respectively. The risk of a circulatory reaction during the first plasma donation was 15.8 times higher than during any other plasma donation. There was a strong trend indicating a decreasing risk for circulatory reactions with increasing age (odds ratio 0.965, p = 0.053, 95%-CI 0.93–1.0). Blood volume and gender were not significant risk factors. The risk for a circulatory reaction was approximately 4-times higher in spring, and 3-times higher in autumn, compared to summer or winter. **Conclusion:** Circulatory reactions in plasmapheresis donors are rare. When donation volume is limited to 650 mL, reactions of hypovolaemic origin are unlikely to occur. The first plasma donation poses the highest risk for a vasovagal reaction.

OS4.6

Notwendigkeit der Bestimmung von Gesamteiweiß (GEW) und IgG im Serum zur Qualifizierung von Plasmaspendern

C. Scheuch[1], K. Lath[1], K.P. Krause[2]
[1]Haema AG, Berlin, D; [2]Haema AG, Leipzig, D

Einleitung: In den Blutspendezentren der Haema AG erfolgt die Qualifizierung der Spender im Rahmen einer Vollblutspende. Entsprechend der Analysenergebnisse und physischen Voraussetzungen sind weitere Vollblut- und Apheresespenden (Plasma-, Erythro-, Thrombozytapherese) möglich. Mit dieser Untersuchung sollte geprüft werden, ob es in Anbetracht der Umsetzung der neuen Richtlinien notwendig ist, die Spender vor der ersten Plasmaspende auf GEW und IgG zu untersuchen. **Material und Methoden:** Es wurden 4335 Erstuntersuchungen auf Gesamteiweiß (GEW) (Biuret- Methode) und IgG (Turbidimetrische Endpunkt-Methode) von Spendern eines Berliner BSZ ausgewertet.

Ergebnisse:
Gesamteiweiß/Serum [g/l] IgG/Serum [g/l]
Medianwert 71,00 10,00
Mittelwert 71,52 10,08
Minimaler Wert 55,0 4,0
Maximaler Wert 90,0 20,6
Standardabweichung 4,25 2,17
Referenzbereich (2s) 63–80 5,74–14,4
Die aus unserer Spenderpopulation ermittelten Referenzbereiche weichen bei IgG von den aus der Literatur bekannten (7–16 g/l) um ca. –1,3 g/l ab.
21 (0,48%) Erstspender wiesen IgG-Werte unter 6,0 g/l auf.
8 Erstspender (0,18%) hatten Gesamteiweiß-Konzentrationen von kleiner 60 g/l im Serum.

Diskussion: Die vorliegenden Analyse des Proteinstoffwechsels dokumentiert, dass ein geringer Prozentsatz von Erstspendern der Haema AG vor der ersten Plasmapherese von den Sollwerten der Eignungsuntersuchungen nach RiliBÄK abweicht. Es ist nicht auszuschließen, dass diese Spender in anderen Einrichtungen im Raum Berlin bereits Plasma spendeten. Der nach links verschobene Referenzbereich für IgG könnte ein Indiz dafür sein. Deshalb sollte die Eignungsuntersuchung anlässlich der Erstspende (Vollblut) bei den Spendern beibehalten werden, die willens und geeignet sind, Plasma zu spenden.

OS4.7

Multicomponent Collection in Two Different Apheresis Systems: Procedure, Donor Data and Donor Regeneration

S. Sipurzynski-Budraß, S. Macher, K. Schallmoser, G. Lanzer
Universitätsklinik Graz – Klinik für Blutgruppenserologie und Transfusionsmedizin, Graz, A

Purpose: The use of automated blood component technology creates new opportunities to tailor and optimize component collections for specific needs. This apheresis technique allows the collection of platelets (plts), red blood cells (RBCs) and plasma in various combinations.Aim of our study was to investigate a possible influence of this special setting on donor data and donor regeneration time. **Methods:** Per apheresis 2 units of plts (6 × 1011) and 1 unit of RBCs (250 mL, Hct 80%) were collected by two devices (Trima Access®, Gambro; Amicus®, Baxter). Each donor (n = 23) underwent the procedure on both apheresis systems with at least 8 weeks (wks) in between. Donor data as blood counts, iron, ferritin and transferrin plasma levels as well as coagulation parameters and plt function (aggregometry, thrombelastogram) were measured before and after apheresis, 48 hours (hrs), 2 wks and 6 wks after procedure. **Results:** All collections were completed and well tolerated. Time of donation was significantly longer by using the Amicus device (77 vs. 89 min). As expected, plts decreased after collection from 284 ± 34 to 200 ± 30 × 106/mL. After 2 wks plts increased up to 341 ± 47 × 106/mL and normalized at 6 wks control. Red cell loss (basal hematocrit of 44.7 ± 3%) was compensated after 6 wks (43.8 ± 2.6%). Starting with a ferritin level of 56 ± 35 ng/mL, it declined to 23 ± 16 ng/mL 6 wks after the first and to10 ± 4 ng/mL 6 wks after the second collection. Some parameters of aggregometry and thrombelastogram were significantly altered, probably caused by elimination of a large amount of plts and dilution. However, there were no signs for increased plt activation due to extracorporal circulation. **Conclusion:** Multicomponent collection in this special setting is a safe and suitable method to collect a double unit of plts and 1 unit of RBC in one procedure. Extracorporal circulation seems to have no influence on donor's coagulation parameters and plt function. Two wks after donation plt counts reached about 120% of the precount, so further plt collections in between may be possible. However, selection of suitable donors and long-term donor surveillance are necessary to make multicomponent collection safe for routine utilization

OS4.8

Introduction of Plasmapheresis Procedures in a Mobile Setup

C. Kreissig, L. Hartmann, H. Eichler
DRK-Blutspendedienst West, Ratingen, D

Purpose: Plasma products from blood group AB donors often tend to be limited whereas RBC components from these donors are less frequently requested. By switching a significant percentage of AB donors from whole blood donation to plasmapheresis, it would be able to cover the need of blood group AB plasma without negatively affecting RBC supply. To reach this goal in a supraregional Red Cross blood service, the plasmapheresis procedure needs also to be introduced to the mobile donation setting. **Methods:** In order to partially switch blood collection technology for defined donors we introduced plasmapheresis as a mobile procedure. MCS plus is used as the cell separation device dedicated for mobile collection of multiple blood components. First, compared to the whole blood donation system, completely different donation logistics had to be built up: Starting with a new donor recruitment strategy including predonation examination, selection of suitable premises and donors, qualification of the collection device for use in a mobile session, validation of the complete process, and implementation of specialized mobile apheresis teams for daily routine. **Results:** In close cooperation with authorities and all other departments of our company we developed a stringent concept for performing mobile sessions of plasmapheresis. **Conclusion:** For efficient use of donor potential and adequat blood supply it is useful to focus on different products for different blood groups. We suggest our newly implemented strategy in performing mobile apheresis donation as a necessary completion of standard whole blood donation. This could serve as a pilot project in establishing strategies of blood component collection for blood services mainly based on mobile sessions.

OS5: Cellular and Gene Therapy

OS5.1

Safety and Efficacy of Therapeutic Early-Onset Granulocyte Transfusions in Pediatric Patients with Neutropenia and Severe Infections

U. Sachs, A. Reiter, T. Walter, G. Bein, W. Wößmann
Justus Liebig-Universität Gießen, D

Background: Bacterial and fungal infections in profound neutropenia after chemotherapy are associated with high mortality despite appropriate antibacterial and antifungal treatment. Granulocyte transfusions are used as a therapeutic addendum, but concern regarding pulmonary reactions often results in delayed use in clinical practice. Accordingly, many patients are already at advanced stages of their infectious disease once granulocytes are transfused. Thus, we conducted a prospective phase II trial to test the safety and efficacy of therapeutic early-onset granulocyte transfusions in immunocompromised children with neutropenia and severe infections. **Study Design and Methods:** Twenty-seven children with hematological disorder or malignancy and severe neutropenia with clinically and/or microbiologically documented severe infection unresponsive to standard treatment were included. They received G-CSF-elicited, cross-matched granulocyte concentrates every other day until complete recovery from infection was documented. **Results:** A medium of two granulocyte transfusions with a medium of 8 × 10E8 granulocytes per kilogram body weight was administered. All transfusions were well tolerated, and no pulmonary symptoms were observed. 92.6% of our patients were able to clear their initial infection, and 81.5% were alive and without signs or symptoms of their infection one month later. All six children with aspergillosis cleared their infection. **Conclusions:** G-CSF elicited, cross-matched granulocyte concentrates are a safe and efficient therapeutic addendum in immunocompromised children with neutropenia and severe infections. Early transfusion of cross-matched granulocyte concentrates can lead to an overall response rate of 92.6% without adverse events. Randomized clinical trials with an early-onset design are required to determine appropriate clinical applications.

OS5.2

Towards Targeted Repair of Human Chromosomal Loci by Use of Single-Stranded Oligodeoxynucleotides

K. Schwarz, F. Radecke, S. Radecke, I. Peter
IKT Ulm, DRK Blutspendedienst Baden-Württemberg, Ulm, D

Purpose: The goal of correcting (point-)mutated genes is currently pursued by two basic strategies which are either viral or non-viral. Using a retrovirus derivative for targeting ('gene replacement'), success at the clinical stage has been reported in treating patients suffering from SCID-X1 or CGD. However, in SCID-X1 patients cases of acute lymphatic leukemia (ALL) developed due to insertional mutagenesis. This highlights the demand for complementing targeting strategies. An alternative is the correction of the defective gene at its chromosomal locus. To this end, long and short double-stranded DNA fragments, chimeric RNA/DNA oligonucleotides (chimeraplasts), triplex-forming oligonucleotides (TFOs), and single-stranded (ss) oligodeoxynucleotides (ODNs) have been designed. Concentrating on ssODNs, studies have established reproducible functionality of this type of correction molecule. However, repair rates are rather low. To elucidate biochemical pathways involved in targeted repair, the work presented set out to investigate whether DNA repair, e.g., mismatch repair (MMR), or a direct incorporation of the correction molecule follows as the step upon the initial interaction. **Methods:** Single-stranded ODNs were directed towards point-mutated enhanced green fluorescence protein transgene loci in HEK-293-derived cell clones. First gene repair assays compared ODNs carrying the canonical termini 5′-phosphate and 3′-OH with their respective variants harbouring non-canonical termini (5′-OH, 3′-H). Second, a protocol was established to allow efficient recovery of integrated short biotin-labelled ODNs from the genomes of corrected cells in order to test directly whether transfected ODNs become parts of the target locus DNA. **Results:** ODNs with canonical termini were about 34-fold more efficient than their counterparts carrying non-canonical termini in a phosphorothioate-modified backbone. Furthermore, biotinylated fragments were successfully recovered from genomic DNAs of gene-corrected cells. **Conclusions:** ODNs are incorporated into a mammalian genome. This unravels one early repair step and also sets an example of genome dynamics possibly relevant to other ODN-based cell techniques.

OS5.3

HLA-B-Associated Transcript 3 (BAT3), a Novel Ligand for the NK Cell-Receptor NKp30, Activates NK Cells in vitro and Prevents Tumor Formation in a Xenograft Model

E. Pogge von Strandmann, V. Rao Simhadri, B. Von Tresckow, S. Sasse, K.S. Reiners, H.P. Hansen, A. Rothe, P. Borchmann, M. Hallek, A. Engert
Universitätsklinikum Köln, D

Purpose: The transplantation of alloreactive NK cells reduces the risk of relapse in acute myeloid leukaemia patients, while improving engraftment and protecting against graft-versus-host disease. This depends on NK cell-mediated suppression of T-cell-mediated graft-versus-host disease by eliminating host DCs (Science 2002;295:2097–2100). Both killing and maturation of DCs by NK cells is dependent on NKp30 function, a Natural Activating Receptor (NCR) expressed on NK cells. The ability to promote NKp30-mediated DC-maturation is confined to NK cells expressing the killer immunoglobulin-like receptor-negative (KIR-) NKG2A(dull) phenotype (Blood 2005;106:566–571). However, so far the cellular ligands responsible for NKp30-activation have remained elusive. The aim of the project presented here, was the isolation of the long sought cellular NKp30-ligand. The molecular knowledge should provide the basis for a better understanding of NK cell-regulation, which is also essential for the development of clinical applications targeting NKp30 on NK cells. **Methods and Results:** Using the Yeast Two Hybrid technique we isolated the putative NKp30-ligand BAT3 (HLA-B-associated transcript 3), that binds directly and specifically to NKp30. We demonstrate by means of laser scanner microscopy, FACS analysis and Western Blotting, that BAT3, which is a nuclear protein, translocates from the nucleus to the cell-surface and is released from the tumor cells in an inducible manner upon incubation with NK cells or exposure to heat shock. Overexpression of BAT3 triggers natural killer cell-mediated interferong (IFNg)-secretion and NKp30-mediated cytotoxicity. Moreover, inhibition of endogenous BAT3 using polyclonal antibodies prevents tumor rejection in vivo. **Conclusion:** Thus, BAT3 is a novel NKp30 ligand, exhibiting a unique mechanism by which a nuclear protein activates NK cells via NKp30-engagement after inducible release to the cell-surface and the cell environment. Potential therapeutic applications using BAT3 for a cellular NK-based therapy of malignant diseases will be discussed.

OS5.4

The Role of Protease-Activated Receptors on Viral-Based Gene Transfer Efficacy

J. Schüttrumpf[1], J. Zou[2], C.F. Freguia[2], S. Baila[2], J. Liu[2], P. Andrade-Gordon[3], V. Arruda[2]
[1]DRK-Blutspendedienst Baden-Württemberg – Hessen, Frankfurt am Main D; [2]The Children s Hospital of Philadelphia, Philadelphia, USA; [3]R.J. Wood Johnson Pharmaceutical Research Institute, Spring House, USA

Adeno-associated viral (AAV)-2 vectors hold promise for the treatment of several diseases and were already tested in clinical Phase I/II studies. Previously, we determined an unexpected inhibitory effect of anticoagulative drugs on AAV-2 and adenovirus mediated gene transfer. Thus we hypothesized that coagulation proteases may influence AAV-2 gene transfer. Cellular responses triggered by proteases are mediated by protease-activated receptors (PAR) and PAR-1 activation by thrombin enhances alphaVbeta5 integrin (co-receptor for AAV-2 and adenovirus)-dependent cellular function. Therefore we sought to test whether PAR activation could modulate AAV-2 and adenoviral gene transfer. AAV-2 vectors were delivered to PAR-1, PAR-2, PAR-4, and beta5 deficient mice. Mice homozygous (−/−) or heterozygous (+/−) for PAR-1 (n = 11 or 18), PAR-2 (n = 13/13), or PAR-4 (n = 8/10) received tail vein injections of AAV-2 vectors expressing coagulation factor IX (FIX) and were compared to littermate controls (+/+). FIX levels among PAR-1 controls were 2-fold higher than in PAR-1 (−/−); $p < 0.02$. Similarly, PAR-4 deficient mice presented 3-fold lower FIX levels than controls (0.4 vs 1.2 μg/ml, $p < 0.05$), while PAR-2 deficiency did not influence gene transfer. Moreover, upon activation of receptors by PAR-1, -2, or -4 -specific peptide agonists in normal C57Bl6 mice, FIX levels increased 1.5 to 5-fold in a dose-dependent manner for PAR-1 and PAR-4. Gene copy monitoring and immunofluorescence staining revealed low vector uptake by livers of PAR knockout mice while PAR activation increased uptake and expression. Interestingly, beta5(−/−) mice showed lower FIX expression than controls (0.5 vs 2.0 μg/ml. $p < 0.0005$; total n = 26). PAR activation or a PAR null allele had a similar effect on adenoviral vector transduction, but no effect on AAV-5 or AAV-8-mediated gene transfer, which use other cellular receptors. Further, the influence of PARs on AAV-2 transduction was not present in beta5 deficient cells or mice, which all suggest a receptor dependent mechanism by PARs. In conclusion, these data demonstrate a novel role of coagulation proteases and PARs on viral vector (AAV-2 and adenovirus)-mediated gene expression and provide an alternative target to modulate gene therapy strategies.

OS5.5

Enhanced Recombinant Expression of FVIII in 293T and Hematopoetic Cells Using an Expression Vector Containing the FXIII 5′ Untranslated Region

S. Heinz, D. Went, D. Bott, E. Seifried, T. Tonn

DRK-Institute for Transfusion Medicine and Immunohaematology, Frankfurt, D

Purpose: Considering the immediate access to the bloodstream and the involvement in coagulation, megakaryocytes and monocytes would be ideal targets for gene therapy of hemophilia A. However, several attempts to show recombinant expression of factor VIII (rFVIII) by primary hematopoietic cells using an ubiquitously expressed CMV-promoter have shown to be ineffective. In part, this failure was attributed to the inefficient transcription from the CMV promoter in hematopoietic cells. This study explores the potential of megakaryocyte and monocyte specific FXIIIA transcriptional elements to enhance the expression of FVIII in hematopoetic cells. **Methods:** The enhancer region (enh), the 5′ untranslated region (5′UTR) both of the FXIIIA were cloned in combination or as a single element in 5′ to 3′ direction of the CMV-promoter into the mammalian expression plasmid pcDNA3.1 upstream of either FVIII B-domain deleted (FVIII-DB) or the full length FVIII (FVIII-FL) cDNA. These vectors were transfected into CD14+monocytes, the megakaryocytic cell line K562 and human embryonic kidney cell line 293T using nucleofection (Amaxa). FVIII expression was analysed by a chromogenic assay and RT-PCR. Transfection efficiency was compared by measuring green fluorescent protein (GFP) expression from a GFP encoding pcDNA3.1 Vector. **Results:** FVIII-DB expression was most effective in K562 cells and primary monocytes when transfected with the 5′UTR containing vector (in mIU/ml: 20 for Monocytes and 150 for K562 compared to 7 and 100 in these cells using the vector without the 5′UTR); the FXIIIA-enhancer element containing plasmid proofed to be equally effective in K562 cells whereas the combination of both, enhancer and 5′ UTR, resulted in reduced FVIII levels compared to the vector with the basal CMV promoter alone. **Conclusions:** The inclusion of the 5′UTR of the FXIIIA gene upstream of the FVIII coding sequence results in a significantly improvement of FVIII expression levels from a CMV driven expression vector in primary monocytes and K562 cells. Further experiments have to rule out if the FXIII 5′ UTR element may be beneficial for hematopoietic lineage restricted expression of in animal models that could ultimately translate into safe gene therapy approaches for hemophilia A.

OS5.6

High Levels of Human Factor IX Transgene Expression in Mice Increase Blood Procoagulant Activity

R. Schwaab[1], J. Grupp[1], T. Albert[1], J. Oldenburg[1], H. Fechner[2], R. Fimmers[1], M. Srour[1]

[1]Universitätsklinikum Bonn, Bonn, D; [2]Benjamin Franklin Hospital, Berlin, D

In gene therapy studies in animals, high levels of FIX expression have already been achieved by our laboratory as well as by others. In the present study, we addressed the question whether such high expression levels of FIX could affect the blood procoagulant status in mice. In order to investigate this aspect, we performed the following experiment: female SCID mice (BALB/C JHanHsd-scid) were injected via tail vein with Doxycycline (Dox)-controlled adenoviral (Ad) vectors for the expression of hFIX. For induction of transgene expression, SCID mice were supplied with drinking water either with Dox (200 µg/ml) or without Dox. Additionally, two control groups of mice were used: one group treated with the same adenoviral vectors, however with integrated luciferase (luc) gene instead of the FIX gene, and one group injected only with saline. Again groups were treated with and without Dox, respectively. For transgene analysis gained plasma was used for the determination of FIX antigen (Ag) and activity as well as D-dimer levels. Mice treated with Ad vectors expressing hFIX and induced with Dox showed a significant increase in D-Dimer levels compared to control mice on day 10 as well as on day 60 postinfection. However, there was no significant increase in D-dimers in mice treated with Ad vectors expressing FIX but not induced with Dox as well as in mice treated with Ad vectors expressing Luc or saline (induced with or without Dox). These results indicate that high expression levels of hFIX increase the blood procoagulant activity in animals (mice), while Ad vectors or Dox alone or in combination do not. To verify correlation of high hFIX-levels and increased blood procoagulant activity, three groups of SCID mice (5–6 mice per group) were injected via tail vein with different amounts of recombinant factor IX. A fourth group of mice (5 mice) was injected with physiological saline (control). Altogether mice received 6 injections in order to keep mice exposed for high doses of FIX during the experiment period, thus maintaining mice in a situation that mimics our previous gene therapy study. Although data were statistically not significant we could show that the increase in FIX activity was paralleled with an increase in the D-dimer levels which therefore supports our gene therapy data. The results reported here indicate that increased blood procoagulant activity could be caused by high expression levels of hFIX in a gene therapy protocol in animals. The outcome of this study should be considered in clinical trials concerning calculations of vector doses and mainly in patients with risk factors that predispose them for venous thrombosis.

OS5.7

Enrichment of Natural Killer Cells and Their Specific Activation in Co-Culture with the Neuroblastoma Cell Line SY5Y

R. Moog[1], U. Schwanke[2]

[1]Universitätsklinikum Essen, D; [2]German Transfusion Service West, Ratingen, D

Introduction: Natural killer cells (NK) play an important role in host defense against viruses, intracellular bacteria and parasites and they spontaneously may lyse tumor cells. It is desirable to use NK capabilities to eliminate neuroblastoma (NB) tumors which account for 10% of malignancies in newborns and in children less than one year of age. In the present study a new attempt was made to condition enriched NK to selectively lyse SY5Y NB tumor cells. **Material and Methods:** NK were isolated from whole blood derived buffy coats (BC, 15 ml, n = 5) using sterile RosetteSep and magnetic activated cell sorting techniques. NK were cultured in a density of 10E + 06/ml in X-Vivo10 medium containing 2% fetal calf serum and 1000 U/ml interleukine-2 for 10 days at 37°C. In parallel SY5Y cells were cultured at 37°C in X-Vivo10 medium without additives. On day 10 NK as well as SY5Y were harvested and the absolute cell count and vitality were determined by flow-cytometry using CD45FITC/CD56 PE/7AAD to identify NK and CD45FITC/CD166 PE/7AAD for SY5Y. Three cytotoxicy assays containing E + 06 cells/ml each were prepared: 100% NK (negative control), NK-in-SY5Y = 10-in-1, 100% SY5Y (positive control) and cultured for 5 days at 37°C. Subsequently, absolute cell count and vitality were assessed again as described above. **Results:** 15.3 ± 4.3 E + 06 NK were isolated from 15 ml buffy coat. Purity and vitality averaged 83 and 99%, respectively. After 10 days in culture cell count and vitality amounted 2.1 ± 0.8 E + 06/ml, 92% for NK and 4.8 ± 1.3 E + 06/ml, 89% for SY5Y, resp. Cytotocity assays exhibited final cell count and vitality as follows: NK 1.9 ± 0.2 E + 06/ml, 88% (negative control), and 1.3 ± 0.8 E + 06/ml, 85% (NK-in-SY5Y = 10-in-1), SY5Y 5.3 ± 1.3 E + 06/ml, 95% (positive control), and 1.4 ± 0.9 E + 06/ml, 0.8% (NK-in-SY5Y = 10-in-1). **Conclusion:** In this study NK exhibited significant cytotoxicy for SY5Y NB cells. Autologous NK cells may be conditioned to lyse NB tumors but this has to be proven in clinical trials in vivo.

OS5.8

Autologous GMP-Compliant Stem Cell Products for Cellular Therapy of Diabetic Peripheral Artery Occluding Disease

M. Gastens, W. Prohaska, B. Stratmann, D. Lammers, S. Kirana, D. Tschöpe, K. Kleesiek

Herz- und Diabeteszentrum NRW, Bad Oeynhausen, D

Purpose: Diabetic foot syndrome (DFS) is a type of peripheral artery occluding disease and appears as late stage complication of diabetic patients. Apart from surgical therapy pAOD patients have been treated by use of autologous bone marrow cells to induce angiogenesis. **Methods and Results:** Using a GMP-compliant production process we manufactured mesenchymal stem cell (MSC) enriched cellular products from bone marrow mononuclear cells (BM-MNC) for the treatment of diabetic pAOD patients. Up to now 11 study

patients have been randomized and selected to the BM-MNC (5), the MSC (5) or the standard care group (1). Two patients were excluded due to low cellularity of BM, one due to withdrawal of patient's consent. Around 45 ml bone marrow were drawn with 885 × 106 total cells. By gradient centrifugation a mean of 260.9 × 106 BM-MNC were isolated containing 1.35% CD34+/lin- and 0.35% CD90+/CD14− cells that were washed and used for treatment of the BM-MNC group. Cultivation enriched CD90+/CD14− cells 27fold to 9.2 × 106 per MSC product. Total number of CFU-F showed a 53fold increase to 6.5 106 MSC per product. In contrast to bone marrow the MSC enriched cell product included 10fold more KDR-positive endothelial progenitors and formed vascular structures in vitro. Application of either cell product to DFS-patients for vascular repair revealed so far no adverse events. First clinical results after 5 month for two patients randomized to the MSC group and one to the standard care group were assessed by TcpO2 and ankle-brachiale index (ABI). TcpO2 as well as ABI appeared enhanced in MSC treated patients: patient 1 MSC TcpO2 8 mmHg/35 mmHg; ABI 0.73/1.31; patient 2 MSC TcpO2 25 mmHg/32 mmHg; ABI 0.64/0.73; patient 3 standard care TcpO2 5 mmHg/5 mmHg; ABI 1.92/1.56. **Conclusion:** GMP-compliant production and enrichment of stem cells with angiogenic properties from small volumes of bone marrow of chronically ill DFS-patients is feasible and first results suggest an improvement of the microcirculation.

OS6: Hemovigilance and Materiovigilance/Quality Management and Regulatory Affairs

OS6.1

European Quality Management in Transfusion Medicine (EU-Q-Blood-SOP-Project)

C. Seidl[1], *E. Schellenberg*[1], *R. Henschler*[1], *A. McMillan Douglas*[2], *C. S. Sibinga*[3], *M. Gorham*[4], *M. Letowska*[5], *J. DeWit*[3], *E. Seifried*[1]
[1]DRK-Blutspendedienst Baden-Würtember – Hessen, Frankfurt, D; [2]AMD, Edinburgh, UK; [3]Sanquin, Amsterdam, NL; [4]NBS, London, UK; [5]IHBP, Warshaw, PL

Introduction: Quality management systems in blood transfusion are of high importance for the safeguard of blood and blood components. The EU-Q-Blood-SOP Project is co-funded by the European Commission and supports the public health program on 'quality and safety of blood' in delivering a practical SOP-based tool that will contribute to the understanding and management of quality processes in blood services. The EU-SOP tool will assist blood establishments in preparing for the inspection of their services related to the implementation of quality relevant elements required by the EU Directive 2002/98/EC and its technical annexes. **Results:** In order to find out the current status of SOPs, their structures and any potential manuals or regulations that are in place in the various participant institutions and countries, including the current inspection practice, a questionnaire has been designed by the project team and has been send-out to the participating blood establishments from 16 EU Member, Acceding or EFTA states. Based on this questionnaire differences and commonalities in the approach to basic structural questions in quality management and specific aspects considering SOPs have been evaluated and summarized in a survey report. It identifies some of the perceived high risk areas in blood collection, preparation, laboratory testing, storage and distribution. 7 of 15 (47%) participating blood establishments considered, that their present SOP system needs to be changed in the light of the European blood legislation, based on Directive 2002/98/EC and its technical annexes. These were mainly participants from the new Member States and Applicant Countries. 4 of 15 (27%) participants (2 from Applicant Countries and 2 from established EU Member States) indicated that their blood establishment is not inspected by governmental authorities. **Discussion:** Currently used standards for quality management systems are heterogeneous. The new EU-SOP methodology comprises precise quality requirements, requisites and quality terms linked to the EU Directives and based on GLP/GMP-standards that have to be specified (filled-out) in order to complete the documents. The results are presented by the project team and advisory board on behalf of the Project's participant (DRK BSDBH, Germany; HBRK, Belgium; NBT, Bulgaria; MOH, Cyprus; VFN, Czech Republic; EBS, Estonia; EFS, France; HNBT, Hungary; BTS, Iceland; NBTS, Ireland; ISS, Italy; IBT, Malta; IHBP, Poland; FMP, Romania; Sanquin, The Netherlands; SNBTS and NBS, United Kingdom). The project is co-funded by the European Commission, Directorate C.

OS6.2

Impact of Demographic Changes on the Blood Supply – Mecklenburg-West Pomerania as a Model Region for Europe

A. Greinacher, K. Fendrich, U. Alpen, W. Hoffmann
Ernst-Moritz-Arndt-Universität Greifswald, D

Background: The population structure in most European countries is currently changing with a shift from younger to older age groups. Little is known about the consequences for blood supply. We analyzed how demography will determine future blood demand and supply in a region where demographic change is particularly dynamic and where detailed donor and recipient data are available. **Methods:** The population of the main catchment area of the University Hospital of Greifswald (415,000 inhabitants) was projected to the year 2015 based on 1-year age groups provided by the population registry, based on 2002 rates assuming: stable death rates and migration patterns. Data on donors and recipients for the years 1996 to 2004 were extracted from the database of the Department of Transfusion Medicine at the Greifswald University. **Results:** Until 2015, the increase in the older population will result in an 11.8–13.9% increase of blood transfusions. In 2004, 39.9% of all RBC were transfused to patients of 70 years and older. In 2015 this age group will require 50.2% of all RBCs. A major finding of our study is that the expected decrease in blood donations that results from a relative decrease in the younger donor population has a higher impact than the increase of blood demand. In 2004 the highest percentage of RBCs was provided by donors between 20 and 24 years of age. Donors in the age group 18–29 years donated 58.4% of all blood units. Assuming constant motivation to donate blood as in 2004, the decrease in the younger population will cause a 27.5–32.6% decrease of blood donations until 2015. **Conclusion:** The increased future demand for blood coincides with a significant reduction in blood donations. From 2008 the shortfalls will grow to 32–35% of the total demand in 2015 in the area studied. The demographic trends will affect many regions in Europe similarly. Coordinated efforts will be required to prevent blood shortages based upon these demographic trends in western societies.

OS6.3

The German Red Cross NAT-Study: Results of Screening More than 30 Million Blood Donations for HIV-1, HCV and HBV

M.K. Hourfar[1], *W.K. Roth*[1], *V. Schottstedt*[2], *C. Jork*[3], *M. Weber-Schehl*[4], *C. Mahnhardt*[5], *U. Mayr-Wohlfart*[6], *K. Gubbe*[7], *V. Brixner*[1], *M. Schmidt*[1], *E. Seifried*[1]
[1]DRK-Blutspendedienst Baden-Würtemberg – Hessen, Frankfurt, D; [2]DRK-Blutspendedienst West, Hagen, D; [3]DRK-Blutspendedienst NSTOB, Springe, D; [4]Bayrisches Rotes Kreuz, Wiesentheid, D; [5]DRK-Blutspendedienst Mecklenburg-Vorpommern, Neubrandenburg, D; [6]Blutspendedienst Baden-Württemberg – Hessen, Ulm, D; [7]DRK-Blutspendedienst Sachsen, Plauen, D

Background: The risk of transfusion transmitted HIV-1, HCV and HBV infections is predominantly associated with donations at an early stage of infection, where diagnostic tests may fail. In 1996 at German Red Cross blood donor services first attempts have been undertaken of shortening this diagnostic window period by means of nucleic acid amplification techniques. Ten years later the most comprehensive set of NAT-screening data in Europe is available. **Study Design and Methods:** More than 30 million blood donations collected from 1997 through 2005 were screened by minipool-NAT, predominantly with pool-sizes of 96 donors. The donations included in the study cover approximately 80% of all the blood collected in Germany during that period. The residual risk of transfusion-associated viral infections was calculated using a model based on back-extrapolation of viral replication rates. **Results:** During the observed time period 23 HCV-, 7 HIV-1 and 43 HBV NAT-only positive donations were detected. This corresponds to a yield rate of 1 in 1,369,203 for HCV, 1 in 4,474,007 for HIV-1 and 1 in 729,138 for HBV. In case of HBV approximately 45% of these donations would also have been detected by additional screening for anti-HBc. **Conclusion:** The risk of a blood recipient becoming infected with HCV, HIV-1 and HBV has reached an extremely low level. Numerous transfusion-transmitted infections could be prevented by early implementation of NAT on a voluntary basis. This observation clearly highlights the benefit of minipool-NAT with poolsizes up to 96 donations. In case of HBV it is assumed, that implementation of anti-HBc screening will further improve blood safety.

OS6.4

Possible Association of Adverse Reactions to Non-Plasma Reduced Pooled Platelet Units and Minor-Incompatible Transfusion

F. Wagner, W. Adamo
DRK Blutspendedienst NSTOB, Springe, D

Purpose: Although minor-incompatible platelet transfusion may cause hemolysis and may have adverse long-term effects, the impact of minor-incompatible transfusions on reported adverse event rate has not been detailed. **Methods:** We checked reports of adverse events to platelet transfusion received at our institution since 2002 for the ABO constellation and relative frequency of reports. In August 2005, we changed from leucocyte depleted pooled buffy-coat derived platelets (PP-NR) to plasma-reduced leucocyte depleted pooled buffy-coat derived platelets (PP-R). The results were compared with those for apheresis platelets (non-plasma reduced) and an RBC preparation checked for selected time frames. **Results:** Overall rates of reported adverse reactions were 3.1/month for PP-NR and 1.9/month for PP-R despite constant rates of sold units. No such difference was found for AP (0.9/month Jan 04 to Jul 05 and 1.6/month Aug 05 to Feb 06). 41 of 134 (30%) evaluable adverse events concerning PP-NR occurred during minor-incompatible transfusion (AP: 5 of 21; 22%), while a single such event was reported for PP-R (1 of 15, 7%). There was a constant overrepresentation of blood group B and AB patients (17% of our donor population) in incidents with PP-NR (2002:31%, 2003:21%, 2004:27%; 2005:23%, all years: 27%) but not PP-R (7%); AP (13%), or RBC units (13%). **Conclusion:** The reduced rate of adverse events observed with plasma-reduced platelet preparations observed in randomized trials seems to hold true in a routine setting. Despite a general recommendation for ABO identical platelet transfusion, there was a striking rate of ABO minor incompatible transfusions among reports of adverse events. The increased rate of blood group B and AB recipients involved suggested that minor-incompatible transfusion of non-plasma-reduced units may be associated with an increased rate of adverse events (these patients are likely to receive O resp. A units due to logistic reasons). This deleterious effect of minor-incompatible transfusion seems have resolved by the introduction of plasma-reduced units.

OS6.5

Platelet Concentrates Containing Resolved Platelet Aggregates Are Not Associated with Significantly More Transfusion Reactions

E. Höbert, B. Rott, E. Hanfland, J. Hoch, J. Oldenburg, U. Harbrecht
Universität Bonn, D

Purpose: Preparation of apheresis platelet concentrates (PC) might be associated with formation of platelet aggregates (PA), which either resolve during storage or persist beyond expiry date. PCs with resolved PA are usually transfused. We investigated whether PCs released for transfusion that contained initially PA were more frequently involved in reports of transfusion reactions compared to PCs without aggregates. Furthermore we calculated the rate of discarded PCs due to persisting PA. **Methods:** We analysed retrospectively our records of non-haemolytic transfusion reactions (NHTR) following transfusions with leukocyte depleted PCs (leukocytes $< 1 \times 10^6$/U) between January 2004 and March 2006 after we had introduced a stratified procedure for aggregates containing PCs. PCs were checked for platelet count after preparation and macroscopically evaluated for aggregates daily by two independent persons. PCs were released for transfusion when aggregates had resolved during shelf life and platelet count was within specification. **Results:** Between 01/2004 and 03/2006 a total of 10815 PC were produced (71% AmicusCrescendo™, Baxter, 29% CobeSpectra™, Gambro.BCT) by double apheresis. 326 (3.0%) initially contained PA, of which 108 (33.1%) had to be discarded due to persistent PA. There were 40 reported NHTRs in 9873 transfused PCs (0.4%). 2/40 PCs (5%) involved in NHTR had initially PA, in contrast to the remaining 38 PCs. Comparison of relations of PCs with PA involved in NHTR (2/40 = 5%) and PCs with PA of all transfused PC (218/9873 = 2.2%) is not significantly different ($p = 0.22$; Fisher's exact test). Only one NHTR report included both bags of a double apheresis PC (without PA) transfused in different patients. **Conclusions:** Although one might speculate that PCs containing resolved PA have for instance higher amounts of cytokines, these products appear not to be disproportionately involved in NHTRs. It is likely that recipient rather than donor properties are causative for PC-related NHTRs, since both bags of a double apheresis PC were involved only once.

OS6.6

Half Year Reviews, a Valuable Tool to Survey Processes as Well as Customer Contentment

A. Markovic, W. Madla, C. Weinstock, H. Fischer, M. Clar
DRK-BSD West Institut Bad Kreuznach gGmbH, Bad Kreuznach, D

Background: The DRK-Blutspendedienst West Institut Bad Kreuznach gGmbH (ITM KH) is a non-profit red cross blood donation service which performs 250.000 donations p. a. These blood donations from unpaid volunteers have to be prepared and tested according national and european regulations to get excellent blood products. The ITM KH also provides immunohaematological services and a continuing education concept for transfusionists and their assistance personnel. **Purpose:** About 15 departments have to work closely together to manage this complex task. To survey processes for efficiency and target-orientation as well as customer contentment, the ITM KH, which is certified by ISO 9001:2000 since 2003, has implemented a valuable tool, the half year reviews. **Methods:** The half year reviews were established for the first time in 2003. Every department had to define and to enhance short-term, medium-term and long-term targets, whose attainments should be reviewed all 6 months. These reviews were categorised into 5 thematic groups: customer, staff member, quality of process/product/service, cost effectiveness, communication. The half year reviews should be concise and realistic, and they should consider measurable and comparable parameters. Key data must be regarded in the previous and the upcoming 6 months. **Results:** Meanwhile we have a 3 year experience with the half year reviews. These reviews, which are written by the heads of the departments together with their staff, sharpen everybody's awareness for customers needs, common targets, evolving changes and the necessity of continuous fine-tuning. **Conclusion:** Half year reviews are a valuable tool to survey processes as well as customer contentment.

OS6.7

A Cost-Effective Strategie for Fast and Rapid Determination of Cell Vitality Parameters in Packed RBC'S

A. Doescher, E.K Petershofen, C. Vogt, C. Grote, T. Mueller
BSD-NSTOB, Oldenburg, D

Introduction: To examine the cell vitality of packed RBC's during storage several parameters like ATP, free Hb or 2,3-DPG are used. Kits are available

Table 1 for Abstract OS6.7

	ATP	2,3-DPG	Plasma Hb	glucose	lactate
linearity (R^2)	0.997	0.994	0.996	0.998	0.995
sensitivity	5 µM	0.5 µM	2.5 mg/dl	0.1 mM	0.25 mM
intra-assay variability (low-range)	4.3%	2.3%	5.1%	1.7%	3.7%
intra-assay variability (high-range)	1.2%	1.4%	n.d.	1.4%	1.4%
hand-on-time* (original assay)	4 h	11.5 h	3.5 h	3 h	3 h
hand-on-time* (modificated assay)	30 min	50 min	20 min	20 min	25 min
costs per sample** (original assay)	3.45	5.18	1.38	0.23	0.59
costs per sample** (modificated assay)	0.22	0.52	0.10	0.05	0.15

but they need either a large sample volume and/or are time consuming. Here we present the modification of commercial testkits for a time- and cost saving detection of ATP; 2,3-DPG; free Hb, glucose and lactate. **Methods:** Samples were analysed a) according to manufactores instructions b) using a modificated version of the test kit and c) if available a second independent method. Kits were minimized to a total volume of 200 µl and tests were performed in microtiter-plates. Each modificated assay was tested for linearity, sensitivity as well as intra- and interassay variability. **Results:** see table 1 *calculated for 96 samples; **Euro **Conclusion:** Performance of test kits in microtiter format is a useful strategy for fast and rapid methods, reliable for high-throughput determination of cell vitality in packed RBC's.

OS6.8

Implementation of an Error-Risk-Management Reporting System (ERMS) at the Red Cross Blood Donor Service Baden-Württemberg-Hessen – First Results

S. Findhammer[1], E. Schellenberg[1], K. Koerner[2], A. Karl[3], M. Wiesneth[2], E. Seifried[1], W. Sireis[1]

[1]DRK-Blutspendedienst Baden-Württemberg, Frankfurt, D;
[2]DRK-Blutspendedienst Baden-Württemberg–Hessen, Ulm, D;
[3]DRK-Blutspendedienst Sachsen, Plauen, D

Purpose: The European Union (EU) Directive on Blood Safety and Quality, implemented on February 2005, requires that Blood Establishments report all serious adverse events related to the collection, testing, processing, storage and distribution of blood and blood components that may have an influence on the quality and safety. The reporting system is designed to identify deviations related to preanalytic, labelling, transport, manufactural and quality control processes to extend the well established hemovigilance reporting system. Deviations from the specifications or incidences, respectively, are reported to the quality management department (QM-D.), where they will be valued with regard to their impact on the safety and quality of the finished medicinal product. **Results:** A total of 421 deviations from specifications were reported to the QM-D per 6 month, which translates to 1 report per 1781 donations (1.5 Mio donations/year). The QM values the reports with regard to their impact on safety and/or quality and makes decisions for further actions. From the total of 421 errors, 3 errors were regarded as serious events directly affecting the patients safety (incorrect specimen labelling (n = 2); false blood group typing (n = 1). 114 reports were related to the product quality, whereby 27 where considered to be severe (industry supplied blood bags did not meet internal specifications). The laboratory as interface between hospital and blood service seems to be especially sensitive for deviations, with 67% of all reporting being related to the preanalytic. **Conclusion:** Taken together, the implementation of a continuous reporting system has proven very valuable in providing safe blood products meeting high quality standards. In addition it is a helpful tool for benchmarking and in developing a learning culture within the blood donor service.

OS7: Apheresis Preparative/Therapeutic

OS7.1

Extracorporeal Plasma Treatment for the Removal of Endotoxin in Septic Patients: Clinical Results of a Pilot Study

S. Bengsch[1], K.-S. Boos[2], D. Nagel[2], D. Seidel[2], D. Inthorn[2]

[1]Universitätsklinikum Jena, D; [2]Klinikum Großhadern, LMU, München, D

Despite the advances in therapeutic approaches in the management of inflammatory conditions the incidence of sepsis is on increase in the intensive care units. In in-vitro experiments we could demonstrate that perfusion of plasma through an anion-exchanger (DEAE-modified cellulose) effectively removes toxins of gram-negative bacteria, i.e. lipopolysaccharides (endotoxin, LPS) as well as of gram-positive bacteria, i.e. lipoteichoic acids (LTA). We investigated in a pilot study whether the use of an apheresis system based on DEAE cellulose is capable to reduce the plasma concentration of endotoxin in patients with severe sepsis. We enrolled 15 intensive care patients with severe sepsis and plasma endotoxin concentrations > 0.3 EU/ml. In addition to standard ICU therapy a total of 83 apheresis treatments were performed. About 1.7 volumes of plasma (6000 ml) were treated at each apheresis session. A significant reduction in plasma endotoxin levels from a median of 0.61 EU/ml to 0.39 EU/ml (−35%) could be achieved (P < 0.001). Long-term comparison of the initial and post treatment levels after a series of 5–6 individual apheresis treatments also showed a statistically significant decline in circulating endotoxin, IL-6, CRP, fibrinogen and an increase in cholesterol levels. Except for a transient and reversible increase of prothrombin time no adverse events were observed in patients undergoing this adsorption apheresis treatment. Our data show that reduction of endotoxin by extracorporeal DEAE cellulose based plasma treatment may prove a promising therapeutic tool for patients suffering from bacterial sepsis and proven endotoxemia.

OS7.2

Transplant-Associated Microangiopathy after Allogeneic Stem Cell Transplantation Following Reduced Intensity Conditioning: Close Association with ABO Incompatibility

N. Worel, G. Leitner, V. Kolovratova, M. Horvath, M. Mitterbauer, W. Rabitsch, H. Greinix, P. Kalhs, P. Höcker

Universitätsklinik Wien, A

Purpose: Transplant-associated microangiopathy (TAM) is a severe complication of allogeneic hematopoietic stem cell transplantation (SCT) associated with high mortality rates. Major risk factors for the development of TAM are toxic effects of high-dose chemo-radiotherapy, heavy pretreatment and the use of unrelated donor (URD) grafts. TAM is reported to occur in about 14% of patients after myeloablative conditioning. To reduce transplant-related mortality associated with allogeneic SCT in patients at risk, reduced-intensity conditioning (RIC) regimens have been introduced. We reviewed data on 112 consecutive patients with a median age of 54 years (18–70) given sibling (n = 54) or URD (n = 57) SCT after RIC with respect to occurrence of TAM. **Methods:** RIC consisted of Fludarabin (90 mg/m^2) and 2 Gy total body irradiation (TBI) or polychemotherapy and 4 Gy TBI. In the majority of patients cyclosporin A (CyA) and mycophenolate mofetil was given for GvHD prophylaxis. Fifty-four patients received an ABO identical and 58 patients an ABO mismatched graft. TAM was defined as > 4% schistocytes in the blood, renewed or prolonged thrombocytopenia, sudden increase in LDH, increased RBC transfusion requirements and decrease in serum haptoglobin. Treatment of TAM consisted of withdrawal of CyA and plasma exchange. **Results:** TAM occured in 11/112 patients (10%) after RIC. The median time of onset was 62 (9–906) days after SCT and was associated with acute GvHD (n = 4), chronic GvHD (n = 3), proteus mirabilis (n = 1) and herpes virus infection (n = 1), severe hemolysis after minor ABO-incompatible SCT (n = 1) and computed tomography proven atypical pneumonia (n = 1). In 9/11 patients with TAM an ABO mismatch was present (p = 0.03), donor source (p = 0.12) and previous autologous SCT (p = 0.09) had no significant influence on the occurrence TAM. A median of 11 (4–30) plasma exchange procedures were performed. Overall, 7 of 11 (64%) patients responded whereas 3 patients died of GvHD and TAM, and another of multi-organ failure. One patient who responded to plasma-exchange died 1 year later of relapse of the original hematologic disease. **Conclusion:** TAM remains a severe complication after allografting. Its incidence and severity is not reduced compaired to myeloablative conditioning. After RIC occurrence of TAM seems to be increased in ABO-mismatched SCT. Wether the use of different cytotoxic agents and immunosuppressants in RIC has an impact on the development of TAM in our patient series remains unclear.

OS7.3

Using a New Certified Irradiation Machine for the Treatment of Chronic GvHD by Extracorporeal Photochemotherapy

H. Ullrich, N. Kröger, A. Zander, J. Schrum, R. Erttmann, P. Kuehnl

University of Hamburg, D

Photopheresis was first published by Edelson for the treatment of cutaneous T-cell-lymphoma. Nowadays one main indication of photopheresis is the prevention and treatment of transplant rejection and of Graft versus Host Disease (GvHD) after bone marrow transplantation. Andreu introduced variations to the original system by using a continuously operating cell separator, applying the 8-Methoxypsoralen (8-MOP) into the leukocyte collection bag and by applying a standardised irradiation dose to all apheresed cells, this procedure is called extracorporeal photochemotherapy (ECPC). In our department of transfusion medicine six patients with therapy refractory chronic GvHD were treated by ECPC. Cell separation was carried out with a Spectra (Gambro BCT), extracorporeal blood volume is thus kept below 300 ml, a good yield and purity of MNC was achieved. 8-MOP was added directly into the mononuclear cell collection bag, the MNC concentrate was then UVA irradiated with a CE certified UVA irradiation machine (Macogenic, Maco Pharma). To ensure continuous standardised irradiation, cells were agitated and kept at constant temperature. Five adult patients and one fifteen year old boy with cGvHD were treated by two aphaereses per week at the start, ECPC and drugs were then gradually tapered according to improvement. Five patients developed cGvHD from acute GvHD after PBSC transplantaion, one had cGvHD after donor lymphocyte infusion one year after the PBSC transplantation. Three patients suffered from mucocutaneous cGvHD and improved after 4–6 ECPC, in all of them drug and ECPC tapering is under way. The 15 year old was transfusion dependent on RBC and platelets until the start of ECPC, even with HLA-antibodies. His platelet count has increased drastically, and he does not need substitution any more. One steroid dependent patient has started tapering without further signs of relapse, one patient with severe gastrointestinal cGvHD has abandoned treatment and died. One 19 year old patient with severe pulmonary and cutaneous improvement has first deteriorated and now suffers from stable disease and is slowly gaining weight. ECPC is a very valuable second line treatment for cGvHD without relevant side effects. Early start of ECPC might lead to faster improvement.

OS7.4

The Mobilization Effect of Platelet Apheresis

H.-G. Heuft, L. Goudeva, J. Martens, A. Schmitt-Thomssen, R. Blasczyk
Medizinische Hochschule Hannover, D

Background: To investigate the mobilization effect of current double and triple platelet (PLT) collection into the donors' peripheral blood pool. **Methods:** A total of 1634 Gambro Trima and Fresenius Comtec PLT aphereses from 710 individual donors were performed. Apheresis standards included mean PLT yields of 2.8 × 10E11 (single), 5.6 × 10E11 (double), and 8.4 × 1011 (triple) within an apheresis time <100 minutes. Donor criteria for single/double PLT aphereses comprehend minimum values for body weight (60 kg) and preapheresis PLT counts >220 × 10E9/L, for triple PLT aphereses 80 kg and PLT counts >280 × 10E9/L. The mobilization effect was determined by the difference (diff) between the donors' actually measured postapheresis PLT counts (Coulter counter) and the postapheresis PLT count prediction (pred) of the cell separator (based on a simple mass balance equation with the number of PLT in the donors' blood pool and the PLT loss in the collect bag). **Results:** (see Table, means, standard deviation) After double or triple PLT aphereses, 22% and 25% more PLT circulated in donor peripheral blood than calculated by the apheresis devices. A correlation analysis including donor age, gender, body weight, total blood volume, PLT precount and PLT loss as well as apheresis time, inlet flow and citrate load revealed PLT loss as the most important mobilizing factor ($R2 = 0.33$, $p > 0.000$). **Conclusions:** PLT apheresis procedures induce a considerable mobilization effect, particularly if higher PLT yields are collected. Current cell separators do not provide a realistic PLT count prediction after platelet apheresis.

OS7.5

Bone Marrow Separation for AB0-Incompatible and Volume-Reduced Transplantation Using a Closed Cytapheresis-System

P. Reinhardt, P. Schauwecker, E. Krug, B. Maccari, H. Schrezenmeier, M. Wiesneth
Institute for Clinical Transfusion Medicine and Immunogenetics Ulm, D

Purpose: Bone marrow (BM) is an important source of hematopoietic progenitor cells (HPC). For small recipients, AB0-incompatible transplants (Tx), cryopreservation or manipulation, the collected BM requires a safe and effective red blood cell- (RBC) and volume-reduction without loss of HPC. **Methods:** 35 BM-aspirates for Tx were analysed retrospectively. Citrate (ACD-A) was added to the collected BM to 10% (vol/vol) and transferred to a BM processing set (Gambro, BCT) in the clean room. The BM was processed on a COBESpectra cell separator using the closed WBC set and the respective BM-setting (all Gambro, BCT), in essence following manufacturer instructions. The original BM was processed >4 times. Enriched MNC fractions were usually sequentially collected in 2 bags. Volume- and RBC-reduction, MNC-, CD34- and CD3-recovery was assessed. **Results:** A volume-reduction was required for every transplant. 27 BM-Tx were AB0-incompatible. 22 Tx were for children weighing 6–38 kg, 40% of processed BM were to be partially cryopreserved. BM volume ranged from 310–2228 ml with an average Hct of 29%, corresponding to 81–624 ml of RBC. Cytapheresis lasted 100–150 min, the initial BM being processed 4 to 16 times (average 8). The volume was reduced in average to 14% (61–359 ml) and a Hct of 6% (RBC 1–29 ml) in collection bag 1; in bag 2 a volume of 34–124 ml (11%) and an average Hct of 5%. The recovery of NC was 34% in bag 1 and 6% in bag 2, for MNC: 52% in bag 1, 9% in bag 2, CD34: bag 1 = 82%, bag 2 = 12% and CD3: bag 1 = 87%, bag 2 = 13%. **Conclusions:** To maintain the Hct between 2–7% in the collected MNC-layer is technically challenging. Processing the initial BM 4–6 times usually allows the recovery of >80% of CD34 and CD3 cells (bag 1), additional processing (bag 2) may be useful as back-up. With continuous monitoring, cytapheresis is an efficient and GMP-compatible technique to reduce RBC and volume of BM-Tx. The reduction achieved is sufficient even for AB0-incompatible Tx of infants or further processing without significant loss of HPC.

OS7.6

Prediction of Graft Cell Dose in Bone Marrow Harvesting for Unrelated HSC

A. Platz[1], M. Punzel[1], R. Wassmuth[2], P. Wernet[1], J. Fischer[1]
[1]Institute for Transplantation Diagnostic and Cell Therapeutics (ITZ), Düsseldorf, D; [2]DKMS Life Science Lab, Dresden, D

Purpose: Bone marrow harvesting is introduced for allogeneic stem cell transplantation for many years. It is still a demanding task to gain a product of high quality and to release the donor as early as possible from the operating procedure. The aim of this investigation is to proof whether routine parameters of quality control have prognostic importance for the amount of collected nucleated cells. **Methods:** Between 1998 and 2006 187 bone marrow transplants were collected from unrelated donors. The collection site was an orthopedic surgery theatre. At each time of production we check blood cell counts of the donor before (PB BMpre) and after (PB BMpost) collection. During collection an intermediate sample (TNCint) is drawn from the product for cell

Table for Abstract OS7.4

A-Type	A-Time (min)	PLT loss ($\times 10^{11}$/A)	PLT_{diff} ($\times 10^9$/L) measured vs pred	PLT ratio measured vs pred	Mobilized PLT ($\times 10^{11}$/A)
Single*	48 ± 12.3	v2.8 ± 0.30	16.2 ± 8.8	1.11 ± 0.06	0.73 ± 0.2
Double**	73.8 ± 14.8	5.52 ± 0.35	29.0 ± 14.8	1.22 ± 0.12	1.53 ± 0.44
Triple***	81.2 ± 16	7.90 ± 0.67	44.3 ± 17.1	1.25 ± 0.14	2.58 ± 0.57

Legend: A = apheresis; Total number of A: n = 1643; * n = 60 (3.7%); ** n = 1132 (69.3%); *** n = 442 (27.0%).

count measure to estimate final product volume and adjust collection duration. Cell counts from the final product (BM) are also performed. Data were prooved by linear regression test and t-test. **Results:** Important relations were found between WBCpre and collected volume under respect of the requested cell count. Here we found a higher volume (500 ml) for donors with WBCpre < -1 standard deviation (SD) when collection volume was normalized for requested NC number. This effect was more explicit in males than in females. The linear regression test showed a relation ($r2 = 0.224$) between WBCpre and zwKM (nucleated cell count TNC). Higher WBC in peripheral blood seems to correlate with a higher TNC count at time of zwKM. **Conclusion:** We could not find really significant data for the prediction of cell and volume outcome in bone marrow transplants inspite of the action performed on the basis of in-process-control. But nevertheless we found a trend if data of donor's preWBC, requested cell count and product's TNCint are available. Therewith adjustment of collection volume and duration are posible.

OS7.7

CD16+ Monocyte Subpopulations Are Differential Regulated after Leukapheresis in Healthy Blood Donors and in Patients with Metastatic Malignant Melanoma

M. Hendelmeier, E. Strasser, M. Erdmann, R. Zimmermann, R. Eckstein

Universitätsklinikum Erlangen, D

Purpose: CD16+ monocytes are elevated in patients with metastatic malignant melanoma. Peripheral blood monocytes are a heterogeneous population and consist of distinct subsets. Monocytes are relatively immature precursors and Dendritic cells (DC) are the terminal stage of monocyte differentiation. Leukapheresis is a stimulus for recruitment of mature and immature myeloid cells in donors and the enrichment of monocyte subsets in apheresis products. The understanding of monocyte heterogeneity may have implications for the development of DC cancer vaccines. **Methods:** 22 blood donors and 18 patients with metastatic malignant melanoma were investigated before and after leukocytapheresis procedures. Monocyte products of patients were compared with the results of the healthy blood donors. The percentage of monocyte subpopulations were investigated by flow cytometry (FACS Calibur, BD). **Results:** The leukocyte concentration of products ranged between $24.3 \times 10e3$ and $111.5 \times 10e3$ WBCs per µl. The mean percentage of CD14-positive cells was 20 percent (range, 11.6% to 31.4%). Subpopulations of CD14-positive and CD33-positive monocytes showed different enrichment in the MNC products. Compared to the initial concentration of CD33dim CD16+ monocytes in donors no cell enrichment in MNC products was found, whereas CD14+CD16+ monocytes in donors were enriched by factor 2 ($4.99\% \pm 2.53\%$ vs. $10.14\% \pm 6.71\%$, $p < 0.0001$). The enrichment of CD14+CD16+ monocytes was even highter (factor 3). The pre- and post-donation counts of CD14+CD16+ monocytes in donors ($n = 22$) differed significantly (4.8% vs. 5.3%, $p = 0.0001$). In patients ($n = 18$) with metastatic malignant melanoma the CD14+CD16+ monocytes increased by 57% ($p = 0.0002$) in the postdonation count. Additionally the CD33dim CD16+ monocytes increased by 40.3% ($p = 0.0002$) whereas the same cell population in healthy blood donors decreased by 12% ($p = 0.079$) in blood counts after apheresis procedure. **Conclusion:** The CD33+CD16+ cells were enriched in the leukapheresis products. CD33dim CD16+ were increased in patients with metastatic malignant melanoma in postdonation counts. These results may suggest a different cell recruitment of monocyte subpopulation in patients with metastatic malignant melanoma compared to healthy blood donors. The leukapheresis procedure itself may stimulate the release of myeloid progenitor cells.

OS7.8

In Process Control of Progenitor Count during Stem Cell Apheresis Shortens Harvesting Duration and Minimizes Required Procedures

J.C Fischer, A. Platz, M. Punzel, P. Wernet

Universitätsklinikum Düsseldorf, D

Introduction: Peripheral blood progenitor cells (PBPC) are mostly collected using a Cobe Spectra (Gambro) apheresis device. Until recently (spring 2006) no collection set was officially introduced, which would allow GMP-grade sampling from the product during apheresis. For this purpose we have been using a locally customized WBC set since November 2000. This enabled us to perform GMP-grade in process control (iPC) of the product itself during collection. Here we present retrospectively analyzed data of 1862 apheresis cycles corresponding to 2475 apheresis procedures performed within the last 10 y. **Method:** Before installation to the cell separator the sample bag of the WBC collection set (No. 7700600, Gambro) was connected to a 8 ml ACDA reservoir (Macopharma) by 3-step sterile docking. This allowed us first to ad additional ACDA to the product during collection without harming the donor and second to perform an iPC consisting of WBC and CD34 cell counting according to the ISHAGE criteria. Apheresis duration was than adapted according to the iPC results. Data were analyzed in respect to gender of the donor, used cytokine and dose, kind of donation (allogeneic ($n = 1427$) or autologous ($n = 1048$)), apheresis duration in terms of fold processed blood volume, number of apheresis within the collection cycle, ratio between harvested and requested progenitor numbers. **Results:** 1227 apheresis cycles with iPC and 635 cycles without iPC were investigated. Successful collection within one apheresis was especially common in allogeneic males, in patients without cytotoxic pretreatment, after introduction of the iPC. Overall the number of apheresis necessary to fulfill the request could be lowered from 1.5 aphereis (mean) to 1.3 per cycle; saving approximately 189 apheresis procedures in the iPC group. Furthermore especially in allogenic male donors ($n = 773$) collection duration could be lowered to less than 3 fold BV processed in 40.3% (compared to 17% before introduction of iPC). **Conclusion:** In process control of PBPC apheresis is feasible and shortens either duration of the harvesting procedure or the number of apheresis necessary for yielding the requested number of progenitors.

OS8: Hemostaseology

OS8.1

Postnatal Treatment of Neonatal Alloimmune Thrombocytopenia (NAIT): What We Know and what We Practice – a Systematic Overview of Controlled Clinical Trials and a Survey of Management Strategies across Canada and Germany

A. Greinacher[1], D. Bassler[2], C. Okascharoen[2], A. Klenner[1], J. Ditomasso[2], V. Kiefel[3], A. Chang[2], B. Paes[2]

[1]Ernst-Moritz-Arndt-Universität Greifswald, D; [2]McMaster University, Hamilton, CA; [3]University Rostock, D

Background: Neonatal alloimmune thrombocytopenia (NAIT) is an uncommon disorder with potentially serious sequelae. Platelet antigen compatible platelet concentrates are regarded as the treatment of choice, but are not immediately available in many centers. Therefore the management of affected infants remains a major challenge. **Objective:** To determine the optimal postnatal treatment of NAIT and ascertain neonatal practices in the management of the condition. **Methods:** We performed a systematic overview of randomized controlled intervention trials (RCTs) in the postnatal management of NAIT. To assess current management strategies, we conducted a survey across neonatal units in Canada and Germany. **Results:** No RCT for the postnatal treatment of newborn infants with NAIT was identified. 106 neonatologists in Canada and 189 centres for neonatal care in Germany were enrolled. The management of NAIT differed substantially between Canada and Germany. Most physicians use a screening threshold for NAIT for preterm infants 30–50 × 109/L (Canada 46.5%, Germany 53.4%). While 42.6% of the physicians in Canada use a trigger of 50–100 × 109/L for screening in term infants, 44% of German doctors use the identical threshold as in preterm infants. In preterm infants, 60.3% of Canadian neonatologists will start treatment for suspected NAIT at a platelet count between 30 and 50 × 109/L. In Germany 31.6% of the physicians commence treatment at this level and more than 20% use a threshold between 10–20 × 109/L. In term infants 6.3% of the Canadian and 16.2% of the German physicians use even lower treatment triggers between 5–10 × 109/L. Ordering and awaiting antigen-negative platelets in the presence of bleeding was considered the therapy of choice by most (60.5%) German physicians, but not by Canadian neonatologists, who preferred treatment with intravenous immunoglobulin (69.8%) and random donor platelets (54.9%). **Conclusion:** There is insufficient evidence from randomized controlled trials to determine the optimal postnatal management of NAIT. Treatment with compatible platelets often diverges from what is theoretically recommended.

OS8.2

High-Prevalence of Prolonged Closure Times in the Presence of Aortic-Valve Stenosis: Association with Perioperative Transfusion Requirements

C. Sucker, M. Kurt, J. Lithmathe, P. Feindt, R.B. Zotz, R.E. Scharf
Heinrich-Heine-Universität Düsseldorf, D

Background: Shear-stress induced acquired hemostatic abnormalities are highly prevalent in patients suffering from severe aortic-valve stenosis. In this study, we determined closure times with a platelet-function analyzer to assess the correlation with perioperative transfusion requirements. **Patients and Methods:** Fifty consecutive patients (mean age [± SD] 68 ± 9 years) admitted for aortic-valve replacement were enrolled. Antiplatelet medication was discontinued at least ten days prior to analysis. Closure times of epinephrin/collagen and ADP/collagen cartridges were determined with a platelet-function analyzer (Dade Behring, Marburg, Germany) and compared to those of healthy control subjects without medication. Multivariate analysis was performed to assess the impact of prolonged closure times on perioperative transfusion requirements. **Results:** Compared to controls, closure times determined with both epinephrin/collagen (210 ± 69 sec vs. 140 ± 50 sec, $p < 0.0001$) and ADP/collagen (145 ± 58 sec vs. 108 ± 45 sec, $p < 0.0001$) cartridges were prolonged in patients with aortic-valve stenosis. Intraoperative transfusion of red-blood cell units was weakly but significantly associated with the closure times determined with epinephrin/collagen ($r = 0.28$, $p = 0.04$,) and ADP/collagen cartridges ($r = 0.28$, $p = 0.04$). Total transfusion requirements of red-blood cell units were associated with ADP/collagen closure times ($r = 0.31$, $p = 0.02$), but not epinephrin/collagen closure times ($r = 0.26$, $p = 0.07$). No association was found with postoperative transfusion of red-blood cell units with both cartridges ($r = 0.07$, $p = 0.62$ and $r = 0.21$, $p = 0.14$, respectively). **Conclusion:** Prolongation of closure times determined with a platelet-function analyzer is highly prevalent in patients with aortic-valve stenosis and appears to reflect shear-stress induced hemostatic abnormalities. Since prolonged closure times are associated with increased perioperative transfusion of red-blood cell units, the assay could significantly contribute to the identification of individuals at risk.

OS8.3

Platelets are Differentially Regulated in Patients with Chronic Inflammation due to Cystic Fibrosis

A. Sturm[1], H. Hebestreit[1], C.P. Speer[1], C. Koenig[1], A. Obergfell[2], U. Walter[2], R. Grossmann[3]
[1]University of Wuerzburg – University Children's Hospital, Würzburg, D;
[2]Institute of Clinical Biochemistry and Pathobiochemistry, Würzburg, D;
[3]Haemophilia Centre, Department of Internal Medicine III, Frankfurt, D

Purpose: Platelets might play a key role in inflammatory disorders due to versatile interactions with the cellular and humoral immune system. In this study we investigated platelet function and activation as well as mechanisms of platelet-leukocyte-aggregate formation in clinically stable patients with cystic fibrosis (CF). **Methods:** Several parameters of platelet function were investigated in 55 patients (16.5 ± 8.9 years) and 55 matched controls (16.4 ± 8.9 years). The percentage of CD62P and PAC-1 positive resting and TRAP-6-activated platelets as well as platelet-leukocyte aggregates were determined by flow cytometry. Soluble markers of platelet activation sCD62P and sCD40L were determined by ELISA. Exocytosis of platelet integrin alphaIIbbeta3 (CD41a-expression) as well as leukocyte expression of PSGL-1 (receptor of CD62P) and integrin alphaMbeta2 were also measured by flow cytometry. **Results:** Platelet activation, measured by PAC-1-binding to resting (5.9% ± 8.8 vs. 12.9% ± 13.5, $p < 0.05$) and activated platelets (31.6% ± 19.5 vs. 42.9% ± 16.0, $p < 0.05$), was decreased in patients with CF. These effects were stronger in patients with higher markers of inflammation. In contrast, proinflammatory platelet functions remained unchanged (CD62P-expression on resting and activated platelets) or were shown to be even increased [soluble CD62P (41.2 ng/ml ± 10.1 vs. 31.4 ng/ml ± 9.8, $p < 0.05$), soluble CD40L (496 pg/ml ± 427 vs. 196 ng/ml ± 183, $p < 0.05$), platelet-leukocyte-aggregates]. **Conclusions:** These data show a differential regulation of platelet function in patients with CF: platelet proinflammatory functions are up-regulated in chronic inflammation, whereas platelet haemostatic function is down-regulated as shown by a decreased activation of the integrin alphaIIbbeta3. The latter effect might partially compensate the procoagulatory alterations caused by acute phase changes in inflammatory disorders.

OS8.4

Heparin-Independent Activation of Platelets by HIT Antibodies: A Common Occurrence

U. Sachs[1], I. Socher[1], A. Giptner[1], S. Jorks[2], G. Bein[1], H. Kroll[2]
[1]Justus Liebig-Universität Gießen, D; [2]Blutspendedienst NSTOB, Dessau, D

Purpose: Heparin-induced thrombocytopenia (HIT) is a potentially life-threatening complication of heparin anticoagulant therapy. It is caused by antibodies elicited by a conformational change in platelet factor 4 (PF4), which exposes neoepitopes resulting from its binding to heparin. HIT antibodies bind to these PF4/heparin complexes and interact with platelet FcgammaIIa receptors, leading to platelet activation, thrombocytopenia, and thrombosis. In the year 2005, 980 specimens were tested by HIPA at Giessen University Hospital. Of 103 that tested positive, 51 (49.5%) caused activation of platelets without the addition of heparin, an observation that was previously anticipated to be due to heparin contamination of the serum. In contrast, evidence has accumulated during the last years that HIT antibodies might be heterogeneous, with some HIT antibodies cross-reacting with PF4 alone, i.e. in the absence of heparin. Such antibodies might be responsible for the progression of HIT after heparin cessation and the delayed-onset type of HIT. Thus, we addressed the question if HIT antibodies can cause spontaneous platelet activation in the absence of exogenous heparin. **Methods:** Sera from 16 HIT patients with strong reactivity in the HIPA assay were treated with 1 USP heparinase I for 60 min at 37°C and re-subjected to HIPA testing. Purified IgG fractions were prepared from all sera and analyzed by HIPA. Presence of contaminating heparin in sera treated with heparinase and in IgG fractions was excluded by a chromogenic anti-FXa assay. **Results:** Following heparinase I digestion, 14 of 16 sera (87.5%) remained reactive in the HIPA in the presence of saline alone (heparinase-insensitive sera). In contrast, two sera (12.5%) lost their reactivity (heparinase-sensitive sera). Purified IgG fractions from all 16 sera were reactive in the HIPA assay when heparin was added to the reaction. In the presence of saline alone, IgG fractions from all 14 heparinase-insensitive sera were still capable of activating platelets in the HIPA. IgG fractions obtained from heparin-sensitive sera were not able to activate platelets in the presence of saline only. **Conclusions:** Platelet activation in the "saline only" reaction of the HIPA can be attributed to the capability of HIT antibodies to induce platelet activation in the absence of heparin in the majority of samples (87.5% in our study). It seems to occur only rarely as a consequence of heparin contamination of the patient's serum (12.5%). The demonstration of HIT antibodies that can activate platelets independent of heparin may provide further insight into pathological mechanisms responsible for HIT and provide clues to a better understanding of delayed HIT.

OS8.5

Dynamics of Platelet Thrombus Formation in Relation to the HPA-1 Polymorphism of Integrin alphaIIb beta3: Quantification under Arterial Flow Conditions

R.E. Scharf, J. Peveling, R. Loncar, A. Beck, V. Aurich, V.R. Stoldt
Heinrich Heine University, Düsseldorf, D

Introduction: Clinical association studies and experimental findings suggest that platelet function and arterial thrombogenesis can be modulated by single nucleotide polymorphisms of platelet membrane glycoprotein receptors. Thus, distinct receptor variants including HPA-1b of integrin alphaIIb beta3 and alpha2 807TT of integrin alpha2 beta1 were identified as risk factors for increased platelet thrombogenicity. **Materials and Methods:** We have used an established perfusion model in combination with confocal laser microscopy and a novel "voxel"-based imaging software to study the dynamics of thrombus formation under flow conditions simulating stenosed arteries. Whole blood from healthy dononors (n = 30), anticoagulated with trisodium citrate (11 mM) and preincubated with mepacrine (10 µM) to render platelets fluorescent, was aspirated through a parallel-plate rectangular perfusion chamber at calibrated flow rates to provide initial wall shear rates of 500, 1,000, or 1,500 sec-1. Prior to perfusion, a glass cover slip coated with fibrillar type I collagen was inserted to form the lower surface of the flow chamber. For 3-dimensional analysis of thrombus growth over time, a series of stacks, i.e. 30 confocal optical sections, from the bottom to the apex of the forming thrombus, were obtained on an area of 26,450 μm^2. Images were analyzed by a "voxel"-based procedure, whereby a voxel is defined by a volume of 0.202 μm^3 (0.45 × 0.45 × 1 [μm^3]). For calibration, fluorescent beads (Invitrogen, Carlsbad, CA, USA) were used. **Results:** At an initial wall shear rate of 500 sec-1, thrombus formation begun after a lag phase of 220 sec. After 420 sec, thrombus volume reached a maximum (mean ± SD, 40,000 ± 4.900 μm^3). Thrombus growth occurred in a 2-step way with an apical growth (height extension) at the interval of 220 to 300 sec, and progression in the plane section at the interval of 300 to 420 sec after perfusion. Platelet aggregate and thrombus formation were completely suppressed in the presence of an anti-alphaIIb beta3 antibody. Interestingly, the HPA-1 polymorphism of alphaIIb beta3 had a significant impact on thrombus growth. Thus, when comparing blood from homozygous carriers of HPA-1b (n = 8) and HPA-1a (n = 8), thrombus formation and progression occured more rapidly with HPA-1b than with HPA-1a platelets, resulting in significantly larger thrombi from HPA-1b than from HPA-1a individuals (p = 0.001). **Conclusion:** The voxel-based analysis of thrombus formation and progression under flow conditions provides a novel technique and can detect phenotypic differences related to the HPA-1 polymorphism of platelet integrin alphaIIb beta3. Specifically, our results confirm in this experimental setting that HPA-1b is a prothrombotic receptor variant.

OS8.6

Incidence and Differentiation of Thrombocytopenia in Pregnant Women Treated with Low-Molecular-Weight Heparin

U. Harbrecht, S. Flommersfeld, E. Forrest, C. Gnida, S. Ohlenforst, B. Rott, H. Seidel, J. Oldenburg
Universität Bonn, D

Purpose: Heparin-induced thrombocytopenia (HIT) is rare during pregnancy, however it is essential to differentiate HIT from pregnancy-related thrombocytopenias in women receiving heparin. The aim of this study was to assess the incidence of thrombocytopenia and of heparin-induced antibodies (HI-Ab) in women receiving low-molecular-weight heparin during pregnancy. **Patients and Methods:** 111 women completed 121 pregnancies and were treated with LMWH or danaparoid (nadroparin n = 101, dalteparin n = 9, enoxaparin n = 9, certoparin n = 6, danaparoid n = 5) during pregnancy and for 4 to 6 weeks after delivery. Reasons for heparin treatment were history of thrombosis (n = 71), inherited/acquired risk factors for thrombosis (n = 31) and/or recurrent fetal loss (n = 19). Development of HI-Ab (HPIA-ELISA, Roche, Germany) was measured in 4–8 week intervals. Platelet count was monitored once a week during the first 6 weeks of LMWH treatment and thereafter every 4–8 weeks. All measurements of HIT-Ab were performed after termination of heparin treatment unless platelet count dropped for more than 50% or thrombocytopenia (<150 G/l) developed. **Results:** Mild thrombocytopenia (range 105–147 G/l) was observed in 8/121 (6.6%) pregnancies. Thrombocytopenia developed during the last trimenon in all but one patient and resolved after delivery in all cases. No underlying disorder (e.g. HELLP) was diagnosed. None of the patients with thrombocytopenia had a positive HPIA-ELISA. In contrast, HI-Ab were detected in 6/121 (5.0%) pregnancies without thrombocytopenia or platelet count drop (>50%). Four patients had low (OD < 1.0) and two intermediate HI-Ab-titres (OD 1.0–2.0; Cut-off-OD 0.43–0.67). In two patients with low titres (OD 0.63 and 0.56) HI-Ab were already present before LMWH treatment and normalised in one of them during LMWH administration. Local allergic reactions to heparin occurred in 7.2% of patients and required change of anticoagulation. **Conclusions:** Mild pregnancy-associated thrombocytopenia without clinical relevance is the predominant aetiology of thrombocytopenia during pregnancy, also in heparin treated patients. Nevertheless, HIT has to be ruled out when thrombocytopenia develops at any time of heparin treatment due to the potentially deleterious consequences of HIT.

OS8.7

Perioperative Haemostatic Management – Thromboelastometry in Cardiac Surgery

M. Reinhöfer, W. Lösche, G. Marx, D. Barz
Universitätsklinikum Jena, D

Background: Cardiac surgical patients consume a much larger fraction of perioperative blood transfusions than the percentage of the surgical population they represent. Haemorrhages after cardiopulmonary bypass (CPB) have a multifactorial aetiology and are attributed to acquired platelet dysfunction, impaired plasmatic coagulation and increased fibrinolysis. The characterization of the haemostatic defects responsible for bleeding is essential for specific treatment and optimal clinical management. Since its first description in 1948, the TEG/ROTEM has been successfully used in the near patient evaluation of haemostasis. Recent years have seen a renewed interest in the technology. In the present study we investigated the possible benefit of ROTEM on perioperative haemostatic management in routine cardiac surgery. **Methods:** Prospectively, 150 consecutive patients undergoing elective cardiac surgery with CPB time of at least 45 minutes were studied (bypass grafting 49%, valve replacement 19%, others 32%). Citrated arterial whole blood samples were analysed by thromboelastometry (ROTEM, Pentapharm Co., Munich, Germany). Measurements were performed at three time points: preoperatively, before induction of anaesthesia (P1); straight after the end of surgery (P2) and after 18 hours postoperatively (P3). Blood loss through the chest tubes, blood product use and other clinical data were recorded. **Results:** CPB resulted in a significant impairment of haemostasis. Postoperative bleeding was clearly associated with long CPB times. In ROTEM a prolongation of clotting time (CT) and clot formation time (CFT) as well as a decrease in maximum clot firmness (MCF) resulted after CPB. Significantly more frequent pathological values with varying quantity in InTEM and ExTEM (30–50% and 11–25%) were observed at time P2. Most of the parameters normalized but did not return to the basal values at time P3. CFT and MCF were very strongly correlated with blood platelet count and fibrinogen level, whereby especially MCF in FibTEM correlated positive with the plasma level of fibrinogen (r = 0.81). Postoperatively thromboelastometric values were correlated with total blood loss and the use of blood and plasma products. **Conclusion:** Our data indicate that ROTEM reflects the alterations of the haemostatic system caused by CPB in standard cardiac surgery procedures. Thromboelastometry assays performed after CPB are useful to predict increased postoperative bleeding tendency and can support early identification and targeted treatment of significant coagulopathy. Further investigations are necessary to evaluate a ROTEM based guideline for perioperative haemostatic management and transfusions of blood products.

OS8.8

Platelet-Derived Microparticles Promote Clot Stability and Enhanced Platelet Adhesion

R. Loncar, D. Dzepina, V. Stoldt, R.B. Zotz, R.E. Scharf
Heinrich Heine University Medical Center Düsseldorf, D

Background: Microparticles (MP) are formed along with membrane remodelling processes of most stimulated eukaryotic cells or are generated upon stimulation including platelets. Recent findings suggest that platelet-derived MP promote hemostasis and thrombosis. In this study, we evaluated the influence of platelet MP on clot stability and their possible role in thrombogenesis. **Methods:** MP were prepared by a previously described method using collagen (Hypertension 2004, 428–433). The influence of platelet MP onto clot structure, determined as platelet contractile force (PCF) and clot elastic modulus (CEM), was evaluated with a Hemodyne haemostasis analyzer. To test the role of platelet MP in arterial thrombogenesis, platelets in anticoagulated whole blood were labelled with the fluorescence dye mepacrine and perfused (shear rate of 1500/s) through rectangular chamber over glass cover slips coated with 0.05 ml of platelet derived MP (600 MP/μm^2). Specific binding of platelets to immobilized MP was evaluated with blood preincubated with abciximab. A fluorescence laser-scan microscope was used for visualization and quantification of platelet adhesion onto MP-coated surfaces at 5 min after beginning of perfusion. **Results:** Mean PCF and CEM in blood of healthy donors (n = 9) were 6.5 ± 3 Kdynes and 12.5 ± 2 Kdynes/cm^2, respectively.

Application of 0.1 ml of platelet-derived MP increased PCF (forces generated by platelets within a clot) without reaching statistical significance (mean increase of 11% as compared to controls without MP). Simultaneously, addition of MP significantly increased CEM as measure of the clot stability from 12.5 ± 2 Kdynes/cm^2 to 22.4 ± 3 Kdynes/cm^2 ($p < 0.05$). After 5 min of perfusion through the rectangular flow chamber, the average platelet adhesion was 48,935 ± 14,600 AU. Preincubation of blood with abciximab inhibited the prothrombotic feature of platelet derived MP (140 ± 80 AU). **Conclusions:** Our experiments demonstrate that platelet-derived microparticles enhance platelet adhesion, support clot stability and, thus, can promote arterial thrombogenesis. These observations may have a clinically relevant impact on thrombotic disorders.

OS9: Virus and Bacterial Testing and Inactivation/Viral Disease

OS9.1

Blood Donor Screening for Influenza Virus Including H5N1– Is It Necessary and Feasible?

M. Schmidt[1], K. Hourfar[1], A. Themann[1], M. Eickmann[2], T. Laue[3], E. Seifried[1]

[1]DRK Institut Frankfurt, Frankfurt, D; [2] Institut für Virology, Marburg, D; Qiagen, Hamburg, D

Background: New emerging pathogens represent an incalculable risk for blood products, because they are not included in current screening procedures. Therefore, the current study focused on the impact of influenza viruses, including avian influenza (H5N1), on blood safety. **Study Design and Methods:** The RealArtTM Influenza RT PCR Kit was used to amplify and detect influenza virus sequences from blood donor samples. We tested 10,272 blood donor samples in mini pools of up to 96 donations. To validate the sensitivity of the assay, routine donor mini pools (90±6 samples per pool) were spiked with H5N1 viruses and were used as positive controls. **Results:** None of the 10,272 clinical asymptomatic blood donors had an influenza viremia. Specificity of the assay was 100% because none of the tested blood donors were found to be positive for influenza virus or for H5N1. The analytical sensitivity was 19.1 PFU/ml and 8.5 PFU/ml for influenza virus and H5N1, respectively. Overall, 1/300 (0.33%) of test results had to be considered to be invalid due to negative results for the internal controls. Identity of virus responsible for the positive result could be further specified with a second NAT for H5N1. **Conclusion:** A non-symptomatic but potentially viremic phase of approximately 1–2 days is assumed for influenza viruses. Therefore it is recommendable that donors who get symptoms such as fever or cough one or two days after their donation, are required to give this information to the blood donor center. In such cases, NAT analysis may be suitable to prevent a transmission of influenza viruses. In case of a worldwide spreading of H5N1, even a rapid implementation of routine-NAT screening for influenza viruses is feasible, in order to guarantee safe blood products especially for immunoincompentent recipients.

OS9.2

Enumeration of CMV Specific CD8+ T Cells by HLA Tetramer-Based Flow Cytometry in Healthy IgG-CMV-Positive Blood Donors

L. Olbrich, J. Miller, R. Repp, M. Gramatzki, A. Humpe

Schleswig-Holstein University Hospital, Campus Kiel, Kiel, D

Purpose: Formation of sufficient numbers of CMV specific CD8+ T cells plays a major role in control of CMV infections in patients after allogeneic stem cell transplantation. Rare data are available on the minimally required number of such cells in patients or in IgG CMV-positive healthy individuals to control infection. We therefore examined the number of CMV-specific CD8+ T cells in 47 CMV-seropositive (IgG) healthy regular blood donors with different CMV-tetramers. **Methods:** EDTA-anticoagulated peripheral blood samples of serologically HLA-typed, CMV-seropositive (IgG) healthy blood donors were stained and analyzed within 24 hours after sampling. Based on beads technology, in a first step the absolute number of CD8+ cells was determined. In a second step, the percentage of CMV-specific cells of the CD8+ cells was evaluated. The absolute number of CMV-specific CD8+ T cells was calculated by multiplying the absolute CD8+ T cell count with the concomitantly obtained proportion of tetramer-binding CD8+ T cells. The following tetramers were applied in FACS analysis: A*0101, A*0201, A*2402, B*0702, B*0801, B*3501, and the respective negative tetramer control. **Results:** In 12 of the 47 analyzed samples a minimum number of 20 CMV specific CD3+CD8+ cells could not be acquired and these samples were omitted in further analysis. For the analyzed 35 donor samples a median number of 22,941 (range: 16,233–44,044) CD3+ cells, of 8,290 (3,620–15,013) CD3+CD8+ cells, and of 117 (20–9,257) CMV-specific CD3+CD8+ T cells were analyzed. The median proportion of CMV-specific CD8+ T cells of all CD3+ T cells was 1.46% (0.19%–66.72%) with a median absolute count of 8 (1–456) cells/μL. 24 samples could be analyzed by at least a second tetramer. The median number of CMV-specific CD3+CD8+ T cells/μL (1, 0.1–17) revealed by the second tetramer was significantly ($p < 0.05$) lower. **Conclusions:** In healthy individuals, the detectable number of CMV-specific CD8+ T cells considerably varies interindividually. Further analyses especially HLA typing of the healthy donors by molecular techniques are needed to elucidate whether the intraindividually different results between various tetramers are caused by serological HLA mistyping, incomplete HLA matching of tetramer and examined individual, differences in recognition of distinct CMV peptides, or by immunodominance between different CMV epitopes and MHC presentation.

OS9.3

Influence of Lyophilization on the Infectivity of Enveloped and Non-Enveloped Viruses in Bone Tissue

A. Pruß[1], C. Uhlenhaut[2], G. Pauli[2]

[1]Charité – Universitätsmedizin Berlin, D; [2]Robert Koch-Institut, Berlin, D

Introduction: Recently reported qualitative experiments proved that retroviral infectivity is not destroyed by lyophilization when applied to systemically infected bone and tendon. The residual infectivity of enveloped and non-enveloped model viruses in freeze-dried bone transplants was determined quantitatively. The results obtained should allow a assessment of virus safety of freeze-dried bone transplants. **Material and Methods:** The lyophilization effect on the infectivity (given as log10 TCID50/mL) of two non-enveloped viruses (Maus Elberfeld virus, MEV, model virus for Picornaviruses like HAV and Poliovirus; Porcine Parvovirus, PPV, model virus for Human Parvovirus B19 and one of the most resistant viruses to physico-chemical inactivation methods) and one enveloped virus (Vesicular Stomatitis virus, VSV, model virus for rabies) was examined for virus-spiked bone material (native human corticalis particles, 0.08–0.8 mm) in comparison to lyophilized virus stock, original virus stock and air-dried virus stock. All experiments were carried out under routine tissue bank procedures for cell free virus stock and for cell associated virus. **Results:** Significant differences were observed regarding the reduction of TCID50 for different viruses. Infectivity of VSV was reduced about 3log10 by lyophilization in presence of bone. The virus titer of MEV was reduced about 6log10 while for PPV no substantial reduction in TCID50 (<1log10) was observed. **Discussion and Conclusion:** Lyophilization is not sufficient as sole inactivation method regarding general virus safety of musculoskeletal transplants. However, reduction of virus infectivity through lyophilization could be used in combination with other inactivation methods such as heat, gamma irradiation or chemical treatment.

OS9.4

In-vitro and In-vivo Evaluation of Platelet Concentrates Treated with Pathogen Inactivation Using the INTERCEPT Blood System

P. Schlenke[1], V. Franck[2], L. Lin[3], W. Hagenah[1], S. Wehmeier[1], T. Wagner[1], H. Kirchner[1]

[1]Universität Lübeck, D; [2]Baxter R&D, Nivelles, B; [3]Cerus Corporation, Concord, USA

Purpose: In Germany, market authorization from the PEI is required before implementation of INTERCEPT Blood System™ in blood centers. We conducted in vitro studies to evaluate the effect of INTERCEPT treatment on apheresis and pooled buffy-coat platelet concentrates (PC) upon storage. In addition, we are performing an in vivo observational study to monitor the frequency of transfusion reactions and to analyse the corrected count increments in transfusion recipients of INTERCEPT treated PC. **Methods:** Twelve units of buffy-coat and apheresis PC were prepared in 35% plasma and 65% InterSol. Each unit was treated with 150 µM amotosalen and 3 J/cm^2 UVA followed by 10 h of compound adsorption. The platelets were stored for up to 8 days and evaluated using a panel of in vitro parameters including: volume, count, pH, lactate, glucose, LDH, CD62 (p-selectin), CO2 and O2. To date, 35 patients have been enrolled in the clinical single-arm, open label observational study. **Results:** The pooled buffy-coat PC (n = 12) contained 3.5 ± 0.4 × 1011 platelets in 341 ± 5 mL. After INTERCEPT processing, the volume and platelet count were 313 ± 6 mL and 3.1 ± 0.3 × 1011, respectively. The pH (22°C) was maintained (6.8 ± 0.1) on day 8 (d8). Glucose decreased to 3 ± 5 mg/dL on d8. CD62 expression (49 ± 5%) and LDH (137 ± 21 U/L) levels were compatible with viable platelet function. Similar results were observed in INTERCEPT treated apheresis PC. Initially, these units contained 3.5 ± 0.4 × 1011 platelets in 290 ± 4 mL. After INTERCEPT processing, the volume and platelet count were 270 ± 4 mL and 3.1 ± 0.2 × 1011, respectively. The pH (22°C) was maintained (6.7 ± 0.1) on d8. Glucose reached the limit of detection (0.1 ± 0.3 mg/dL) on d8, although other measurements (O2, CO2, lactate) indicated active metabolism. On d8, the CD62 expression (55 ± 8%) and LDH (127 ± 22 U/L) levels were consistent with viable platelet function. A detailed interim evaluation of the clinical results is still ongoing. A total of 230 platelet transfusions have been given. No serious adverse events related to the use of INTERCEPT treated PC have been reported. In addition, the frequency of transfusion reactions were reduced in comparison with previous published data obtained from conventional PC. **Conclusions:** The results demonstrated that storage of INTERCEPT treated buffy-coat or apheresis PC up to 8 days is feasible. Other ingredients in the additive solution InterSol, such as acetate, could have provided an alternative energy source to glucose. The clinical study is currently underway. Preliminary evaluation showed an overall low frequency of transfusion reactions and to date no INTERCEPT related serious adverse events have been reported.

OS9.5

Safety and Efficacy of Intercept Treated Apheresis Platelet Concentrates for Pediatric Patients Used in Routine: An Interim Report

G. Stiegler[1], V. Witt[2], P. Mörtl[1], G. Leitner[1], P. Höcker[1]
[1]Medizinische Universität Wien, A; [2]St. Anna Children Hospital; Wien, A

Purpose: We initiated an observation study to evaluate 500 transfusions of Intercept treated (IT) apheresis platelet concentrates (PC) to pediatric patients. Our first aim was to examine the safety and efficacy of IT PCs. Secondary, we gained experience with the adoption of the production of IT PCs into our routine workflow. Third, we compared the corrected count increments (CCI) and the incidence of transfusion reaction of IT PCs and not-IT apheresis PCs in patients who received both products during the same time period. **Methods:** PCs for IT were collected with the Amicus (Baxter) with an InterSol fraction of 60%. Randomized quality control measures were performed: residual Amotosalen, hem agglutinin titers, and sterility testing (BacTalert, BioMerieux). When indicated, PCs were gamma irradiated and/or plasma depleted. Patients at the age of 0.5–18 years were eligible for this open labelled, controlled study and received both, IT-PCs (group A) and not-IT-PCs (group B). Platelet counts before and one hour after transfusion, bleeding score, and adverse events were documented. **Results:** 94% of the PCs fulfilled the pre-treatment criteria for IT. IT started median 9 hours (4–20) after apheresis. Incubation in CAD took 8.5 hours (4.5–10.5). Platelet concentration was not changed by IT (before 1280G/L, ±304; after 1259G/L, ±291, $p > 0.02$). The PC volume was reduced from 304 ml (±11) before IT to 272 ml (±22) afterwards ($p < 0.02$). Thus, platelet dose was 3.88×10^{11} (±0.9) before the IT, and 3.43×10^{11} (±0.7) thereafter ($p < 0.02$). The working time needed for the IT was 20–25 minutes for each PC. Residual Amotosalen was 0.26 µM (±0.22). Hem agglutinin titers were <1:32 in all measures, and no bacteria were detected. 86 pediatric patients with haemoto-oncological disorders (mean 11.2 years, ±5.45) received both, 135 PCs from group A and 323 PCs from group B. PCs were transfused prophylactic (88%) or in case of bleeding (12%). There was no difference in the bleeding score between both groups ($p > 0.02$). Transfusion adverse events occurred less frequently in group A (1/135) than in group B (10/323, $p < 0.02$). Events comprised febrile (A:1, B:3) and allergic reactions (B:7). The platelet pre-counts were similar in both groups (A: 14G/L, ±6; B: 15G/L, ±8, $p > 0.02$). The CCI differed significantly (A: 9, ±10; B: 14, ±15; $p < 0.02$). **Conclusions:** The IT causes a platelet dose loss of 12% due to the PC volume loss. Transfusion of IT PCS results in a smaller CCI as compared to not-IT PCs possibly due to the impact of InterSol, Amotosalen, and UVA illumination on platelet function. Dose reduced PCs and low CCI may lead to an increased need for platelet transfusions. However, IT PCs provide effective haemostasis. The small hem agglutinin titers indicate that IT PCs can be used for blood group unequal transfusions without further manipulation. Acute transfusion reactions are significantly reduced when IT PCs are used due to the low amount of plasma. Transfusion of IT-PCs to pediatric patients is save and effective.

OS9.6

Clinical Significance of Bacterially Contaminated Platelet Concentrates

S.-B. Nicol, J. Brachert, S. Hartmann, T. Montag
Paul-Ehrlich-Institut, Langen, D

Background: In bacterially contaminated platelet concentrates (PCs), there is a difference between the contamination rate and the infection rate, i.e. only 10 to 20 percent of PCs containing bacteria are leading to transfusion-transmitted bacterial infections in the recipients. This phenomenon is not understood up to now, although antibiotic treatment of a certain percentage of patients can explain it partly. **Material and Methods:** PCs were contaminated with a representative spectrum of different bacteria species respectively bacteria strains following "real life" conditions, i.e. they were inoculated under aseptic conditions with 10 colony forming units (cfu) per platelet bag corresponding to 0.03 cfu per ml. Thereafter, the platelet bags were stored at 22.5°C under agitation. In a high frequency, samples were drawn from the bags in order to characterise the growth kinetic of the given bacteria strain. **Results:** Strong differences in growth behaviour of bacteria in platelet concentrates were observed. Some of the bacteria examined (e.g. strains of Staphylococcus epidermidis, Streptococcus pyogenes, Klebsiella pneumoniae, Escherichia coli) were growing up from 0.03 cfu/ml up to 10^{8-9} cfu/ml within 24 to 48 hours. Several strains of Propionibacterium acnes are not able to proliferate in PCs after contamination with 0.03 cfu/ml. Applying higher initial bacteria counts for contamination (e.g. 10 cfu/ml corresponding to ca. 3000 bacteria per bag), they strains grew up to high numbers. Similar growth properties were observed applying a strain of Pseudomonas aeruginosa, which usually did not grow up in PCs following inoculation of up to 1000 cfu/ml (corresponding to 3×10^5 per bag) into platelet bags. One strain of Klebsiella pneumoniae showed strong differences in its growth in PCs from different donors. In some PCs, the Klebsiella strain remained in an enormous prolonged lag phase of up to 3 days before starting their proliferation. Thereafter, it grew up rapidly to 10^{8-9} cfu/ml. **Conclusions:** The categories established in clinical microbiology for assessment of bacteria concerning their clinical relevance (pathogenic, apathogenic, facultative pathogenic) are not valid for bacteria contaminating blood components. For instance, Pseudomonas aeruginosa usually possesses a high pathogenic potency, e. g. in hospital infections. On the other hand, imagining a strain of Pseudomonas aeruginosa which remains in the very low count of 10 to 100 bacteria per bag (0.03 to 0.3 cfu/ml) after contaminating a platelet concentrate, the probability of a transfusion-transmitted infection is very low if not excluded. Contrariwise, a clinical relevant infection of the recipient after transfusion of a PC containing 10^8 cfu/ml of the usually apathogenic bacterium Propionibacterium acnes is very likely. In conclusion, there is a strong need for working out criteria for assessment of clinical relevance of bacteria as blood contaminants.

OS9.7

Monitoring of the Photochemical Pathogen Inactivation Procedure for Platelet Concentrates by PCR and Bioanalyzer

K. Janetzko
University of Heidelberg, Mannheim, D

Purpose: Photochemical treatment has been developed to inactivate pathogens by forming adducts between a reactive substance and nucleic acids.

Previously we could demonstrated that the DNA modifications inhibit the polymerase chain reaction (PCR). With mitochondrial DNA (mtDNA) as an abundant template in platelet concentrates we established a PCR system including qualitative evaluation of results on agarose gels in order to monitor the photochemical treatment (PCT). For a higher standardization of the procedure and a quantitative evaluation of PCR results we introduced the Bioanalyzer 2100 system. Thereby we will be able to monitor PCT by means of an failed or passed algorithm. **Methods:** Platelet concentrates were prepared from pools of 4 ABO-matched buffy coats (BC-PC) according to routine blood bank manufacture procedures, treated with the PCT using the INTERCEPT Blood System for platelets. Platelet mtDNA was prepared using the Qiagen Mini Blood Kit. Primers were designed within the Cytochrome C oxidase I and the 16S region of mtDNA. Duplex PCR was performed using a standard PCR cycler. The amplification products were afterwards analysed by the Bioanalyzer 2100 system (Agilent Technologies, Waldbronn, Germany). **Results:** The PCR inhibition assay is suitable to reflect the PCT process. Amplicons <150 bp used as an internal control could be amplified irrespective from the PCT procedure, whereas amplification of larger PCR products (>1,200 bp) was significantly inhibited by PCT. By using the Bioanalyzer system the amplification products could be detected as peaks in the corresponding size range. Integration of peak areas for the small and the large amplicons in samples before and after PCT enabled us to define a cut-off value indicating successfully performed PCT. **Conclusions:** The PCR inhibition assay in combination with evaluation of results by the Bioanalyzer system has the potential to monitor the success of the PCT by a failed or passed algorithm on the basis of a defined cut-off level. The system is suitable to be integrated into a quality control laboratory with lower costs compared to quantitative RealTime PCR.

OS9.8

Detection of Bacteria in Platelet Concentrates Prepared from Spiked Single Donations Using Cultural and Molecular Genetic Methods

M. Störmer[1], U. Cassens[2], K. Kleesiek[1], J. Dreier[1]
[1]Herz- und Diabeteszentrum Nordrhein Westfalen, Bad Oeynhausen, D; [2]Klinikum Dortmund, D

Purpose: Depending on the blood component, bacteria show differences in their growth kinetics. Owing to the storage at 22°C, platelet concentrates (PCs) seem to be more prone to bacterial multiplication than red cells. Knowledge of the potential for bacterial proliferation in blood components is therefore essential before considering the implementation of a detection strategy. Bacterial growth in the different blood components obtained from deliberately contaminated whole blood (WB) units and the efficacy of bacterial detection using real-time RT-PCR were determined. Cultivation served as the reference method. **Methods:** One of four WB units was spiked with 1 CFU/mL Staphylococcus epidermidis or Klebsiella pneumoniae, kept for 15 hours at room temperature and component preparation was processed. Sampling was performed during the whole separation process from each blood component for sterility testing. Nucleic acids were extracted using an automated high-volume extraction method based on magnetic separation technology. **Results:** The 15-hour storage of inoculated WB revealed an insignificant increase in bacterial titer. Using RT-PCR: No bacterial growth was detected in RBC or plasma units. Klebsiella pneumoniae showed rapid growth in the pooled PC and could be detected immediately after PC preparation. Staphylococcus epidermidis grew slowly after a long lag phase and could be detected 24 hours after separation. **Conclusions:** These experiments show, that sampling is suggestive 24 hours after preparation of PCs at the earliest, to enable bacterial propagation and to minimze the sampling error. This pre-enrichment should enable the vast majority of contaminated PCs to be detected using current methods.

Poster Sessions

PS1: Stem Cells, Gene Therapy, Regenerative Medicine

PS1.1

Tumor Screening of Donor Look-Back Samples by Electron Spin Resonance Spectroscopy (ESR/EPR)

G. Matthes[1], I. Eichhorn[2], K. Schnurr[3]
[1]Universitätsklinikum Leipzig AöR, Leipzig, D; [2]DRK-Blutspendedienst Baden-Württemberg, Baden-Baden, D; [3]MedInnovation GmbH, Wildau, D

Purpose: Blood donor screening does not include tumor marker. Approximately 1 of 8.000 donors reports a tumor diagnosis post donation. There is no early tumor marker available for blood donor screen-ing at the time of blood donation. To test a possible early tumor marker, look back samples (LBS) from donors with a post-donation report of cancer were analyzed. **Methods:** ESR/EPR tumor marker test detects active malignant processes all cancer types, with a high diagnostic sensitivity. 133 LBS from 57 donors with post-donation report of cancer, and 284 healthy donors were investigated. **Results:** Diagnostic sensitivity was 100% for all LBS <6 & 9 months before tumor diagnosis, 83% for LBS <12 months, 78% for LBS <24 months, 67% for LBS <36 months. There are time periods of active and silent tumor activity for prostate, breast, kidney, and bladder cancer. In all healthy donors could not be obtained any abnormalities. **Conclusion:** Malignant processes can be detected from 0.2–31 months before clinical diagnosis. Analysis of all look-back samples has shown that for cancer types breast, prostate, colon, skin, stomach, rectum, sarkoma already 9 months before clinical diagnosis a tumor can be detected by a positive ESR/EPR tumor marker test.

PS1.2

Comparison of Adhesion Molecules Expression on Granulocytes Produced by Apheresis Including G-CSF Administration and Apheresis without G-CSF

A. Beloiartsev, H. Thude, T. Lorenzen, S. Rummler, D. Barz
Transfusion Medicine Institute, University of Jena, D

Purpose: The use of granulocyte colony stimulating factor (G-CSF), administered to donors, improves the yield of granulocytes collected. Until now it is unclear whether apheresis procedure in combination with prior G-CSF stimulation induces modification in the expression of granulocyte adhesion molecules, which control the granulocyte function. This study was performed to analyse changes by apheresis procedure in adhesion molecules expression on granulocytes received from donors, treated either with or without G-CSF. **Methods:** Granulocyte concentrates of 57 individuals produced by apheresis were enclosed in the study. 37 of them had undergone G-CSF treatment before apheresis (group 1) and 20 donors received no G-CSF (group 2). The expression of 8 adhesion molecules (CD62L, CD162, CD44, CD58, CD18, CD11a, CD11b, CD11c) were detected on freshly isolated granulocytes before and after G-CSF stimulation respectively (in vivo), as well as on granulocytes from apheresis concentrate (in vitro) using flow cytometry analysis. **Results:** The granulocyte expression of CD18 and CD11b remains unchanged after G-CSF treatment, measured in vivo. The in vitro measured expressions in group 1 showed an increase in CD44 (272%), CD58 (172%), CD18 (10%) and CD11b (22%) expression and a decrease in CD162 (−3%), CD11a (−7%) and CD11c (−14%) expression. The expression changes in group 2, also measured in vitro, showed an enhancement in CD162 (13%), CD44 (199%), CD58 (258%), CD11a (21%), CD11b (8%) and CD11c (12%) expression and a decline in CD62L (−14%) and CD18 (−2%) expression. The expression changes, declared in percents, related to the expression value before G-CSF stimulation in group 1 and to the expression value before apheresis in group 2 respectively. **Conclusion:** Our results demonstrate no high expression changes of such important functional molecules as CD11a, CD11b, CD18 and CD44 in donor blood after G-CSF treatment. In addition, the difference between in vivo and in vitro measured expressions by non stimulated individuals suggest, that the apheresis procedure influences the granulocyte adhesion molecules expression, which should be analysed more closely.

PS1.3

Clinical Efficiency of Granulocytes in Neutropenic Children

F. Heinemann, S. Rummler, K. Althaus, T. Lorenzen, F. Zintl, D. Barz
Universitätsklinikum – Institut für Transfusionsmedizin, Jena, D

Background: Granulocytes are an important component of human immunity. For this reason we transfused 134 granulocyte concentrates (gc) to 26 severely neutropenic children with apparent infection or proven sepsis while receiving adequate antibiotic therapy. All patients underwent a haematopoietic stem cell transplantation or intensive chemotherapy. **Aims:** The aim of this study was to analyse the clinical effect of transfusions of granulocytes at children. **Methods:** The granulocyte concentrates (gc) were collected with Spectra Gambro BCT. using the PMN version 7.0 in manual operation. The maximal blood flow was 65 ml/min. For anticoagulation and acceleration of sedimentation we never used more than 550 ml of a mixture of 33% sodiumcitrate (50 ml) – 6% HES 450/0.7 (500 ml) per apheresis. The granulocytes were collected from male donors only. The pretreatment of donors has been carried out with 263ìg Lenograstim 6 till 12 h before donation. 134 gc were collected from 59 donors. We transfused with a maximal transfusion rate of 1 × 1010 granulocytes/m^2 body surface of patient and hour as soon as possible after collection and irradiation. **Results:** We managed to collect a gc of 287 ml in 123 minutes with a processed whole blood volume of 6808 ml. The gc yielded 4.33 × 1010 leukocytes, 83% out of these are neutrophile granulocytes, 9.61% are lymphocytes, 14.18 × 1010 are platelets, 20.41 × 1010 are red blood cells with a haematocrit of 0.658 per unit. All data are showing mean values. Transfusion success per unit gc was different according to the different transplantation procedures. If the patients had no tranplantation leukocytes increased about 361%, platelets about 46% and CRP decreased about 9%. If they had an allogenic transplantation leukocytes increased about 69%, platelets about 44% and CRP decreased about 0.5%. After autologous transplantation the leukocytes increased about 495%, platelets 21% and CRP decreased about 2%. In regard to the transplanted material patients who underwent a bone marrow transplantation show a leukocyte increase about 90%, platelet increase about 58% and a CRP decrease about 3% per unit gc. Patients who underwent a stem cell transplantation had an leukocytes increase about 130%, platelets increase about 23% and CRP decrease about 6%. 15 out of 26 treated patients survived and received 37 out of 134 gc of the study. **Conclusions:** The granulocyte transfusions result in a clear increase of leukocytes, especially granulocytes, and platelet and a decrease of CRP. Transfusion success is related to the transplantation procedure like allogenic or autologous and bone marrow or stem cell transplantation.

PS1.4

Impact of rhG-CSF Administration and Peripheral Blood Stem Cell Donation on Normal Donors Quality of Life and Health Status

N. Worel, G. Leitner, K. Baumgartner, P. Kalhs, M. Horvath, H. Greinix, P. Höcker
Universitätsklinik Wien, A

Purpose: Mobilized allogeneic peripheral blood stem cells (PBSC) are increasingly used as graft source instead of bone marrow. Although the short-term safety profile of rhG-CSF seems acceptable, minimal data exist regarding long-term safety. We therefore reviewed data of 163 sibling donors (M/F 92/71) with respect to side effects of rhG-CSF, adverse events of collection and late effects. **Methods:** For follow-up we assessed peripheral blood counts, electrolytes and total protein levels on days 1, 7, 30, 100, 365 after donation and than yearly for 5 years. Influence of rhG-CSF and PBSC donation on quality of life (QoL) and health status were assessed by a questionnaire in a cross-sectional study. Additionally donors were asked about infections, diseases and operations since donation. Written informed consent was signed before PBSC mobilization and collection. Donors had a median age of 40 yrs (11–72) at PBSC collection. A questionnaire to assess QoL and health status was sent to 151 donors a median of 4 yrs (0.2–11) after donation. **Results:** The main adverse events related to rhG-CSF and donation were bone pain and myalgia (42%), flue like symptoms (21%), citrate toxicity (11%) and fatigue (12%), respectively. Follow-up of laboratory parameters showed a decrease of platelets during early post-donation period and a peak value on day 30. White blood cells decreased within 7 days, returning to normal on day 30. 64% of donors responded the questionnaire and reported a good to very good actual QoL in 90%, and a good to very good actual health status in 94%, respectively. Donors reported no influence of rhG-CSF and PBSC donation on QoL and health status in 71 and 73%, 24% reported a positive, while 5 and 3% reported a negative influence. Events were listed up in infection/disease (10%), operation (15%) and medication (19%) since PBSC collection. Two donors had to be hospitalized within 2 weeks after donation due to severe enteritis and subarachnoidal haemorrhage. The latter never had platelet counts <100 G/L after PBSC donation and recovered without neurological deficit. Two donors, had died at the time of the survey, one of squamous cell cancer (51 yrs) 6 months after donation and one of diabetic renal failure (49 yrs) 14 months PBSC collection. **Conclusion:** The short-term safety profile of rhG-CSF and donation seems acceptable. Although reported events in medical history after PBSC donation could not be associated with rhG-CSF and collection procedure, a regular follow-up for at least 5 years should be considered.

PS1.5

Regulation of the First Steps in Mesenchymal Stem Cell Engraftment

B. Rüster[1], S. Göttig[1], R. Ludwig[2], R. Bistrian[1], E. Seifried[1], J. Gille[2], R. Henschler[1]

[1]Institut für Transfusionsmedizin und Immunhämatologie, Frankfurt, D;
[2]Zentrum der Dermatologie und Venerologie, Frankfurt, D

Objective: MSC are a promising candidate cell therapeutic to alleviate GVHD, increase allograft survival, improve stem cell engraftment, or to mediate tissue re-organisation after ischemic lesions such as myocardial infarcts or stroke. To understand and subsequently optimize the benefits of MSC in transplantation, we investigated their performance in the first 24 h after transplantation in mice. **Methods:** MSCs were isolated from patients undergoing hip replacement. Passages 4 to 9 were used, which showed unimpaired tri-lineage differentiation. Flow cytometry and RT-PCR were employed to measure adhesion molecule expression, a parallel plate flow chamber system was used to investigate the interaction of MSC and endothelial cells in vitro, and immunodeficient NODSCID mice or C57BL/6 P-selectin −/− mice were used to assess their in vivo behaviour. Intra-tissue visualization of MSC was performed using fluorescence microscopy of cryosections to investigate their extravasation potential in different organs. **Results:** (1) MSCs expressed adhesion molecules of only two of the three main families shown to be relevant for regulated homing behaviour: Whereas MSCs expressed beta1 integrins VLA-4, VLA-5, and chemokine receptors CXCR4 and CCR6, none of the known selectins/ligands (L-selectin, P-selectin glycoprotein ligand (PSGL)-1, CD24) were detected on MSCs. (2) Trypsinization did not negatively affect expression or presence of homing receptors on MSCs. (3) Using in vitro shear stress studies, we could show that both VLA-4/V-CAM1 and endothelial P-selectin are involved in interaction of MSCs with endothelial cells. (4) Transplanted MSCs also rolled on endothelium in vivo in a P-selectin dependent manner as shown by intravital microscopy, remained intravascular in the lung, spared the bone marrow, and extravasated into different organs including spleen and liver. **Conclusion:** Establishment of clinical studies with MSCs will be facilitated through pre-clinical investigations of MSC preparations which demonstrate regulated and organ-selective homing function in test animals.

PS1.6

Optimized Proliferation and Differentiation of Human Mesenchymal Stem Cells Cultured upon Extracellular Matrix Proteins

U. Lindner, B. Driller, P. Behrens, F. Böhrnsen, J. Kramer, J. Rohwedel, H. Kirchner, P. Schlenke

Universiät Lübeck, D

Purpose: Human bone-marrow derived mesenchymal stem cells (MSCs) are an important source for tissue engineering. For the repair of extended tissue lesions like bone replacement huge amounts of cells with maintained differentiation capacity – manufactured under GMP conditions – are required. In-vitro expanded human MSCs show a limited proliferation life span and a loss of differentiation potential during the culture period. We investigate the influences of basement-membrane extracellular matrix (bmECM) proteins, being part of the bone-marrow microenvironment, on in-vitro life span, proliferation and differentiation of human MSCs. **Methods:** MSCs were isolated from bone marow of patients undergoing hip replacement. Cells were seeded on bmECM proteins laminin, collagen IV, fibronectin, and ECM-gel for five passages. Proliferation capacity and viability were determined via flow cytometry. Quantative analysis of differentiation potential for the three "classical" lineages (osteoblastes, adipocytes, chondrocytes) were performed using staining procedures, fluorometric (alkaline phosphatase (ALP)) and photometrical (Glyco-saminoglycan (GAG)) assays. Cells were characterized using flow cytometry for MSCs-phenotyping, STRO-1 and ALP-antigen expression as well as by morphological analysis. **Results:** After five passages, MSCs seeded on laminin and ECM-gel showed an over 100 fold higher replication activity compared to those grown on plastic. Furthermore the multilineage differentiation potential was maintained to a greater extent. Although MSCs cocultured with collagen IV did not reach an "ECM-gel-like" growth rate, the ALP-activity level and GAG-content in late passages was up to 2 fold higher compared to ECM or laminin expanded cells. In long-term investigations (up to ten passages) we observed, that under collagen IV treatment a population of small cells with high replication activity and differentiation potential was selected. More spindle-shaped cells appeared in protein-treated cultures, while more flat-cells, indicating cell senescence, were found on plastic surface cultures. Protein surfaces have also effects on the STRO-1 expression (up to 80% in late passages). **Conclusions:** Culturing MSCs on bmECM proteins leads to higher growth rates, suggesting that these natural matrices have a direct effect on replicative capacity. Simultaneously, the multilineage differentiation potential is maintained to a higher extent. Thus, MSCs cultured on bmECMs proteins will probably be a valuable tool for tissue engineering and regenerative medicine.

PS1.7

Human AB-Serum as well as Thrombin-Activated Platelet-Rich Plasma are Suitable Alternatives to Fetal Calf Serum for the Expansion of Mesenchymal Stem Cells

A. Kocaömer, S. Kern, H. Klüter, K. Bieback

Institut für Transfusionsmedizin und Immunologie, Mannheim, D

Purpose: Mesenchymal stromal cells (MSC) are currently in focus regarding their clinical potential in cell therapy and tissue engineering. However, protocols for clinical-scale production of MSC use culture media supplemented with Fetal Calf Serum (FCS) which poses a potential risk for infections as well as immunological reactions. Our goal was to develop a standardized isolation and expansion protocol for MSC which does not depend on FCS as a supplement. We chose both pooled human AB-Serum (AB-HS) and thrombin-activated Platelet-Rich-Plasma (tPRP) as alternatives and studied their effect on adipose tissue-derived MSC. **Methods:** MSC isolated from adipose tissue (AT) of 10 donors were cultured under three different conditions: 1) 10% FCS, 2) 10% AB-HS (pool of 5 AB donors), 3) 10% tPRP (pool of 6 AB donors). Colony-forming units were counted and cumulative doubling rates determined while MSC were maximally expanded. The differentiation capacity toward the adipogenic, osteogenic and chondrogenic lineages was assessed as well as cell surface markers analyzed with flow cytometry at an early passage and late passages. **Results:** MSC of all culture conditions displayed fibroblastoid morphology, however, differences in growth pattern and adhesion were evident. Both AB-HS and tPRP induced a 20–23% higher growth compared to FCS, attaining a cumulative population doubling rate of 40 at passage 8, compared to 31 with FCS ($p < 0.001$). Growth of AB-HS and tPRP cells leveled off after 40–50 population doublings (P8–P10). Colony numbers were comparable (1 CFU/1000 cells), whereas colony sizes were much larger for AB-HS and tPRP. Cells of all culture conditions consistently differentiated towards all three mesenchymal lineages at passages 1 and 7. Cell surface marker expression was characteristic for MSC and comparable for all culture conditions with the exception of a distinct CD45+, CD14+ side population at early passages for AB-HS and tPRP cells ranging from 5–30% depending on the donor tissue. **Conclusions:** We show that pooled human AB-Serum and thrombin-activated Platelet-Rich-Plasma are clinically safe alternatives to FCS. These human sources are better characterized regarding potential infectious threats, while providing a higher proliferation rate and retaining differentiation capacity and mesenchymal stem cell marker expression throughout long-term culture. We propose AB-HS as first choice in replacing FCS in GMP-compliant manufacturing processes based on the ease of preparation and identical effectiveness in MSC isolation and expansion.

PS1.8

The Small GTPase Rho is a Molecular Target to Engineer MSC in Order to Improve Their Migration Function

R. Richter, B. Grace, B. Rüster, E. Seifried, R. Henschler
Institut für Transfusionsmedizin und Immunhämatologie, Frankfurt, D

Objective: MSC are increasingly used in clinical trials as a cellular therapeutics to improve hematopoietic regeneration after stem cell transplantation, to alleviate GVHD, or to stimulate tissue regeneration e.g after myocardial infarction. We have previously described that MSCs lack transwell migration capacity as well as detachment function on activated endothelial cells under shear flow, whereas they at the same time display highly prominent actin stress fibers. We therefore set out to engineer MSC to achieve more flexible cytoskeletal structure. **Methods:** MSC were isolated form adult patients undergoing hip surgery. Passages 5–9 of these cells were analyzed in these studies. The cultured cells were identified as MSCs by their intact tri-lineage differentiation into osteoblasts, chondrocytes and adipocytes. Modulation of Rho activity was achieved through microinjection of cDNAs encoding dominant negative or constitutively active isoforms of Rho GTPases. Transmigration was assessed in Transwell chambers. For fractionation, plasma was diluted in 0.1% trifluoro-acetic acid (TFA), sterile filtered and subjected to a 10 × 250 mm Reverse Phase HPLC column. Elution was performed with 80% Acetonitril, 0.1% TFA. 4 ml fractions were collected starting from min 10. **Results:** Overexpression of dominant active Rac1, or the specific inhibitor of Rho, C3 transferase caused reduction of actin stress fibers and formation of lamella-like protrusions on the cell membrane of MSC. Inhibition of Rho by addition of the cell-permeable Rho inhibitor C2I–C3 resulted in a 5–10 fold higher efficiency to induce transmigration of MSCs against gradients of the growth factors PDGF and b-FGF, or the phospholipids lysophosphatidic acid (LPA) or sphingosine-1-phosphate (S1P). Plasma, in our experiments, was found to contain the most efficient activity for induction of MSC transmigration. Fractionation of plasma by reverse phase chromatography revealed one predominant activity improving transmigration of MSCs. Interestingly, the efficiency of the plasma activity could not significantly be improved by inhibition of Rho, disclosing the possibility that plasma contains Rho inhibitors. **Conclusion:** We conclude that MSCs can be engineered to respond to chemotactic stimuli by suppression of the small GTPase Rho using soluble inhibitors of by cDNA transfection. Furthermore, plasma itself possibly contains Rho inhibitors which can be employed to engineer MSC transplants towards cells with a migratory phenotype prior to infusion.

PS1.9

Myeloid Progenitors of Pro-Angiogenic Cells Circulate in Blood and Target Tumors

E. Deak[1], S. Göttig[1], B. Rüster[1], E. Seifried[1], J. Gille[2], R. Henschler[1]
[1]Institut für Transfusionsmedizin und Immunhämatologie, Frankfurt, D; [2]Zentrum der Dermatologie und Venerologie, Frankfurt, D

Objective: Angiogenesis has been shown to be a prerequisite for tumor growth and metastasis, and a number of anti-angiogenic molecular therapies have been developed to suppress tumor growth. Pro-angiogenic bone-marrow derived progenitor cell populations (BM-PCs) which home to tumors have been shown to be suitable cellular vectors to efficiently eradicate tumors by suicide gene therapy (De Palma, Nat Med 14:1193, 2003; De Palma, Cancer Cell 8:211, 2005). We therefore asked which type of HPCs may be mobilized to blood, and whether they have the capacity to form pro-angiogenic cells in solid tumors or to metastases. **Methods:** The Lewis Lung Carcinoma (LLC) and the highly metastatic melanoma B16 (B16–F10) cell lines were established in C57/BL6 mice. Transplantation of CD45.1 and CD45.2 mouse strains, and of donor bone marrow cells from beta-actin/GFP C57/BL6 mice was used to follow bone marrow origin of the BM-PCs. Flow cytometric analysis and cell sorting were used to enumerate and to purify BM-PCs, and immunohistochemistry to follow the intra-tissue localisation of bone-marrow derived cells with proangiogenic phenotypes. **Results:** We found incorporation of bone-marrow derived cells into both LLC tumors and B16 metastases in C57/BL6 mice within a period of ~ 9–20 days. Tissue localization of migrated BM-PCs in the tumors was confirmed using immunohistochemistry of CD45 (BM-PCs) and CD31 (endothelial cells) antigens. Flow-cytometric analysis demonstrated the presence of the pro-angiogenic tie2-exppressing monocytes (TEMs, CD45+tie2+) and endothelial progenitor cells (EPC), which were CD45+ VEGFR2+. Both populations co-expressed CD11b/Mac1. In their blood, tumor-bearing mice showed increased numbers of myelopoietic colony-forming cells (CFCs) and lineage marker (lin)- Sca1+ progenitor cells. Flow cytometric cell sorting identified a population of lineage marker (CD4, CD8, CD45R0, TER119, CD166)-negative, CD11b+VEGFR2- cells from bone marrow as a precursor for EPCs in clonogenic assays, which during culture generate CD45+VEGFR2+CD11b+ EPCs. In contrast to the lin- CD11b+VEGFR2- HPCs, both CD45+VEGFR2+CD11b+ EPCs and CD45+tie2+CD11b+ TEMs isolated from the tumors were found to be non-clonogenic in these progenitor assays. **Conclusion:** Myeloid lin- progenitors circulate in the blood of tumor-bearing mice, and are a potent source for tumor-infiltrating pro-angiogenic cells. Tumor-bearing mice show enhanced mobilization of these myeloid progenitors, resulting in accumulation of pro-angiogenic TEMs and EPCs in tumors. BM-PCs generated from lin- progenitors, could thus be an attractive cellular therapeutic to target the tumor vasculature.

PS1.10

Monocytes Mimic Endothelial Progenitor Cells

E. Rohde, C. Malischnik, D. Thaler, T. Maierhofer, W. Linkesch, G. Lanzer, C. Guelly, D. Strunk
Medizinische Universität Graz, Graz, A

The generation of endothelial progenitor cells (EPC) from blood monocytes has been propagated as a novel approach in the diagnosis and treatment of cardiovascular diseases. LDL uptake and lectin binding together with endothelial marker expression are commonly used to define these EPC. Considerable controversy exists regarding their nature, in particular, because myelomonocytic cells share a number of properties with endothelial cells (EC). This study was performed to elucidate whether the commonly used endothelial marker determination is sufficient to distinguish supposed EPC from monocytes. We measured endothelial, hematopoietic and progenitor cell marker expression of monocytes before and after angiogenic culture by fluorescence microscopy, flow cytometry and real-time RT-PCR. The function of primary monocytes and monocyte-derived supposed EPC were investigated during vascular network formation and EC colony forming unit (CFU-EC) development. Monocytes cultured for 4–6 days under angiogenic conditions lost CD14/CD45 and displayed a commonly accepted EPC phenotype including LDL uptake and lectin binding, CD31/CD105/CD144 reactivity and formation of cord-like structures. Strikingly, primary blood monocytes already expressed most tested endothelial genes and proteins at even higher levels than their supposed EPC progeny. Neither fresh nor cultured monocytes formed vascular networks but CFU-EC formation was strictly dependent on monocyte presence. LDL uptake, lectin binding and CD31/CD105/CD144 expression are inherent features of monocytes making them phenotypically indistinguishable from putative EPC. In consequence monocytes and their progeny can phenotypically mimic EPC in various experimental models. These data question the nature of the enigmatic blood-derived EPC. Additional experiments are needed to clarify the role of myelomonocytic cells or their cytokines during vascular and organ regeneration.

PS1.11

Differences in the Transmigration of Different Dendritic Cells

A. Moldenhauer[1], M. AS Moore[2], K. Schmidt[1], H. Kiesewetter[1], A. Salama[1]
[1]Charité – Universitätsmedizin Berlin, D; [2]Sloan-Kettering Institute, New York, USA

Background: Several methods exist for the generation of dendritic cells (DCs). However, little is known about the transmigration capacities of these cells. **Methods:** We studied the transmigration of DCs derived from hematopoietic progenitor cells (HPC), peripheral blood monocytes and leukemic cells. **Results:** DCs from monocytes and leukemic cells could be generated within one week, whereas DCs from HPC required two weeks for maturation. All DCs generated showed similar morphologic features and allostimulatory capacities, but their transmigration capacities varied. HPC-derived DCs showed the highest migratory response to macrophage inflammatory protein (MIP) 3a (32.2 ± 11.7%) and b (45.5 ± 16.6%). Monocyte-derived DCs were equally attracted to MIP-3b (23.5 ± 3.2%) and stroma-derived factor (SDF) 1a (25.8 ± 6.6%). Few leukemic DCs migrated in response to SDF-1a (9.2 ± 3.7%) and almost none to MIP3b (5.7 ± 1.3%). Other chemoattractants tested were MIP-1a, MIP-3a and RANTES. Replacement of fetal bovine by human serum did not change the overall migratory capacities of the DC's, but was observed to influence its responses to certain chemokines like RANTES and MIP3b. **Conclusion:** Our findings suggest that HPC and monocyte-derived DCs can be administered subcutaneously and intravenously, and that leukemic DCs should be injected into the lymph node.

PS1.12

Regulating MHC Expression for Cellular Therapeutics

C. Figueiredo, P.A. Horn, R. Blasczyk, A. Seltsam
Medizinische Hochschule, Hanover, D

Purpose: HLA polymorphism is the most relevant barrier to the development of cell-based therapies for regenerative purposes. To overcome this limitation, we used RNA interference (RNAi) to specifically knock down HLA class I transcripts. **Methods:** Regions susceptible to the action of small interfering RNAs (siRNAs) were identified in HLA-A heavy chain and â2-microglobulin (â2m) transcripts to achieve a gene or class I specific HLA silencing, respectively. Lentiviral vectors were designed to express short hairpin RNA sequences (shRNA) targeting HLA-A heavy chain or â2m constitutively or controlled by a doxycycline-inducible promoter system. The level of HLA suppression in HeLa cells, B-LCLs and peripheral blood monocytes was detected by flow cytometry, real-time RT-PCR and Western Blot. The capacity of this silencing approach to resist IFN-ã-mediated HLA class I up regulation was tested in stimulation assays. Complement-dependent cytotoxicity assays were performed to evaluate the protective effect of HLA suppression against immune response. CD8+ T cell response was tested in proliferation and IFN-ã secretion assays. **Results:** The transduction of inducible RNAi cassettes containing the sequences for shRNAs targeting â2m suppressed HLA class I expression by up to 90% in HeLa, B-LCLs and primary monocytes in a fully reversible manner. Similarly, conditional delivery of short hairpin RNA targeting HLA-A heavy chain transcripts silenced HLA-A expression by up to 90%. It was shown that HLA silencing was maintained even under inflammatory conditions. In cytotoxicity and proliferation assays, it was demonstrated that HLA class I knockdown was effective in preventing antibody-mediated cell lysis, CD8+ T cell response and interferon-gamma secretion, while the residual HLA expression in HLA-silenced cells was protective against NK cell-mediated lysis. **Conclusion:** We demonstrate the feasibility of controlling HLA expression by genetically modifying cell-based therapeutics to overcome the limitations of immunological rejection, bringing cellular therapies closer to reality.

PS1.13

TLR7 Ligands Induce Higher IFN-Alpha Production in Females

H. Hackstein, B. Berghöfer, T. Frommer, G. Haley, L. Fink, G. Bein
Justus-Liebig Universität Giessen, D

Background: IFN-alpha exercises multiple immune modulatory and antiviral activities and has been suggested to play a critical role in the pathogenesis of systemic lupus erythematosus (SLE), an autoimmunedisease afflicting with nine times higher incidence primarily women. IFN-alpha is realesed in high amounts by plasmacytoid dendritic cells (pDCs), a rare population of 0.5% of peripheral leukocytes, upon stimulation with TLR7 and TLR9 ligands, a novel class of synthetic immune adjuvants in clinical application. **Methods:** Blood samples of three independent groups of healthy human individuals ($n1 = 120$; $n2 = 101$; $n3 = 123$) were incubated with synthetic TLR7 and TLR9 ligands and then analyzed for IFN-alpha and TNF-alpha production. PDC numbers in male and female whole blood samples were measured by flow cytometry. X-inactivation status of TLR7 gene was evaluated by single cell PCR of sorted pDCs and monoclonal B-cell lines with subsequent RFLP-analysis. The impactof supplemented exogeneous 17fÒ-Estrogen and estrogen receptor antagonist on IFN-alpha and TNF-alpha production was measured by independent experiments. **Results:** Our study revealed a capacity of female PBL to produce significantly higher IFN-alpha levels after TLR7 stimulation ($p1 < 0.0000001$; $p2 < 0.0000001$; $p3 < 0.0001$) compared to male PBL. In contrast, no sex-differences were evident after TLR9 stimulation. TNF-alpha production after TLR7 stimulation and also total pDC numbers were not different between females and males. X-inactivation escape of the TLR7 gene in monoclonal B-cell lines, and single pDCs indicated regular silencing of one TLR7 allele in females. Exogenous 17fÒ-Estrogen and estrogen receptor antagonism did not indicate a significant role on TLR7-induced IFN-alpha production. **Conclusion:** Our data revealed for the first time a profound sex-dependent pathway of TLR7-induced IFN-alpha with higher production in female blood samples. These findings may explain the higher prevalence of SLE in females and the reported decreased therapeutic efficacy of synthetic TLR7 ligands in male individuals.

PS1.14

High Throughput Minor Histocompatibility Antigen Prediction

D.S. DeLuca, B. Eiz-Vesper, C. Bade-Doeding, R. Blasczyk
Hanover Medical School, Hanover, D

Purpose: The search for minor histocompatibility antigens (mHags) has implications not only for preventing graft versus host disease, but also for therapeutic applications involving leukaemia-specific T cells. In the context of hematopoietc stem cell transplantation, any polymorphic gene can potentially be an mHag-source, with the additional requirement that the polymorphism leads to a differential T cell epitope expression. **Methods:** We have filtered over 18,000 entries which represent protein variations in NCBI's dbSNP polymorphism database describing 15,000 genes which could potentially encode minor antigens. Almost a thousand of these genes contain null allele variants, having important implications because the whole protein sequence is allogeneic (whereas a single nucleotide polymorphism results in a single amino acid difference). Additionally, our group has produced an expression profile of graft versus leukaemia-specific genes using affymetrix DNA chips. **Results:** Of the resulting 500 GvL-specific genes, 235 were found to be polymorphic. Of the 28,000 theoretically possible nonamers, 131 were predicted to be both processed by the immunoproteasome as well as presented by clinically relevant HLA alleles. These peptides, encoded by 40 genes, represent the most likely candidates to produce a leukaemia-specific alloreactive T cell response. **Conclusions:** The fully automated nature of this system is necessary to regenerate results in response to an ever-increasing pool of biological data.

PS1.15

Influence of the Citrate Concentration in Platelet Concentrates by Trima Accel (Gambro BCT)

K. Althaus, S. Rummler, T. Lorenzen, S. Straube, G. Nowak, D. Barz
Universitätsklinikum Jena, D

Background: Platelets in citrated PCs are hypofunctional platelets with reduced reaction time. We supposed less functional and metabolic alterations with higher citrate concentration. The PADA (Platelet ADhesion Assay) is a test to assess attributes for PC by analysis of the adhaesivness of platelets for testing particles via fibrinogen at low shear rates. The measurement is the adhesion index (AI). PADA is a comparable platelet function assay like accepted CD 62 expression for routine assesment in quality control. **Aims:** Our goal was to find an optimal citrate concentration for in vitro storage conditions. **Methods:** 10 donors are recruited among a pool of regular apheresis donors. Single donor platelet concentrates are collected by the Trima Accel. PC are collected four times from each donor with different anticoagulation protocols: 1. 1:8 (one part sodium citrate and 8 parts whole blood (wb)); 2. 1:9; 3. 1:10; 4. 1:11. Platelet function assay PADA, pH, glucose and LDH are measured on day of preparation and day 7 of storage according to the instructions and by standard in-house methods. Citrate concentration is measured on the day of preparation by a photometrical test. **Results:** The table below indicates the results of AI, PLT count, pH, LDH and glucose. The mean citrate concentrations in PC were: 1:8 : 23.5, 1:9 : 21.5, 1:10 : 16.2 and 1:11 : 14.2. **Conclusions:** Citrate concentration may be the cause for different metabolic and functional alterations in PC. 1:11 is our standard anticoagulation protocol in routine. This appears not to be the optimum. Short storage time of platelet concentrates provides good platelet function in all types of preparation. Metabolic parameters do not influence the adhesion ability in our concentrates.

ACD-A: WB	/	1:8 Day 1	1:9 Day 1	1:10 Day 1	1:11 Day 1	1:8 Day 7	1:9 Day 7	1:10 Day 7	1:11 Day 7
AI	/	45	41	42	49	23	27	20	12
PLT	$\times 10^9$	988	1171	1083	1088	1071	1205	1201	1112
LDH	µmol/l	2.3	2.6	2.8	2.5	3.0	3.2	3.0	3.0
Glucose	mmol/l	23.1	20.6	19.2	18.9	17.0	15.3	14.6	14.0
pH	/	6.98	7.12	7.13	7.04	6.90	6.96	7.02	7.15
citrate	mmol/l	23.5	21.5	16.2	14.15	/	/	/	/

PS1.16

Prophylactic Red Blood Cell Exchange for Prevention of Severe Hemolysis after Minor ABO-Incompatible Stem Cell Transplantation Following Reduced-Intensity Conditioning

N. Worel, G. Leitner, M. Horvath, M. Mitterbauer, W. Rabitsch, H. Greinix, P. Kalhs, P. Höcker
Universitätsklinik Wien, A

Purpose: In about 20% of allogeneic stem cell transplantation (SCT) minor ABO incompatibility does exist. This is accompanied with the risk of severe hemolysis especially during hematopoietic regeneration. The risk of hemolysis increases if peripheral blood stem cells are used instead of bone marrow (BM) and a graft-versus-host disease (GvHD) prophylaxis without methotrexate (MTX). As we have observed lethal hemolyses in patients undergoing minor ABO mismatched SCT following reduced intensity conditioning (RIC) we decided to perform prophylactic red blood cell exchange (RBCX) in all consecutive patients undergoing RIC prior to SCT with a minor ABO incompatible donor. **Methods:** From April 1999 to March 2006, 112 consecutive patients underwent SCT with a sibling (n = 55) or unrelated donor graft (n = 57) after RIC. GvHD prophylaxis consisted of CyA and mycophenolate mofetil (MMF). Fifty-four patients had an ABO-identical donor, 33 received an ABO-minor/bidirectional and 25 an ABO-major incompatible graft, respectively. RBCX was perfomed between day -5 and -1, removing 1 time patients RBC mass to reduce his remaining RBCs to about 40%. Packed RBCS of group 0 were used as exchange fluid. **Results:** So far, 20 patients underwent prophylactic RBCX before SCT. The procedure was tolerated well in 16 (80%) patients, 2 developed citrate toxicity and 2 nausea and hypotension during treatment leading to discontinuation of RBCX in the latter patients. Whereas 18 patients did not experience any signs of hemolysis after minor ABO incompatible SCT, 2 showed a marked increase in lactic dehydrogenase and serum bilirubin levels without a drop of hematocrit levels below 28% during hematologic recovery. Six of 20 patients with prophylactic RBCX died between 4.3 and 29.2 months after SCT of GvHD and infection (n = 3), invasive aspergillosis (n = 1) and relapse of hematologic disease (n = 2). One patient rejected his graft within 1 month. The other 13 (64%) patients are in continuous complete remission a median of 13.9 months (1.2 to 36) after SCT. **Conclusion:** RBCX is a save and well tolerated procedure to prevent severe hemolysis by elimination of the majority of incompatible recipient RBCs as demonstrated by our data. Whether a more intensive immunosuppression can overcome the risk of hemolysis without affecting the establishment of donor chimerism remains unclear. Nevertheless, close monitoring of patients at risk between days 5 and 15 after SCT is recommended.

PS2: Blood Component Production, Infectious Safety, Immunohematology

PS2.1

The Greifswald Blood Donor Study (GREBDOS): A Tool for Comparing Blood Donors with the General Population

N. Lubenow, U. Konerding, U. Alpen, K. Bezold, W. Hoffmann, T. Kohlmann, A. Greinacher
Universität Greifswald, D

Purpose: Few data for comparing blood donors with the general population exist. This makes it difficult to outline strategies for blood donor motivation. We report the design and first results of a major study comparing the population of blood donors with the general population within the same region: The Greifswald Blood Donor Study (GREBDOS). **Methods:** GREBDOS is linked to the cross-sectional Study of Health in Pomerania (SHIP) performed with 4 310 persons representative of the Western Pomerania population in the age from 20 to 80 years in Germany. In SHIP characteristics of the socio-economic situation, the subjective health status, and the health related behaviour as well as laboratory parameters were obtained. In GREBDOS over 12 months each 6th person enrolling for blood donation was asked to participate in the study. If this person refused or had already participated, the next 6th person was asked. Complete participation comprised 1) to fill in a structured questionnaire which contained a selection of questions posed in SHIP and 2) to give a blood sample. To provide the opportunity for correcting selection biases due to multiple donations the number of donations given within the study interval was recorded for each participant after the study. **Results:** In total 4,014 persons were asked to participate in the study. Of these 535 had already taken part. Of the remaining 3,479 persons 2,596 (74.6%) participated. Of these 128 did not fulfil the requirements for blood donation. From the remaining 2,468 participants 2,407 (97.5%) questionnaires and 2,406 (97.5%) blood samples were obtained. Uncorrected for multiple donations the participants' mean age was 30.2 years (SD = 10.3) and the number of females 1,234 (50.0%). **Conclusions:** GREBDOS is the first major population based study providing an empirical base for analyzing characteristics of blood donors in comparison with the general population. The expected results may become instrumental for planning future donor recruitment programs. Moreover, these results might help to assess the extent to which blood samples gathered in blood donation centres can be used as reference information for clinical and epidemiological studies concerned with blood laboratory parameters.

PS2.2

Evaluation of a Novel Internal Controlled Broad-Range Real-Time Polymerase Chain Reaction Assay for Sensitive Detection of Bacterial Contamination in Platelet Concentrates

M. Danzer, B. Fiedler, K. Hofer, H. Polin, C. Gabriel
Red Cross Transfusion Service of Upper Austria, Linz, A

Purpose: In the present study, a 16S rDNA real time polymerase chain reaction (PCR) assay was developed and evaluated for screening of bacterial contamination in platelet concentrates (PCs). PCR amplification of bacterial 16S rDNA was performed in a LightCycler 2.0 with a set of universal primers. Detection was carried out with the aid of 7 fluorescence resonance energy transfer (FRET) hybridisation probes. Based on melting temperature shifts and different LightCycler dyes, gram positive/negative bacteria and a discrimination of groups can be achieved. **Methods:** Half logarithmic diluted ATTC reference material of P. aeruginosa (n = 84) and S. aureus (n = 84) were tested to determine the detection limits by Probit analysis. The existence of cross-contamination was assessed by testing alternating high titre bacterial- positive and -negative samples. The specificity of the real-time assay was determined by testing 100 PCs, all negative tested by BacT/ALERT. In addition, a Panel of 20 selected bacteria were diluted at the detection limit und tested in duplicate. **Results:** The respective 95% detection limits (and 95% CI) on the ATTC reference material was 5.2 (10.2–3.9) cfu/ml for P. aeruginosa and 16.8 (44.1–11.4) cfu/ml for S. aureus. Based on the bacterial panel, no significant differences in sensitivity for gram positive and gram negative bacteria were found. The sensitivity of E. faecalis was probably twofold lower as compared to the other strands. No cross contamination was observed. 99 of 100 culture negative PCs were bacterial PCR-negative. One positive result from the specificity testing could not be clarified, but was identified as low level E. coli contamination from enzymes in the assay. **Conclusions:** This real-time PCR assay enables the detection of more then 250 bacteria in PCs. The turnaround time of 3–4 hours is much shorter than an automated culturing system or semi-automated bacterial detection system. The method allows rapid detection of low initial numbers of bacteria before transfusion of PCs.

PS2.3

Haemocompatibility and Performance of P-CAPT™ PRION Reduction Filters

M. Cardoso[1], C. Sumian[2], I. Walicka[2], J. Lathrop[3]

[1]MacoPharma, Langen, D; [2]Macopharma, Tourcoing, F; [3]Arc, Rockville, USA

Purpose: Transmissible Spongiform Encephalopathy (TSE) diseases, also known as prion diseases, are neurodegenerative illnesses including variant Creutztfeldt-Jakob Disease (vCJD). Three probable blood transfusion transmitted cases of vCJD have recently been reported in the UK. The P-CAPT™ Prion Removal Filter (MacoPharma), incorporating PRDT affinity ligands for the selective adsorption of prions, has been developed to remove infectious prions potentially present in leucodepleted red cell concentrates. The studies described in this abstract were designed to demonstrate the reproducibility of the filtration process and to determine the filter and kit specifications required to obtain optimal prion removal. Evaluations were conducted to demonstrate if exposure to the P-CAPT™ filter has any deleterious effect on the quality of red blood cell concentrates and whether the filter complies with user operational and processing requirements. **Methods:** The efficiency of the filter in terms of prion removal was measured under different flow rate conditions. Red blood cell concentrates stored in both SAGM and plasma were treated with the MacoPharma P-Capt™ filter. 42-day stability of the red cell concentrates in SAGM and 28 day stability of the red cell concentrate in plasma were evaluated at pre-determined time points by measuring grams haemoglobin per unit, haematocrit, $K+$ (mmol/l) haemolysis (%), and other parameters. **Results:** The final filter and kit configuration was determined that maintains the flow rate permitting optimal prion removal for leucodepleted red cell concentrates. For all RBC parameters measured with the P-CAPT™ filter, including haemolysis ($< 0.8\%$), pH, and grams hemoglobin per unit, the results were within the routine specifications acceptable to the UK blood services (Guidelines for the Blood Transfusion Services in the UK "Red Book") and met the Council of Europe Guidelines (Guide to the preparation, use and quality assurance of blood components). **Conclusion:** These results indicated that red blood cell stability is not adversely affected by exposure to the P-CAPT™ filter. The filter appears to be compatible with use for removal of TSE infectivity and is suitable for use in the production of red cell concentrates in a routine blood processing setting.

PS2.4

Specific Anti-B19 Antibodies and B19 Infectivity in Parvovirus-B19-DNA-Positive Donors and Risk of Transmission

M. Schmidt[1], M.D. Giambattista[2], P. Caillet-Fauquet[3], E. Seifried[4], K. Hourfar[4], R. Laub[2]

[1]DRG Baden-Württemberg – Hessen, Frankfurt, D; [2]Central Department for Fractionation, Red Cross, Bruessels, B; [3]Université Libre de Bruxelles, Bruessels, B; [4]DRK Institut Frankfurt, D

Background: NAT-based studies have led to growing recognition of the risk of transmission of human Erythrovirus B19 (a human parvovirus) by blood or blood products. Since April 2000, all donations have been screened by semi-quantitative Real-Time MP-NAT. The only positive donations released are ones having a B19 concentration below 105 IU/ml. In estimating the transmission risk, parameters like infectivity and specific serology (IgG and IgM) are of high interest. **Methods:** Seventeen donors with an initial B19 level higher than 105 IU/ml were monitored for 1 year. Every donor was interviewed for clinical symptoms. Samples were collected and screened for B19-DNA and specific IgM and IgG antibodies. Two different serological ELISAs were used to identify anti-B19 specific to linear and conformational capsid epitopes. A new infectivity test based on an adherent hepatocarcinoma cell line was used in parallel to determine B19 infectivity. **Results:** No good correlation was found between clinical symptoms and viral load. In about one-half of the donors, the B19-DNA load decreased rapidly during the first 12 weeks by more than 5 logs and then stabilized at a low background level for 1 year. In the other donors (where the initial B19-DNA load was lower), a slow 2–3-log reduction was measured. All donors actively developed anti-VP antibodies. Despite the presence of abundant anti-B19 IgG antibodies, B19 infectivity persisted in several cases. **Conclusions:** This follow-up study shows that a low B19-DNA concentration can persist and be detected in plasma samples for over a year. In some donors B19 antibodies are present but fail to neutralise the B19 infectivity determined on hepatocarcinoma cell cultures. Because these donors may be infective despite low virus concentrations, it is necessary to reassess the strategy of discarding only donations with a high level of B19. More investigations are required to understand the immune dysfunction observed in these donors.

PS2.5

Hepatitis E Virus Infection – Exotic 3rd World Disease or a Possible Threat to Blood Transmission in Germany?

G. Caspari[1], W. Jilg[2]

[1]Berlin, D; [2]Institut für Med. Mikrobiologie und Hygiene, Regensburg, D

Purpose: Hepatitis E virus (HEV) infection is well known as a cause of waterborne epidemics of hepatitis in the Far East and Mexico. Infections in Germany were considered to be imported from endemic regions. We analysed whether HEV could possibly be transmitted through blood transfusion in Germany. **Methods:** Literature search. **Results:** Viremia in HEV infection is limited, and HEV infection was considered to be prevented by a six-months donor deferral if the donor returned from malaria-endemic regions (which largely overlap with HEV-endemic regions). However, besides HEV genotype 1 and 2 which cause epidemics of hepatitis E in the Indian subcontinent and Mexico, there are two additional genotypes (3 and 4) which infect different animals (mainly swine) and may be transmitted to humans as a zoonosis. Autochthonous infections of humans with these viruses were described in case reports from many European countries, the US and Japan. They are underdiagnosed as foreign travel is still considered a prerequisite for HEV diagnosis by many physicians. Several transfusion- associated hepatitis E transmissions have been described in Japan. Recently, the first case of a transfusion-transmitted hepatitis E has been reported from England. **Conclusions:** Research into the distribution of zoonotic HEV infection is urgently needed. A clearer picture of how HEV infection may be transmitted to humans is necessary to establish possible deferral criteria for blood donors. Of special interest is the behaviour of HEV in pools of plasma inactivated by the solvent/detergent procedure, because there is neither a virus envelope nor are there relevant concentrations of anti-HEV antibodies in the plasma pool. It would be a catastrophy if HEV were able to contaminate anti-D immunoglobulin for pregnant women because HEV mortality in this group is especially high.

PS2.6

2D-DIGE Analysis Reveals Only Minor Modifications of the Plasma Protein Profile in Lyophilized SD-Pathogen Inactivated Plasma

A. Greinacher[1], L. Steil[1], E. Hammer[1], T.Q. Phong[1], M. Kalus[2], E. Scheel[2], H. Mertens[2], J. Bux[2], U. Völker[1]

[1]Ernst-Moritz-Arndt-Universität Greifswald, D; [2]DRK Blutspendedienst NRW, Hagen, D

Purpose: Logistics and handling of plasma are still major challenges for providing plasma. Storage of plasma requires $-30°C$ and especially in case of emergency transfusion the thawing process is time consuming. An interesting new product is SD-treated, lyophilized fresh frozen plasma (LyoPlas, DRK-Blood Service West, Hagen, Germany), which allows storage from $+2$ to $+25°C$ and reconstitution for transfusion within a few minutes. While these characteristics are very interesting, processing of the product may cause structural modifications leading to loss of function or formation of neoepitopes. We applied functional assays and proteomic technologies for assessing the protein composition of LyoPlas. **Methods:** The reconstituted products and the starting plasma pool were assessed by standard clotting assays. In addition LyoPlas samples of two batches were collected at 4 different steps during the production process. These samples were analyzed by two-dimensional differential in gel electrophoresis (2D-DIGE) to reveal changes in protein composition and protein spots displaying processing-dependent changes in abundance were identified by mass spectrometry. **Results:** Beside the known reduction in plasmin inhibitor and protein S, LyoPlas showed no significant differences compared to untreated pool plasma by clotting assays (PTT 36.1 + 1.1 s; FV 94.9 + 7.5%; FVIII:c 0.72 + 0.02 IU/mL; FXI 72.6 + 5.8% [mean+SD, n = 61]). 2D-DIGE analysis allowed quantitative comparative monitoring of a set of about 500 spots per sample. The statistical analysis of the spot patterns revealed 30 protein spots that displayed changes in intensity. For most of those target proteins (e.g. fibrinogen gamma chain, apolipoprotein A-IV, serotransferrin) an enrichment during the SD-treatment was observed, whereas the influence of lyophilization was only minor. Process induced degradation of proteins was not detected. **Conclusions:** Processing of human plasma by SD-treatment and lyophilization does not cause major alterations in protein composition. This was shown by means of functional clotting assays and proteomic technologies, which will probably develop into important tools for transfusion medicine to assess the impact of manufacturing and pathogen inactivating procedures on the integrity of blood derived therapeutics.

PS2.7

A Novel System for Monitoring and Documentation of the Plasma Freezing Process

R. Knels[1], F. Reinhardt[2], C. Pollmer[1]

[1]DRK-Blutspendedienst Sachsen gGmbH, Dresden, D; [2]DRK-Blutspendedienst Sachsen gGmbH, Plauen, D

Purpose: Freezing of human plasma is a critical step for the quality of this product. By an audit at our Blood Center (BSD) the authorities demanded a better monitoring of the freezing process. **Methods:** In accordance to the change control procedure of the BSD first we compile the design qualification with following parameters to acquire: position of the plasma, point of start and finish, freezing overall time, point of unloading, runback sole temperature during freezing and storage in the freezer. Further we wanted to develop a mechanism to control the time between collection and freezing. For freezing plasma the BSD uses Hof-freezers (Hof Sonderanlagenbau GmbH, Germany) with integrated relays. To monitor the points of start, finish and unloading we wanted to send the point of circuit switching of these relays and the measurement results of the runback sole temperature from the integrated sensor to an external computer. To monitor the temperature and other technical details we use equipment and the software "Almemo" from Ahlborn Mess- und Regelungstechnik GmbH, Germany. Finally we have to give all information to the blood bank software BAS/400, because the last requirement was that the plasma cannot be cleared directly for distribution in case of any deviations. **Results:** First we connected the sensor and the relays with Almemo and control the input and the consistence of data. We found that the relays for the finish point information what result in blinking of a green lamp will not work, if we use the overnight storage modus of the freezer. The solution was building in a next relays by Hof. In the next step our software engineers create a module for the BAS/400 for the data input from "Almemo", the appraisal of the results and blocking of the distribution in case of deviations. For monitoring the position first we read a barcode on the plate and then in connection with the measuring of the weight the donation number of the plasma. After finish the acquisition of the plasma data, we "give" the plates to a freezer (reading of plates and freezer barcodes). The last step was to create an interchange protocol between the Windows based "Almemo" and the DB2 based BAS/400 on IBM i-series. **Conclusion:** After implementation and validation the monitoring and documentation of the freezing process working well, easy, without wasting time and in accordance with GMP.

PS2.8

Effect of Gamma Radiation with 30 Gy on the Coagulation System in WBC-Reduced Fresh Frozen Plasma

V. Weisbach, J. Strobel, B.E. Hahn, R. Eckstein

Universitätsklinikum Erlangen, D

Purpose: The effect of gamma radiation with 30 Gy on the coagulation system in WBC-reduced fresh frozen plasma (FFP) has not been elucidated previously. **Methods:** In 74 FFP units which had been stored for 352 ± 103 (range 241 to 646) days below −30°C, we determined the following parameters immediately after thawing and after gamma radiation with 30 Gy: Prothrombin time (PT), activated partial thromboplastin time (aPTT), thrombin time (TT), anti-thrombin III (ATIII), protein C, protein S, von Willebrand Factor antigen, ristocetin cofactor, plasminogen, Alpha- 2-antiplasmin, the coagulation factors fibrinogen, FII, FV, FVII, VIII, FIX, FX, FXI, FXII, FXIII, parameters of activation of the coagulation system FXa, FXIIa, D-Dimer, fibrin-monomer, thrombin antithrombin complex (TAT), prothrombin fragment 1 + 2 (F1 + 2), plasmin antiplasmin complexes (PAP), platelet factor 4 (PF4), FVII activity ratio was assayed to quantify activation of FVII. **Results:** The results are shown in the table (only significant changes are shown). FV, FVII, FIX, FX, FXII showed very similar results compared to FII. **Conclusions:** Gamma radiation of WBC-reduced FFPs with 30 Gy results in a significant but weak activation of the coagulation system in FFPs.

	Before radiation	After radiation	p-value
Prothrombin time (%)	89.8 ± 8.2	90.7 ± 8.0	0.002
APTT (seconds)	35.0 ± 4.1	34.4 ± 4.1	<0.0005
Fibrinogen (mg/L)	257 ± 35	261 ± 35	0.003
Factor II (%)	95 ± 9	98 ± 9	<0.0005
Factor VIII (%)	118 ± 31	116 ± 32	0.02
ATIII (%)	98 ± 8	99 ± 8	<0.0005
FVII activity ratio	1.19 ± 0.29	1.31 ± 0.34	<0.0005
FXIIa (ng/mL)	0.81 ± 0.50	0.90 ± 0.51	0.006
F1 + 2 (nmol/L)	1.19 ± 0.20	1.24 ± 0.20	<0.0005
PAP (ng/mL)	16.2 ± 11.5	20.2 ± 12.0	<0.0005
Prot. S, free antigen (%)	98 ± 15	101 ± 17	0.009
Plasminogen (%)	92 ± 14	94 ± 15	0.007

PS2.9

Using Osmotic Fragility with an Optimised Approximation in Quality Control of Red Blood Cell with SAGM and PAGGS-M

T. Schulzki, S. Heer

Regionaler Blutspendedienst SRK, Chur, CH

Purpose: To find out the usefulness of osmotic fragility(OF) for quality control of red blood cell storage we implemented the method in a evaluation of MCV by two methods and used it in an evaluation of the additive solution PAGGS-M. The mathematical approach to use OF and a comparison of the results between the two additive solutions are shown. **Methods:** MCV was measured with an Sysmex® analyzer and calculated from micro hematocrit. A complete (12 tubes) OF was done and an double curve approximation of the results was calculated (sum of two distributions). In contrast to the work of Epps("Chemistry and Physics of Lipids 74 (1994) 163–174") we used a lognormal distribution in combination with another lognormal and/or normal distribution. The concentration of NaCl-solution to achieve a certain rate of hemolyis (5%, 50%, 95%) was calculated and used to compare products. Some metabolites and electrolytes completed the design, also spontaneous hemolysis during storage and pH. **Results:** The approximation works fine when it is fine tuned by parameters of the loss function. MCV as calculated by Sysmex® and hematocrit show different results for both of the additive solutions. OF 5%-hemolysis rises in SAGM-during storage but stays the same for PAGGS-M. With 50%-hemolysis the results are more constant for both, showing a little more resistance for PAGGS-M during storage. A derived value (5%-hemolysis–95%-hemolyis), shows more clearly the ongoing changes. The data are completed with the other parameters measured and they show a rise of osmotic active substances intracellular, not readily exchanging with diluent. **Conclusion:** The results show the reason because in certain papers OF seems to be of no use in judging product quality: the 50%-hemolysis seems to be rather constant, but especially the 5%-hemolysis for SAGM and the 95%-hemolysis for PAGGS-M show significant changes during storage. Together with data from the two ways to measure the MCV and some metabolite and electrolyte data processes in the erythrocyte can be explained much better. Lactate seems to accumulate in the red cells and might be the main reason for the high OF 5%-hemolysis in SAGM. OF with the approximation routine used seems to be a valuable tool in validation procedures of products, but to time consuming for daily routine. A re-stricted test might be of value in routine quality control.

PS2.10

Quality Aspects Using Different Methods for Erythrocyte Preparation

U. Seyfert, T. Speer, S. Zewinger
Klinkum – IHT, Ludwigshafen, D

Erythrocytes may be prepared during collection using apheresis technology or processing of whole blood. **Material and Methods:** We investigated the influence of additive solutions (SAG-M; PAGGS-M), irradiation (30 Gy), continuous and non continuous apparative erythrocytapheresis (Haemonetics; Baxter), washing procedures by technicians versus apparative washing (Haemonetics) in cryopreserved erythrocyte concentrates on quality assurance of red cells. We compared 10 different groups (n = 15–20 each group) and performed measurements of haemoglobin, haematocrit, haemolysis, potassium, ATP, leucodepletion, osmolarity (cryopreserved red cells) using commercially available test kits. Weekly controls over the storage life were performed. **Results:** There was an increase in haemolysis of the red cells after whole blood collection and after erythrocytapheresis but <0.8% of red cell mass at the end of storage times. A similar increase was found in the irradiated groups (SAG-M-, PAGGS-M whole blood, apheresis groups) at day 20 (medians between 77 and 139.9 mg/dl free hemoglobin). There was a significant increase of potassium release in the irradiated SAG-M (41 mmol/l) versus the PAGGS-M group (65.5 mmol/l) at day 20. There were moderate differences of free hemoglobin levels at the end of storage life using SAG-M (139.9 mg/dl) versus PAGGS-M (116.3 mmol/l) whole blood. Erythrocyte concentrates produced during a continuous apheresis procedure had higher ATP levels at the end of storage life (466 vs. 380 umol/l; p = 0.01). Apparative washing procedures producing cryopreserved red cells result in higher ATP levels (616 vs. 383 umol/l; automation vs. control). **Conclusion:** The effects of additive solutions, irradiation and automatisation on quality assurance of red cells produced during whole blood collection or apheresis technology are important from a clinical point of view. There is need for further improvements of additive solutions and preparation technology.

PS2.11

Osmotic Resistance of Red Blood Cell Concentrates Is Maintained during Storage for 27 Days

I. Trestyanszki[1], T. Volgmann[2], T.H. Müller[2]
[1]DRK-Blutspendedienst NSTOB, Bremen, D; [2]DRK-Blutspendedienst NSTOB, Springe, D

Purpose: The stability of red blood cell membranes exposed to hypotonic NaCl solutions has been proposed as a quality parameter of red cell preparations. The conventional determination of the osmotic resistance by visual evaluation is, however, tedious and subjective. The purpose of this study is the development and evaluation of an objective method to measure the osmotic resistance. **Methods:** Samples from red blood cell preparations (50 μL) were added to a series of 12 NaCl solutions (103–240 mosmol/L; 1.0 mL each) to incubate at 22°C for 12 h. An aliquot of the supernatant was transfered to a 96-well microtiter plate to measure the OD values at 540 nm. The mean osmotic resistance was calculated from the inversion point of the OD vs. log(dNaCl) curves. Red blood cells concentrates in SAGM prepared by standard procedures from whole blood collections were stored at 4 + 2°C. **Results:** Highly reproducible measurements of the osmotic resistance (intra-assay CV < 2.0%) are ensured by the photometric detection of the extent of haemolysis. The mean osmotic resistance in mosmol/L and its ratio to the individual initial value was evaluated for 10 red blood cell concentrates during the storage for 27 days (see Table). The osmotic resistance was not affected by the storage of red blood cell concentrates for at least 27 days. The inter-individual variation in the osmotic resistance was maintained during this period. **Conclusions:** A simple and rapid method for reliable measurements of the osmotic resistance of red blood cell preparations has been established. The storage of red cell concentrates in SAGM for up to 27 days did completely preserve this parameter of membrane stability.

stored for:	72–96 h	11–12 d	20 d	27 d
mean ± SD	169 ± 11	171 ± 11	170 ± 13	169 ± 13
(min–max)	(153–188)	(155–187)	(152–191)	(150–190)
ratio ± SD		1.01 ± 0.02	1.00 ± 0.02	1.00 ± 0.02

PS2.12

DGTI Workshop 2005 for the Molecular Diagnosis of Red Blood Cell, Platelet and Granulocyte Alloantigens

H. Kroll[1], S. Mutz[2], C. Gassner[3], F.F Wagner[4], S. Jorks[5], G. Bein[2]
[1]Red Cross Blood Transfusion Service NSTOB, Dessau, D; [2]Institute for Clinical Immunology and Transfusion Medicine, Giessen, D; [3]Central Institute for Blood Transfusion and Immunological Department, Innsbruck, A; [4]Red Cross Blood Transfusion Service NSTOB, Springe, D; [5]Red Cross Blood Transfusion Service NSTOB, Dessau, D

Purpose: Molecular typing of alloantigenic polymorphisms on red blood cells, platelets and granulocytes has become routine in immunohaematologic laboratories. Frequently, commercial assays are used. However, some laboratories use their own protocols with a low grade of interlaboratory standardisation. We therefore performed external proficiency testing in collaboration with the members of the Section Immunohematology/Gene technique of the German Society of Immunohaematology and Transfusion Medicine (DGTI). **Methods:** In the 2005 workshop, a total number of 54 laboratories participated in different categories: red blood cells 46, platelets 45, granulocytes 11. Blood donors were carefully selected according to their ABO, RHD, RHD zygosity, RHCE, KEL, FY, JK, MNSs; HPA-1, -2, -3, -4, -5, -9, 15 and HNA-1a, -b, -c, 4a alleles. Genomic DNA was isolated from peripheral blood leukocytes by standard procedures. The selection of the typing method was left to participants. Results were reported on standardised questionnaires. **Results:** The error rates were as follows: Red blood cells: AB0: 5/504 (1.0%), RHD: 7/240 (2.9%), RHD zygosity: 3/72 (4.2%), RHCE: 6/960 (0.6%), KEL: 0/456 (0.0%), FY: 2/456 (0.4%), JK: 2/456 (0.4%), MNSs: 2/552 (0.4%). Platelets: HPA-1: 30/720 (4.2%), HPA-2: 11/704 (1.6%), HPA-3: 11/688 (1.6%), HPA-4: 3/528 (0.6%), HPA-5: 16/704 (2.3%), HPA-9: 1/48 (2.1%), HPA-15: 17/656 (2.6%). Granulocytes: HNA-1a: 1/66 (1.5%), HNA-1b: 1/66 (1.5%), HNA-1c: 1/48 (2.1%), HNA-4a: 0/30 (0.0%). Samples from donors with the alleles weak D type 1, weak D type 2, RhCw induced the highest number of mistypings. Compared to the previous year the FY*X and FY*null alleles were correctly typed by almost all laboratories. 34 participants (63.0%) could be certified in all workshop categories. **Conclusions:** Genotyping as a standard technique for the determination of red blood cell, platelet and granulocyte alloantigens has reached a high level of quality. However, some mistypings still occurred. Our analysis demonstrates that high quality genotyping can only be established and maintained by external proficiency testing.

PS2.13

RHMOD Phenotype Caused by Double Heterozygosity for Two New Alleles of the RHAG Gene

E.A. Scharberg[1], *H. Tsuneyama*[2], *K. Ogasawara*[2], *M. Uchikawa*[2], *H.H. Keller*[3], *E. Richter*[1], *P. Bugert*[1]

[1]DRK-Blutspendedienst Baden-Württemberg-Hessen, Baden-Baden, D; [2]Japanese Red Cross Tokyo Blood Center, Tokyo, Japan; [3]SRH Klinikum Karlsbad-Langensteinbach, Karlsbad-Langensteinbach, D

Purpose: The Rh associated glycoprotein (RhAG) is essential for the expression of Rh antigens. Individuals with homozygous mutations of the RHAG gene, which encodes the RhAG, can show a complete absence (Rhnull phenotype of regulator type) or modified expression of all Rh antigens. We report a case of a patient with extremely decreased expression of all Rh antigens caused by double heterozygosity for two different missense mutations of the RHAG gene. **Methods:** The Rh phenotyping was performed in the gel technique using monoclonal (IgM) test sera in direct spin test and polyclonal Rh sera in indirect antiglobulin test. The agglutination tests were performed with untreated and enzyme treated (bromelain and papain) red cells. All exons of the RHCE and RHAG genes were analysed by amplification from genomic DNA and direct sequencing. **Results:** Untreated red cells of the patient showed negative and very weak positive results with monoclonal Rh reagents. Enzyme treated cells tested with monoclonal sera and untreated red cells tested with polyclonal reagents in indirect antiglobulin test reacted positively revealing the R1R2 phenotype. Analysis of the entire RHCE gene showed the expected CcEe specific nucleotide sequences and no additional mutations. Sequencing of the RHAG gene showed heterozygosity for a missense mutation 269G > T in exon 2 and a missense mutation 560G > A in exon 4. The mother of the patient had a normal expression of all Rh antigens (R1R2) and a missense mutation 269G > T in exon 2, the father had also a normal expression of Rh antigens (R1r) and a missense mutation 560G > A in exon 4. **Conclusions:** Double heterozygosity for two new alleles 269G > T (exon 2) and 560G > A (exon 4) of the RHAG gene revealed a unique genetic background for a patient with an Rh mod phenotype with extremely weak expression of all Rh antigens. The associated amino acid substitutions Gly90Val and Gly187Asp are located in the predicted membrane-spanning domains of the RhAG glycoprotein.

PS2.14

Rapid Detection of Platelet Antibodies Using a Simple Antigen-Specific Particle Assay (ASPA)

O. Meyer[1], *A. Agaylan*[1], *H.-H. Borchert*[2], *T. Aslan*[1], *S. Bombard*[3], *H. Kiesewetter*[1], *A. Salama*[1]

[1]Charité, Universitätsmedizin Berlin, D; [2]Freie Universität Berlin, D; [3]DiaMed AG, Cressier s/Morat, CH

Purpose: The clinical significance of platelet antibodies is reflected by their association with autoimmune thrombocytopenia, alloimmune thrombocytopenia, drug-induced immune thrombocytopenia, and neonatal alloimmune thrombocytopenia. However, the antigen-specific assays currently used for characterization of platelet-reactive auto- and alloantibodies are too technically complex and impracticable for most routine laboratories. Here, we describe a novel antigen-specific particle assay (ASPA) for platelets similar to that of red blood cells. **Methods:** Platelets were solubilized and then incubated with red-dyed polystyrene particles coated with monoclonal antibodies to platelet glycoprotein complexes GPIIb-IIIa, GPIb-IX, and GPIa-IIa. These particles were directly tested for coating with autoantibodies, indirectly tested for serum autoantibodies, or alloantibodies against HPA-1a or HPA-5b. Serum samples from healthy blood donors (n = 100) served as negative controls. The sensitivity of the ASPA was evaluated using WHO standards for the detection of alloantibodies against HPA-1a and HPA-5b. **Results:** Negative reactions were clearly distinguishable from positive reactions. Both WHO-standards reacted specifically positive as well by the ASPA and by the MAIPA. In all cases with alloantibodies, the results of the ASPA were largely in concordance with those obtained by the standard monoclonal antibody-specific immobilization of platelet antigen assay (MAIPA). **Conclusion:** The new antigen-specific particle assay is reliable, yet less complex and time-consuming than the currently available assays, and it can be implemented in any routine laboratory.

PS2.15

Detection of a Novel CD36 (GPIV) Gene Variant Causing an ALLO-Immuniation. A Case Report

X. Duc Nguyen, H. Klüter, P. Bugert

Institut für Transfusionsmedizin und Immunologie Mannheim, D

Case Report: A full-term male baby was delivered without complications from a healthy mother. Generalized petechiae has been observed since birth. The blood count showed a thrombocytopenia with 5.000 plt/μL. Haemoglobin, leucocytes and coagulation screening tests were normal. According to the symptomatic signs, neonatal alloimmune thrombocytopenia (NAIT) was suspected. Maternal serum, EDTA-blood of the child and the father was collected for further investigations. Because of the petechiae and thrombocytopenia, the baby received a pooled platelet concentrate resulting in a sufficient increment. Investigations on platelet antibodies were immediately performed. **Results:** Additional to HLA antibodies, specific antibodies in the maternal serum against GPIV (CD36) of the father could be detected by SASPA (simultaneous analysis of specific platelet antibodies). Interestingly, this antibody did not react with GPIV of platelets of healthy blood donors. A specific antibody against a polymorphism of GPIV was suspected and thus CD36-expression on maternal and paternal platelets as well as sequencing of CD36 of both parents was performed. Both showed a normal expression of CD36. Sequencing of CD36 revealed a heterozygosity in exon 14 at position 1585 (T > C) leading to an amino acid replacement (Phe459Leu) in the father. Accordingly, a PCR-SSP based genotyping was performed. The result confirmed this mutation in the father but not in the child with suspect NAIT. In addition, we genotyped the elder brother of the child and siblings of the father as well as 500 healthy blood donors. We found this CD36-polymorphism in the child's brother and two siblings of the child's father, but not in any of 500 healthy blood donors. **Conclusion:** We identified a novel CD36 gene variant which represents a private antigen proved to cause an allo-immunisation. The role of this allo-antigen with regard to NAIT remains unclear.

PS2.16

Real-Time Analysis of HPA-1a Antigen-Antibody Interaction by Surface Plasmon Resonance Technology

I. Socher[1], *C. Andrei-Selmer*[1], *G. Bein*[1], *H. Kroll*[2], *S. Santoso*[1]

[1]Clinical Immunology and Transfusion Medicine, Giessen, D; [2]German Red Cross Blood Service NSTOB, Dessau, D

Neonatal alloimmune thrombocytopenia (NAIT) is induced by maternal immunization against a fetal human platelet alloantigen (HPA). In about 75% of serologically verified NAIT cases alloantibodies (alloabs) against HPA-1a are responsible. Here, we studied the real-time binding characteristics of different HPA-1a alloabs by surface plasmon resonance (SPR) technology. In comparison to most other techniques, SPR allows direct measurement of antigen-antibody interaction without any washing procedure. Integrin alphaIIbeta3 was purified by affinity chromatography from platelets from HPA-1aa or -1bb donors, and immobilized onto CM5 biosensor chip by amino coupling. Monomorphic monoclonal antibody (mab) AP3 (anti-alphaIIbbeta3) or polymorphic mouse and human anti-HPA-1a mabs (SZ21 and 2E10) were injected serially into the reaction chamber. Real-time antigen-antibody binding characteristics (association-dissociation) were recorded and analyzed by Kinject software (Biacore). Mab AP3 showed similar binding characteristics with HPA-1a and -1b isoforms (control experiment). In contrast, mab SZ21 dissociated more rapidly from HPA-1b than from HPA-1a, indicating its preferential binding to HPA-1a. Similarily, human mab 2E10 (originally derived from a NAIT mother) bound to HPA-1a, but not to HPA-1b. Furthermore, we tested various HPA-1a alloabs from mothers with NAIT (n = 10) and from patients with PTP (n = 3). Anti-HPA-1a alloabs from NAIT patients bound to HPA-1a antigen with different binding characteristics. In the control experiment, no association with HPA-1b was detected. Vice versa, HPA-1b alloabs interacted specifically with HPA-1b antigen. Interestingly, HPA-1a from PTP patients showed specific binding to HPA-1a, but not to HPA-1b. These results indicated that SPR technology may represent a useful technique for direct analysis of platelet alloab binding characteristics. This information may help to improve the diagnosis of antibody mediated thrombocytopenia and the understanding of the pathomechanism of this disease.

Symposium

S1: Hemostaseology

SH1.1

Hemotherapy with Recombinant Factor VIIa in Patients with Bleeding Complications: An Update

R.E. Scharf, A. Gerhardt, R.B. Zotz
Heinrich-Heine-Universität Düsseldorf, D

This review will summarize our current experience in the hemotherapy with recombinant factor VIIa (rFVIIa) for bleeding control and also discuss future directions. The use of rFVIIa has been approved for treatment of hemorrhagic episodes in hemophiliacs with inhibitors to factors VIII or IX, in patients with congenital FVII deficiency, and in patients suffering from Glanzmann's thrombasthenia (an inherited platelet disorder characterized by a deficiency or defect of GPIIb-IIIa). In the past few years, the mechanism of action for rFVIIa was clarified in detail. An analysis of published data provides evidence that hemotherapy with rFVIIa can be considered as an established, safe, and effective treatment. The product appears to be free of antigenicity and without risk of viral transmission. However, the potential thrombogenicity of rFVIIa requires precaution and needs further evaluation in appropriate clinical trials. After becoming available, rFVIIa has also been increasingly used outside the labelled indications for acute treatment of life-threatening bleeding episodes when respective standard therapy regimen failed. In a randomized controlled trial, treatment with rFVIIa within four hours after the onset of intracerebral hemorrhage was shown to limit the extension of hematoma, to reduce mortality, and to improve functional outcomes. Another clinical study demonstrated that adjunctive therapy with rFVIIa for bleeding control resulted in a significant reduction in RBC transfusion in patients with severe blunt trauma but not in those with penetrating trauma. However, only a few randomized double-blind, placebo-controlled trials have been conducted with rFVIIa so far. Thus, conclusive evidence of its effectiveness from controlled clinical trials is not yet available. Most of the published studies are reports on single cases or small series. These include reports on the use of rFVIIa in the treatment of bleeding complications in patients with hepatic failure, liver transplantation, von Willebrand disease, various platelet disorders including thrombocytopenia, congenital or acquired coagulation factor deficiencies, drug-induced bleeding, neonatal bleeding, and in individuals without any pre-existing coagulation disorder but with acute diffuse life-threatening bleeding triggered by surgery or trauma. Larger randomized controlled trials are required to assess the efficacy, safety, and dosage of rFVIIa in these currently "off-label" clinical applications. Direct comparisons and pharmacoeconomic data are needed to determine the exact position of recombinant factor VIIa in relation to conventional hemotherapy regimen.

SH1.4

Response to Anti CD20 Monoclonal Antibody Rituximab and Epitope Mapping of Inhibitory Antibodies in Patients with Acquired Haemophilia

M. Krause[1], C. Kessel[1], C. Königs[1], I. Scharrer[2], E. Seifried[3], W. Kreuz[1]
[1]J.-W.- Goethe University of Frankfurt, D; [2]J.Gutenberg University, Mainz, D; [3]Institute of Transfusion Medicine, Frankfurt, D

Introduction: Acquired haemophilia (AcH) is associated with the development of polyclonal autoantibodies against FVIII, which affects directly the A2 or C2 domains of the FVIII molecule. Immunomodulatory therapy regimes with normalization of FVIII levels and elimination of the inhibitor are reasons for the treatment in patients with AcH. The aims of the present study were to localize the inhibitor epitopes on the FVIII domains, and the response to Rituximab. **Patients and Methods:** In five pts (2 females, 3 males; age: 64–81 yrs) the inhibitor titer was from 9 to 156 BU and FVIII activity was <1% to 6%. Rituximab was administered at a dosed 375 mg/m^2 once weekly for 4 weeks in combination with prednisone therapy (1–1.5 mg/kg). Random peptide phage display libraries were used to identify peptide sequences specific for inhibitors. The short peptide sequences allow the mapping of conformational epitopes on the surface of the FVIII molecule. **Results:** In all pts we documented complete remission (CR). Inhibitor titers were 0 BU,and FVIII activities were normalized. The time to response (CR) was much longer in two pts, who showed higher inhibitor titers (50 BU;188 BU and 23 or 32 weeks) comparend to pts with lower inhibitor titers (9 BU;22 BU;29 BU and 2, 4 or 5 weeks). With a median follow up of 22 months, long-term CR was achieved in two female pts; one pt relapsed 19 months after CR. Another pt died in septic shock 8 weeks after begin of therapy with Rituximab. In one male with inhibitor titer from max. 50 BU we identified epitopes in the A1 and A2 domain of FVIII, and in the other pts the peptide sequences map to epitope on the C2 domain of FVIII. **Conclusion:** Limited by the small number of pts, the therapy with rituximab shows high response rates and seems to be effective in the elimination of inhibitors against FVIII in our pts with AcH. The mechanism of response to autoantibodies against FVIII by the specific immunomodulatory therapy is still unclear in pts with AcH.

SH1.5

The Impact of Combined Polymorphisms of Integrin αIIbβ3 (HPA-1) and Integrin α2β1 (α2 807 C/T) on Platelet Adhesion

L. Robert, V. Stoldt, R.B. Zotz, R.E. Scharf
Heinrich Heine University Medical Center, Düsseldorf, D

Purpose: Platelet adhesion to subendothelial matrices plays a crucial role in the arrest of posttraumatic bleeding but also in pathological conditions such as thrombosis. Recent studies clearly demonstrated that integrins, especially α2β1 (GPIa-IIa) and αIIbβ3 (GPIIb-IIIa), are intimately involved in occlusive thrombus formation at the site of endothelial lesions. Previously, we provided experimental evidence that platelet adhesion onto immobilized fibrinogen and collagen is modulated by these platelet receptor polymorphism. Actually, we examined the functional synergism of HPA-1 and 807 C/T polymorphisms on platelet adhesion using an in vitro system simulating arterial flow conditions. **Methods:** The relationship between "prothrombogenic" (HPA-1b/1b + α2 807TT) vs. "wildtype" (HPA-1a/1a + α2 807CC) combination of polymorphisms was evaluated using anticoagulated blood obtained from donors (n = 18) with respected combination of polymorphisms. Platelets in whole blood were labelled with a fluorescence dye and platelet adhesion onto collagen-coated glass cover slips was assessed in a rectangular chamber under arterial flow conditions (shear rate 1500 s^{-1}). A laser-scan microscope was used for visualization and quantitation of platelet adhesion after 15 sec, 1 min, and 5 min of perfusion. **Results:** During perfusion, platelet adhesion onto collagen linearly increased with exposure time. The "prothrombogenic" (HPA-1b/1b+ α2 807TT) genotype combination enhanced platelet adhesion onto immobilized collagen in the range from 20%-106% compared to the "non-thrombogenic" (HPA1a/1a+ α2 807CC) combination. A maximal difference was observed after one min of perfusion. **Conclusions:** In this study, we found certain functional linkage between HPA1 and 807CT polymorphism. The "prothrombotic" genotype combination showed a higher platelet adhesion activity under arterial flow conditions compared to the "nonthrombotic" genotype combination. Our data support the contention that genetically determined variants of platelet integrins are risk for arterial thrombogenesis and thus confirm the hypothesis derived from clinical association studies.

Technical Session I

TS1: Automatisation and Data Management

TS1.1

Blood Bags with Integrated RFID-LABELS to Provide a Complete Traceability from Production to Patient: First Routine Experiences and Future Prospects

T. Wagner[1], J. Zimmermann[2], G. Schwondra[3], U. Ockenfuss[4], M. Behague[2], W. Kaufmann[3], G. Lanzer[5]

[1]Medizinische Universität Graz, A; [2]MACO Pharma, Lille, F; [3]Siemens AG Österreich, Wien, A; [4]Schweizer Electronic AG, Schramberg, D; [5]Medizinische Universität Graz, A

Background: The aim of this project is to develop a range of RFID tags for both tracing of blood products from donor to recipient and close temperature monitoring. It will increase safety due to reduction of mistaken identity of blood bags and pilot tubes as well as blood products and patients. To achieve quality objectives of a 100% reliability rate RFID tags have to be adapted to the harsh process requirements including pasteurisation, centrifugation and irradiation. **Methods:** Different passive RFID-labels (Omron®, Infineon®) were attached to the RBC container beneath the primary label directly before the pasteurisation step took place. With the use of proper hard- and software different test points were defined to analyze correct function of the tags. The blood containers were shipped to our department and subsequently used in our routine setting. Critical step with respect to tag survival are centrifugation (~ 4000 g) and irradiation (30 Gy). **Results:** A total of 1466 RFID-labelled RBC units were tested. After centrifugation as many as 99.12% worked correctly. Only 13 tags lost their functionality. Another 10 tags broke down during shelf live. All tags worked after being exposed to a single irradiation dose, but lost their function after 10 consecutive irradiation doses. Interestingly, 1.36% was reported defect but found ok when retested. Therefore, proper training of each individual involved is a critical step to assure success. Summary: In this first pilot study we were able to demonstrate the blood product applicability of standard passive RFID-labels. The use of temperature-monitoring RFID-labels which meet our defined specification requires development of reliable electronic components, novel interconnection solutions and a modified battery technology. This process is largely completed and first tests using active RFID will start soon. The results of this project will help to improve quality, reduce wastage due to improper storage and avoid incorrect transfusions.

TS1.2

Restzellzählung im Plasma am Durchflusszytometer (FacsCalibur) – eine testbezogene interne Qualitätskontrolle

B. Brys[1], B. Baumann-Baretti[2], K.-P. Krause[3]

[2]Haema AG, Leipzig, D; Haema AG, Berlin, D; [3]Haema AG, Leipzig, D

Ziel: Die Restzellzählung im Plasma wird am Durchflußzytometer Facs Calibur (BD) mit dem Testkit Plasma Count (BD) durchgeführt. Zu diesem Test wird bis zum jetzigen Zeitpunkt kein Qualitätskontrollmaterial angeboten. Bei Einführung des Tests wurden verschiedene Möglichkeiten zur internen Qualitätskontrolle geprüft. Ziel war es, eine Kontrollprobe mit extern deklarierten Zielwerten zu finden. **Material und Methode:** Es wurden die im Einsatz befindlichen Hämotologiekontrollen zur Testung modifiziert, da deren Konzentrationsbereiche nicht im Bereich der Restzellmessungen im Plasma liegen, indem Verdünnungsreihen erstellt und getestet wurden. Das getestete Hämatologiekontrollmaterial in verschiedenen Verdünnungsstufen führte bei Messungen für WBC und RBC zu reproduzierbaren Ergebnissen. Die Ergebnisse der Messung des Hämatologiekontrollmaterial für PLT waren nicht reproduzierbar, so dass ein Aliquot eines Thrombozytenkonzentrats in gleichen Verdünnungsstufen eingesetzt wurde. So können aus einer Probe die 3 zu prüfenden Parameter getestet werden. Für die Kontrolle sind die Zielwerte vorgegeben, die durch die deklarierten Werte (WBC, RBC) der Hämatologiekontrolle bestimmt sind. Ausgangswert der PLT-Werte ist der aktuell gemessene Wert des Thrombozytenkonzentrats. Diese interne Kontrolle wird in jeder Testserie eingesetzt. **Schlussfolgerung:** Es wurden Kontrollproben aus den vorhandenen Hämotologiekontrollen für die Restzellmessung WBC und RBC im Plasma und für PLT aus dem Aliquot eines Thrombozytenkonzentrates entwickelt; sie ermöglichen eine Kontrolle der täglichen Serie zur Restzellzählung im Plasma.

TS1.3

TaqMan NADIS Enables Full Monitoring of NAT Screening and Production of NAT Reagents

M. Schmidt, A. Themann, V. Brixner, E. Seifried, K. Hourfar

DRK Institut Frankfurt, Frankfurt, D

Background: Since 1997 all donations from German Red Cross Blood Donor Service Frankfurt and several customers from central Europe were screened by real-time in-house MP-NAT for HIV-1, HBV and HCV. Additional testing for HAV and B19 started in 2000. With the increasing number of tests there was the need for a software solution to monitor the complete NAT-testing process. **Methods:** A special software program (TaqMan Nucleic acid Amplification Detection and Information System) was developed that allows documentation of the NAT-testing process. Barcode data from all tested samples were transferred to the TaqMan NADIS program and were compared with a working list. After pooling and extraction of nucleic acids an automated assignment of pool-extracts to specific positions on PCR-microtiter plates is performed. After the PCR-setup, the virus-specific thermocycler-program is started automatically by scanning of the microtiter plates' barcode. The TaqMan-NADIS program allows sample tracking at every stage of the NAT-testing process. An additional characteristic of the software is the batch management feature which allows barcode-controlled production of NAT reagents. All NAT assays are composed of three different components (master mix, internal controls and positive controls). TaqMan NADIS controls daily the correct linkage of all components, the expiration date of all assays and the residual number of reagents. **Results/ Conclusions:** More than 600,000 samples were tested with the TaqMan NADIS program since 2005. TaqMan NADIS is a stable program, as no system errors occurred during the described time period. The development of the TaqMan NADIS program enables a fully barcode-controlled NAT-testing process as well as batch management of NAT reagents and a direct link to different customer-specific LIMS systems. The NADIS software built the foundation for a CE certification process, which should be completed this year.

TS1.4

Online-Anbindung von Blutmischwaagen an Blutbank-EDV mit Hilfe Fresenius Donationmaster Net Release 1.3.0.4

K. Wedekind[1], S. Kolb[2], K.-P. Krause[3]

[1]Haema AG, Berlin, D; [2]Fresenius HemoCare, Bad Homburg, D; [3]Haema AG, Leipzig, D

Einleitung: Gestiegenen Anforderungen der Behörden und die Notwendigkeit einer voranschreitenden GMP-gemäßen Erfassung aller Herstellungsschritte bei der Produktion von Erythrozytenkonzentraten macht eine lückenlose Dokumentation der Vollblutentnahme erforderlich. Zur Online-Anbindung der Blutmischwaagen existieren verschiedene Kommunikationssysteme. Dazu gehören u.A. das Auslesen mit Hilfe von Speicherkarten, kabelgebundene Mischwaagenlösungen und die DECT-Funkverbindungen. Es gibt vielfältige Vorteile der DECT-Kommunikation im Vergleich zu den anderen genannten Varianten: Einige Vorteile sind:

- sofortige Auswertbarkeit von Entnahmedaten (online)
- DECT Standard: geschütztes Frequenzband, verschlüsselte Datenübertragung
- freie Platzierung der Mischwaagen und des angeschlossenen PC im Spendesaal
- Reichweite im Raum bis zu 100 Meter
- Für den mobilen Einsatz (Außenabnahmen) geeignet
- Geringer Installations- und Administrationsaufwand

Diese Form der Anbindung passt am besten zu den von uns gestellten Anforderungen. Beim Einsatz der aktuell verfügbaren Softwarelösungen traten verschiedene Probleme auf:

- Probleme bei Kommunikation zwischen Waage und Software
- Fehlende Entnahmedaten
- Zusammenbruch der DECT-Verbindungen zwischen Waage und PC

Die Aufarbeitung der Probleme war mit erhöhtem Arbeitsaufwand verbunden. Daten mussten manuell nachgetragen werden, Mischwaagen wiederholt am Tag initialisiert werden. Nach Diskussion der Probleme mit dem Hersteller wurde ein Feldtest mit einer neuen Softwareversion durchgeführt. **Material und Methode:** Zum Einsatz kamen das CompoGuard Blutmischwaagensystem (Version 1.3.0.4) von Fresenius mit DECT-Fixed Part und die dazugehörige Donationmaster Net Software (Release 1.3.0.4). Geprüft wurde die Rate an Ausfällen bzw. die Konsistenz der Datenübernahme von der Mischwaage zum EDV-System. **Ergebnisse:** Die Installation der Software verlief ebenso leicht, wie die der vorherigen Softwareversionen. Das System unterstützt die Windowsbetriebssysteme Win 9x, Win NT, Win 2000, Win XP. Ein Wechsel der blutmischwaagen-internen Software war notwendig. Spendeprogramme, Barcodelisten oder anderen definierte Parameter standen nach der Aktualisierung der Software unverändert zur Verfügung. Der Feldtest mit der neuen Software-Version lief in unserem BSZ über drei Monate. In diesem Zeitraum traten keine auffälligen Netzwerkprobleme oder damit verbundene Beeinträchtigungen in der Online-Auswertung mehr auf. Alle Blutmischwaagen laufen sehr stabil im DECT-Netz, der aktuelle Waagenstatus (Spende, Online, Offline) kann jeder Zeit eingesehen werden, die Online-Datenübernahme war fehlerfrei, die Performance war sehr gut. **Zusammenfassung:** Das CompoGuard Blutmischwaagensystem mit DECT-Funknetzwerk (Release 1.3.0.4) garantiert eine sichere und routinetaugliche GMP-gerechte Anbindung der Mischwaagen an ein EDV-System.

TS1.5

Tecan Te-PoolSafe Balance Module Allows Monitoring of the Pooling Process for NAT-Testing

M.K. Hourfar[1], M. Koller[2], R. Kehrli[2], E. Seifried[1], M. Schmidt[1]
[1]DRK-Blutspendedienst Baden-Württemberg, Frankfurt, D; [2]Tecan Schweiz, Männerdorf, CH

Background/Aims: Most countries that have implemented NAT-screening of blood donations perform testing in minipools. However, documentation of the pooling process until now has been incomplete. Therefore our aim was to establish and validate technical improvements that allow process control and full documentation of the pooling process, leaving blood banks confident that the appropriate amount of plasma has been pipetted from every sample to the pool. **Methods:** A fast and very sensitive balance module with a 16-position holder for pooling tubes has been developed, which can be easily integrated into Tecan Freedom EVO Clinical and Genesis RSP liquid handling platforms. A novel software monitors and evaluates every single dispense from primary samples to the sample pool to confirm liquid arrival. The weighing accuracy of the Te-PoolSafe option is approx. 3 mg per dispense. The Tecan Te-PoolSafe option was evaluated by creating 50 minipools of poolsizes from 6 to 96 donations each using plasma samples which were previously used for routine-NAT testing. **Results:** A total number of n = 20,012 blood donations were tested on a Tecan's Genesis RSP and a Freedom EVO Clinical pipetting system. 99.6% (19,932) of all dispenses were within the acceptance criteria of ± 5% (equivalent to ± 5 ml). The Te-PoolSafe module detected 0.4% (80 of 20,012) mispipettings successfully, which were outside of the acceptance criteria. 53 of 80 mispipettings with a volume below 95 ml were not detected by the clot-detection of the pipetting platform, but most probably a large fraction of these samples would have been excluded by visual inspection of the archive plates. Visual inspection of the corresponding primary tubes showed blood clots, short sample or no apparent cause. The remaining 27 of 80 mispipettings were higher than 105 ml. The average deceleration of the pooling process was determined with about 25%. **Conclusions:** With the novel Tecan Te-PoolSafe liquid arrival check system for the first time complete and consistent process documentation of pooling for NAT-testing is feasible. It enables blood banks to monitor and to compare every single dispense made with predefined, required volumes. **Results:** can be transferred to the laboratory information management system (LIMS) for automated selective exclusion of inaccurately dispensed samples. Mispipetted samples can be separately re-pipetted. The additional safety by implementing the Te-PoolSafe module, however, is associated with a deceleration of the pooling process. Nonetheless, the minor deceleration of the pooling process is acceptable, as overall process safety can be further increased.

TS1.6

Highly Sensitive and Fully Automated HBV DNA Extraction with the Qiagen BioRobot MDx to Indentify Chronic HBV Carriers

M.K. Hourfar, V. Brixner, E. Seifried, M. Schmidt
DRK-Blutspendedienst Baden-Württemberg, Frankfurt, D

Background and Objectives: The German Advisory Committee Blood and official authority (the Paul Ehrlich Institute) recommended that anti-HBc repeat reactive multiple time donors should be screened additionally by HBV individual donation (ID)-NAT (95% sensitivity less than 12 IU/ml) and for anti-HBs. Because of an estimated pre-valence of 1.9% of anti-HBc repeat reactive donations, a fully automated DNA extraction system was implemented into blood donor screening. **Study Design and Methods:** A modified Qiagen BioRobot MDx extraction protocol was developed for highly sensitive HBV ID-NAT testing. Samples were extracted overnight by vacuum extraction. After extraction, the working list was transferred to a software which was used to monitor the amplification steps and supports the evaluation of the in house NAT. Finally, all results were transferred to a LIMS system. **Results:** The validation of BV ID-NAT (24 replicates of 6 different concentrations) yielded a 95% analytical sensitivity of 8.6 IU/ml (range 6.7 IU/ml to 14.3 IU/ml). 6 out of 2000 anti-HBc reactive samples, found to be HBV-DNA positive with the BioRobot MDx, could be confirmed by a manual extraction procedure. The DNA concentration was between 3 IU/ml and 33 IU/ml. The fraction of invalid test results was in an acceptable range. **Conclusion:** The implementation of fully automated and highly sensitive HBV DNA extraction with Qiagen BioRobot MDx was feasible. Up to 96 ID-NAT examinations per run can be performed without the need for additional personnel. The sensitivity of <10 IU/ml complies with the requirements of the German regulatory authority for the safety of blood products. Our experience demonstrates that the DNA extraction with the Qiagen BioRobot MDx allows highest sensitivities and efficient reduction of labor associated with HBV detection.

TS1.7

2 Years Experience on Residual Cell Enumeration with BD Plasma Count Kit for QC Testing of Fresh Frozen Plasma

B. Lambrecht[1], U. Bauerfeind[1], H.-P. Spengler[2], F. Nauwelaers[2], H. Mohr[1], T. Müller[1]
[1]DRK BSD NSTOB, Springe, D; [2]BD Biosciences, Erembodegem, BE

Purpose: A fully automated single tube flow cytometric assay was used for the simultaneous quantitation of residual cells in FFP. Previous validation proved that the assay was linear and precise within the range of interest. For routine testing the method was set up in the quality control lab. Performance was evaluated during a 2 year period. **Methods:** Test frequency was 1% of all FFP units (vol.: 200–340 mL). Simultaneous determination of WBCs, RBCs, and PLTs by a single tube absolute count assay (Plasma Count kit) was performed one day after donation before freezing the FFP unit. A FACSCalibur with automated sample loader and Multiset software for automated data acquisition and analysis were used routinely. Additionally, 176 samples measured over a selected time period were re-evaluated by CellQuest Pro software (BD Bioscience, Heidelberg, Germany). **Results:** Altogether 5 operators tested on 108 days 2666 samples during a time period of 2 years. In 35 cases we found OOS (out of specification) results. Exact numbers are shown in table 1. Multiset and CellQuest Pro software reveal comparable results. **Conclusions:** Use of the BD Plasma Count Kit represents a simple and reliable way to determine residual cells in plasma by flow cytometry. Evaluation of analysis software demonstrated that results were independent of the software used.

Table 1. Results from QC routine testing of FFP over a two year period

Cell type	Specification limits (cells/µL)	Max. found (cells/µL)	OOS (n)	OOS (%)
rWBC	<5	196	31	1.2
rRBC	<6000	3960	0	0.0
rPLT	<20000	28952	4	0.15

Poster

P1: Stem Cells

P1.1

Feasibility and Safety of Endothelial Progenitor Cell Mobilisation in Patients Suffering from Critical Ischemia of Lower Extremity

C. Kreissig, I. Rehfeld, H. Eichler
Institute of Transfusion Medicine Breitscheid, Department of Hemapheresis and Cell Therapy, Ratingen, D

Purpose: Transplantation of CD34+ peripheral blood or bone marrow stem cells is a well established procedure in various hemato-oncologic diseases. The CD34+ cell compartment not only contains hematopoietic but also endothelial progenitor cells (EPC). The therapeutic potential of EPC has already been evaluated in preclinical studies by using animal models. To date several clinical studies are ongoing to evaluate feasibility and safety of autologous EPC application in patients suffering from ischemia of extremities, myocardial infarction, or impaired cardiac function. **Methods:** In cooperation with a vascular surgery center we are performing a phase 1 trial on patients with critical ischemia of lower extremity grade III or IV. They undergo G-CSF mobilisation for 5 days (12 µg/kg BW per day) followed by a single leukapheresis. Apheresis products are positively selected for cells expressing either CD34 (Isolex 300i, n = 4) or CD133 antigens (CliniMACS, n = 5). The selected cell fraction is cryopreserved, and injection of thawed autologous progenitors is performed either intravasculary, e.g. during angioplasty, or intramusculary. **Results:** Up to now 9 patients were treated. G-CSF mobilisation and apheresis procedure were well tolerated by all patients without significant side effects (maximum CALGB grade 1), and a sufficient mobilisation efficiency was observed. Peripheral blood CD34+ cell counts reached 20 to 215 progenitors per µl. Therefore, 0.5 to 2.4 × 10E6 CD34+ cells could be applicated intraarterialy and/or intramusculary to study patients. **Conclusion:** G-CSF mobilisation and collection of EPC by leucapheresis proved to be a feasible and safe procedure in our patients suffering from critical ischemia of lower extremity. In principle, such patients showing high grade arterial stenosis could represent a high risk population due to increasing blood viscosity during G-CSF mobilisation. On the other hand, we did not yet observe severe side effects during mobilisation or leucapheresis. Further investigations have to confirm these preliminary observations.

P1.2

Prediction of G-CSF Mobilisation Efficiency in Allogenic PBSC Donors

I. Rehfeld
Institut für Transfusionsmedizin, Ratingen-Breitscheid, D

Purpose: For clinical transplantation, harvest of bone marrow (BM) got mostly displaced by peripheral blood stem cell (PBSC) collection. In the allogenic setting little is known about the role of adhesion molecules in the context of good and poor mobilizing donors. As a large hemapheresis centre, performing 120 to 150 unrelated peripheral blood stem cell collections per year, we want to identify parameters predicting the mobilization efficiency of G-CSF application in healthy volunteer donors. **Method:** The cell surface antigens CD45, CD11a, CD49d, CD49e and CD54 were quantified on peripheral blood samples from healthy donors (n = 10). Samples were taken each prior to lenograstrim application and after 4 days drug stimulation. After checking for leukocyte and CD34 counts the blood samples were stained with PC 5 or FITC labeled antibodies (Beckman Coulter). RBC were lysed by NH4CL. For flow cytometric analysis 10,000 leukocytes and 200 CD34+ cells were examined for each sample. Coexpression of the different adhesion molecules CD49d, CD49e, CD54, and CD11a on leukocytes and CD34+ were analysed. Poor mobilizing donors were defined by <40 CD34+ cells per µl. **Results:** A negative correlation with the mobilization efficiency could be observed for CD49d expression: high expression of CD49d antigens on leukocytes (≥15%) prior to lenograstrim application resulted in bad mobilization efficiency. **Conclusion:** Our results suggests that the CD49d integrin on leukocytes might be a useful indicator for identifying poor mobilizers on date of donor's physical examination. Further validation with a larger numbers of donors are needed to proof these preliminary observations.

P1.3

Monitoring of Engraftment and Relapse after Allogeneic Hematopoietic Stem Cell Transplantation Based on Lineage Specific Short-Tandem-Repeat Chimerism

M. Marx[1], P. Schauwecker[1], B. Höchsmann[1], S.V. Harsdorf[2], D. Bunjes[2], H. Schrezenmeier[1], M. Wiesneth[1]
[1]Institute for Clinical Transfusion Medicine and Immunogenetics, University of Ulm, D; [2]Department of Internal Medicine III, University of Ulm, D

Purpose: Short-Tandem-Repeat (STR) analysis of hematopoietic chimerism after allogeneic hematopoietic stem cell transplantation (HSCT) has been widely used for monitoring of engraftment and residual disease. Occasionally a mixed chimerism is observed first only in either granulocytes or lymphocytes. This study evaluates association of lineage specific mixed chimerism with relapse or graft rejection. **Methods:** Peripheral blood granulocytes and lymphocytes were separated by Ficoll density gradient. DNA was isolated according to a standard procedure (Qiagen, Germany). For chimerism analysis, different microsatellite loci were amplified by fluorescent PCR primers. The PCR products were separated by capillary electrophoresis using a 310 ABI Prism Genetic Analyzer (Applied Biosystems, USA). **Results:** Diagnostic impact of separate analysis of granulocyte and lymphocyte mixed chimerism was retrospectively studied in 1581 analyses from 298 lymphoid and myeloid leukemia patients after HSCT. In 75 (25%) patients mixed chimerism was first detected in only one of the lineages. Analysis of mixed chimerism after short-term (day < 100 after Tx) and long-term follow-up (day > 100) resulted in different interpretation. Lineage specific short-term observation of mixed granulocyte or lymphocyte chimerism in 12 patients showed no significant correlation with relapse of malignant disease or graft rejection, but mixed chimerism in lymphocytes indicated an association with viral infection in 7 out of 9 patients. Long-term follow-up of mixed chimerism in 39 patients with relapse of AML showed mixed chimerism first in lymphocytes (n = 34) and in only few cases first in granulocytes (n = 5). 15 patients with relapse of CML demonstrate same frequencies of first occurrence of mixed chimerism in lymphocytes (n = 7) and granulocytes (n = 8). In patients with relapsed acute (3) or chronic lymphocytic leukemia (4) mixed chimerism was always detected first in lymphocytes. **Conclusions:** Lineage specific chimerism, like granulocyte or lymphocyte based, is highly informative and increases the sensitivity for monitoring of engraftment, residual disease or leukemic relapse after allogeneic HSCT. Short-term mixed chimerism in lymphocytes is highly associated with virus infection whereas long-term mixed chimerism in lymphocytes indicate relapse of lymphoid as well as of myeloid leukemia.

P1.4

Optimum Storage Conditions of Cord Blood Units Prior to CD34(+) Isolation

A. Moldenhauer, J. Wolf, G. Habermann, G. Genter, H. Kiesewetter, A. Salama
Charité – Universitätmedizin Berlin, D

Purpose: Varying opinions exist regarding the storage conditions of cord blood prior to cryopreservation. Most experts recommend storage at room temperature and cryopreservation within the first 24 hours following delivery of the baby. However, the optimum storage conditions remain unknown. **Methods:** Cord blood units (n = 40) were stored for 24, 48 and 72 hours at room temperature (RT) and at 4°C. Following storage, CD34(+) cells were isolated and analyzed for their cell count, flow cytometry profile, apoptosis rate, colony-forming capacity by methylcellulose assays, and transmigration capacity in response to stroma-derived factor 1. Where possible, a direct-paired comparison was performed (n = 15). **Results:** The cell counts of peripheral blood mononuclear cells (MNC) were generally 10-fold higher in cord blood units stored at RT than in those stored at 4°C, resulting in a 10-fold increase in the number of isolated CD34(+) cells. There was no difference in the frequency of CD34(+) cells following immunomagnetic isolation (>95%) or in the frequency of CD133(+) and CD45(+) cells. At 48 hours, the apoptosis rate was lower at RT than at 4°C (37.7 ± 7.4 versus 49.9 ± 4.2%). The plating efficiencies (PE) were highest following storage for 48 hours (RT 14.7 ± 3.6%, 4°C 16.3 ± 4%), independent of the temperature. Storage times of 24 and 72 hours resulted in PEs with an average below 10%. The cells stored at RT for 48 hours were observed to have the highest transmigration capacity (54 ± 11.9% versus 4°C 10.7 ± 2%). Migration of CD34(+)cells stored for 24 hours was lower than those stored for 48 hours. The transmigration capacity after 24 hours showed no temperature-dependent difference (RT 24.6 ± 7.1 versus 4°C 36.1 ± 10.2%). **Conclusion:** Our data indicate that cord-blood units should be stored for 48 hours at room temperature before CD34(+) isolation.

P1.5

Variable Quality of Collected Cord Blood Units – Does it Depend on Donor Related Factors?

E. Strasser, A. Fischer, V. Weisbach, J. Zingsem, J. Ringwald, R. Eckstein

Universitätsklinikum Erlangen, D

Purpose: Cord blood (CB) samples showed variable product quality concerning the sample volume (minimum 60 mL) and the leucocyte count. Compliance with these quality criteria is required for a successful stem cell transplantation. Only few data were available concerning donor related factors, which may impact on product quality. **Material and Methods:** Product data of 689 CB units (WBC, nucleated cells, CD34-positive cells, CFUs and hematocrit) were statistically analysed (Windows SPSS 13 program) and compared to age and weight of the pregnant women, weight increase during pregnancy and deviations from the calculated delivery date as well as maturity and sex of the newborn. **Results:** Some of the major findings were that pregnant women with an age below 30 years showed significantly lower CD34-positive cells in CB harvests compared to older women. In male neonates higher CB product volumes (78 ± 22 vs. 61 ± 20 mL, $p = 0.018$) were found compared to females, when the age of the mother was less than 30 years, a higher weight increase during pregnancy appeared or in case of a delayed delivery. The volumes of CB products spread between 42 mL and 118 mL in male and between 36 mL and 114 mL in female neonates. Altogether 44% of these samples did not comply with the minimum volume of 60 mL or the minimum leucocyte count of 600.000 WBC per millilitre. Significant differences of CB-sample volumes were found depending on the weight (less than 75 kg vs. more than 75 kg) of pregnant women (67 ± 26 mL vs. 74 ± 28 mL, $p = 0.048$) and in delayed pregnancy (less than 7 days vs. 7–21 days) of the pregnant women less than 30 years (86 ± 18 mL vs. 76 ± 11 mL, $p = 0.029$). **Conclusions:** This study found that age and weight of the pregnant women as well as the sex of the newborn may impact on product volume, total number of CD34-positive cells and product hematocrit. Further research on that subject may help to identify donor preselection criteria that may help to reduce the proportion of cord blood units of insufficient quality.

P1.6

Erythroid Progenitors Express TNFa and Its Receptors in vitro

I. Dorn, P. Lazar, S. Boie, S. Malchow, P. Langentrassen, H. Kirchner, J. Luhm, P. Schlenke

UK S-H, Campus Lübeck, D

Purpose: In the past, we established an in vitro model of human erythropoiesis for basic research in the broad field of red blood cell development. Using gene arrays, we identified TNFa and its receptors as possible candidates with an influence erythroid maturation. In the present study the expression and function of TNFa and its receptors during in vitro erythropoiesis was investigated. **Methods:** After leukapheresis, human CD34+ cells were isolated using an immunomagnetic technique. Purified cells were cultured over 21 days in a three-phase liquid assay (d1–7: SCF, TPO, FLT3-L; d8–14: SCF, EPO, IGF-1; d15–21: EPO). Cell growth and differentiaton was evaluated by flow cytometry (staining against CD34, 45, 36, and glycophorin A (GPA)). Cytospin preparations were stained by Pappenheim. RNA of different culture days was isolated. A RT-PCR for TNFa, TNF-RSF 1a (TNF-R1) and TNF-RSF 1b (TNF-R2) was established and performed using I Cycler of BioRad. Results were normalised on GAPDH. Furthermore RT-PCR was performed after incubation of cells in the presence of antibodies against TNF-R1 and 2 (Acris). TNFa in culture supernatants was quantified by ELISA (Bender MedSystems). **Results:** The established assay showed all stages of human erythropoiesis. On d21 cultures consisted of about 32% normoblasts and 55% reticulocytes. Whereas purified stem cells expressed TNFa RNA only to a minimal degree, TNFa RNA increased continiously during in vitro erythropoiesis, with a maximum reached on d15 (58fold compared to d1). On this day about 95% cells expressed CD36 and GPA and were mainly at the stage of poly- and orthochromatic erythroblasts. TNF-R1 mRNA was mainly detected between d1–d7, where only stem cells and non-erythroid cells could be observed. In contrast to this, TNF-R2 could be detected during the entire time of the culture with a clear increase after addition of EPO. By inhibition of TNF-R1, TNFa mRNA increased 150fold and also an increase in TNFa protein concentration could be observed. This was associated with a decreased proliferation and increased differentiation. By blocking TNF-R2 no increase in TNFa RNA could be detected. **Conclusions:** Although TNFa is discussed as being a negative regulator of erythropoiesis, erythroid progenitors themselves seem to produce TNFa and differ in TNF receptor expression. Furthermore, we could show that inhibition of TNF-R1 resulted in an higher TNFa production, associated with an reduced proliferation and enhanced differentiation of erythroid cells. The underlying mechanisms remain unclear. Further experiments and analyses at the protein level should reproduce and expand our preliminary results.

P1.7

Clinical Validation of Autologous Peripheral Blood Stem Cell Grafts

B. Wagner, P. Schramm, G. Wittmann, W. Schramm, H. Ostermann

Kliniken der Universität München, D

Purpose: High-dose chemotherapy (HDT) and autologous peripheral blood stem cell transplantation (APBSCT) have been well established mainly for the treatment of lymphoma and myeloma. Hence we intended to clinically validate our measurements for quality control. **Patients and Methods:** We retrospectively analysed 104 patients (69 males, 35 females) at stem cell harvest and HDT/APBSCT. PBSC were mobilized by chemotherapy and rHuG-CSF. After completion of apheresis CD34+ cells were quantified by flow cytometry. The apheresis products were frozen in DMSO using a controlled-rate liquid nitrogen freezer and stored below −150°C. Fresh and thawed material were analysed for blood count and colony-forming cells. HDT before APBSCT was done according to different protocols including rHuG-CSF after transplantation. **Results:** 104 patients were subjected to 137 leukapheresis procedures to receive 127 times HDT/APBSCT. A median peripheral blood CD34+ cell count of 47/μl yielded a median of 6.0*10E6 CD34+ cells/kg body weight (BW) and 4.9*10E5 CFU-GM/kg BW. CD34+ progenitor cell counts in peripheral blood were strongly correlated with the yield of CD34+ cells ($r^2 = 0.947$) and CFU-GM ($r^2 = 0.768$) in the apheresis product. Threshold peripheral blood counts for the collection of 2.0 and 5.0*10E6 CD34+ cells/kg BW were identified at 20 and 60 CD34+ cells/μl, respectively. Following 127 HDT the APBSCT comprised in the median 4.8*10E6 CD34+ cells/kg BW and 4.0*10E5 CFU-GM/kg BW. Median time to engraftment (leukocytes > 1/nl) was 10 days (range 7–29) and (platelets > 20/nl) 11 days (range 5–54), respectively. 108 febrile episodes (median duration 5 days) occurred. Mucositis requiring total parenteral nutrition (TPE) and/or narcotic analgesics occurred in 66 and 62 episodes, respectively. Median hospital length of stay was 24 days. Each HDT/APBSCT required in the median 2 (0–27) red blood cell concentrates (RBC) and 3 (0–39) platelet concentrates (PC). To assess the effect of CD34+ cell dose and engraftment 3 subgroups were formed: the particular times to engraftment in the low dose (<2.0*10E6 CD34+ cells/kg BW), intermediate dose (2.0–5.0*10E6 CD34+ cells/kg BW) and high dose groups (>5.0*10E6 CD34+ cells/kg BW) were 14.6, 11.0 and 10.8 days (leukocytes > 1/nl) and 22.0, 12.5 and 11.3 days (platelets > 20/nl), respectively. Likewise cell dose affected the occurrence and duration of febrile episodes, the number of PC transfused and the length of hospital stay, but not the demand of RBC, TPE or narcotic analgesics. In this respect our data confirm 2.0*10E6 CD34+ cells/kg BW as a minimum dose for APBSCT. **Conclusion:** The clinical validation of graft quality was successful demonstrating the safety of HDT/APBSCT.

P1.8

Ex vivo Expansion of Mesenchymal Stem Cells for Regenerative Therapy: Impact of Stem Cell Source and Plating Density on Efficacy of ex vivo Expansion

M. Rojewski, T. Becker, G. Baur, M. Wiesneth, H. Schrezenmeier
Universitätsklinikum Ulm, D

Purpose: Mesenchymal stem cells (MSC) are functionally characterized by their multilineage differentiation potential and their immunomodulatory properties. Use of MSC in clinical studies in various regenerative and immunomodulatory settings require efficient large scale ex vivo expansion. Here, we compare efficacy of different sources to establish MSC lines in primary cultures and the role of culture conditions on MSC expansion in secondary cultures. **Methods:** MSC were isolated by plastic adherence for 24 hours of bone marrow (BM) aspirates (n = 31), trabecular meshwork (n = 7), CD34 negative fraction of BM (n = 1) or PBSC after G-CSF (n = 28), therapeutic leucozytapheresis (n = 9) and buffy coat (n = 23). Kinetics of expansion was analysed by plating cells at different initial cell densities and counting total cell number of viable cells. **Results:** Isolation of MSC was successful when BM aspirate (28/31 assays), trabecular meshwork (7/7) or CD34 negative fraction of BM was used as source, independent from further processing like preselection by agglutination (12/14) or dilution. In contrast, isolation of MSC from peripheral blood derived material (therapeutic leucozytapheresis, PBSC after G-CSF, BC) was not successful (0/50 assays) and processing by Ficoll (n = 6), agglutination (n = 8), wash steps with PBS (n = 6), or cell sorting (n = 5) showed no effect for any source. In order to optimize conditions for ex vivo expansion, MSC from BM were plated at initial densities of 3, 10, 30, 100, 300, 1000, 3000, and 10000 cells/cm^2 culture area in secondary cultures. Expansion factors after 21 days of culture were 6545, 3063, 1161, 358, 202, 58, 21, and 7, respectively (representative exp.). It is crucial to start secondary cultures at low plating densities in order to obtain sufficient numbers of MCS for clinical application within a reasonable time period. Expansion factors of senescent MSC were lower, but even at higher passage numbers the expansion factor was still dependent on the initial seeding density. **Conclusions:** We demonstrate that BM aspirate is a readily accessible source for isolation and ex vivo expansion of MSC. Efficacy of establishment of MSC from BM was not improved by preselection methods. In contrast, peripheral blood even with various preselection techniques is not suitable for MSC generation. A low plating density is essential to assure sufficient harvest from secondary cultures within a reasonable time. We will present additional data on the impact of various cell culture media and culture supplements.

P1.9

Precursor Cells in Inflamed Synovial Tissue

M.B. Fischer, B. Rüger, D. Hollemann, G. Yanagida
Medizinische Universität Wien, A

A population of CD34 positive endothelial precursor cells, lacking the mature endothelial cell marker CD31, but co-expressing CD133 and VEGFR-2 could be found within the synovial tissue. A second population of CD34 positive precursor cells expressing the chemokine receptor CXCR4, the receptor for SDF-1, was found. The chemokine SDF-1 plays a central role in the selective homing and recruitment of circulating stem cells. These two populations of precursor cells are found in cell clusters surrounded by a third population of STRO-1 positive, alpha-smooth muscle actin (SMA) positive mesenchymal progenitor cells in areas of vasculogenesis. STRO-1 and alpha-SMA double positive mesenchymal progenitor cells resemble a population of pericyte precursors that stabilize newly formed vessels by preventing vessel pruning. Single CD133 positive precursor cells were found in the lumen of blood vessels and in perivascular areas. These results indicate an important role of peripheral precursor cells in the induction of new vessel formation and tissue repair.

P1.10

Precursor Cells in Inflamed Muscle Tissue

M.B. Fischer[1], D. Hollemann[1], J. Wanschitz[2]
[1]Medizinische Universität Wien, A; [2]Medizinische Universität Innsbruck, A

Bone marrow derived circulating precursor cells can colonize peripheral tissue to mediate new vessel formation and to contribute to significant tissue repair, however, the exact phenotype of the different population of precursor cells is still an enigma. Here we can show that CD133 positive precursor cells were significantly expressed in inflamed muscle tissue of patients with dermatomyositis, polymyositis and inclusion body myositis as compared to age matched healthy individuals. The numbers of CD133 positive precursor cells correlated with the density of inflammation. Confocal laser-scanning microscopy revealed co-expression of CD34 and MyoD on CD133 positive precursor cells, indicating that these cells are myogenic precursor cells (satellite cells) ready to induce tissue repair. An additional population with CD133, CD34 and VEGFR-2 expressing endothelial precursor cells was found, giving clear evidence for vasculogenesis in inflammatory myopathies. Our result demonstrate thc involvement of myogenic and endothelial precursor cells in the repair processes of peripheral tissue.

P1.11

Impact of ABO-Mismatch in Allogeneic Blood Stem Cell Transplantion (SCT)

K. Hölig, A. Haack, L. Lerche, K. Theuser, G. Ehninger, M. Bornhäuser
Universitätsklinikum Dresden, D

Background: There are conflicting data in the literature regarding the influence of ABO-mismatch on the outcome of allogeneic SCT. Some studies show a difference between standard and reduced-intensity (Fludarabine-based) conditioning regimens, others report on differences regarding the incidence of Graft versus Host disease (GvHD). **Patients and Methods:** The aim of our study was to evaluate if ABO-incompatibilities between donor and recipient (ABO-mismatch) affect the prognosis after allogeneic SCT with standard or reduced-intensity conditioning regimen. Furthermore we evaluated the role of ABO-mismatch in the development of acute and chronic GvHD. 580 patients (348 men and 232 women) with 1st allogeneic SCT between 30.10.1995 and 28.07.2005 were included in the analysis. 188 patients underwent HLA-identical sibling transplantation and 359 received hematopoetic stem cells from HLA-matched unrelated donors. The stem cell source was bone marrow in 80 and peripheral blood stem cells in 485 cases. The median follow up period was 47.6 months (12–118 months). Statistical analysis was performed with SPSS-Software (Kaplan-Meier analysis and Chi-Quadrat-test). **Results:** 278 (48%) patients received ABO-identical grafts, in 302 (52%) received ABO-mismatched grafts (134 minor, 148 major and 20 bidirectional incompatibility). Kaplan-Meier analysis of overall survival after SCT was not statistically different between ABO-identical, minor, major and bidirectionnally mismatched transplantations. There were also no differences in survival time according to ABO-matching in patients with standard conditioning regimen. After reduced-intensity conditioning there was a trend (p = 0.0570) towards a negative association of survival with major-ABO-incompatibility. The incidence of acute GvHD was not significantly different between ABO-matched or any group of ABO-mismatched transplantations (p = 0.759). There was also no correlation between the incidence of chronic GvHD (limited or extensive) and ABO-matched or mismatched transplantation (p = 0.856). **Conclusions:** The results of this single-center analysis do not support the hypothesis that ABO-mismatch between donor and recipient might be a significant risk factor for survival or incidence of GvHD after allogeneic SCT. In patients undergoing reduced-intensity, Fludarabine-based conditioning and SCT with ABO-major-mismatch a negative prognostic influence cannot be ruled out completely.

P2: Cellular and Gene Therapy

P2.1

Closed System Immunomagnetic CD34+ Enrichment of Frozen/Thawed Human Cord Blood Hematopoietic Progenitor Cells Significantly Reduces the Frequency of Engrafting Cells in a NOD-SCID Mouse Model

S. Gerodez[1], *K. Bieback*[1], *K. Eckert*[2], *H. Eichler*[3]
[1]Institut für Transfusionsmedizin und Immunologie, Mannheim, D; [2]Berlin, D; [3]Ratingen, D

Purpose: Cord blood is a useful source of Hematopoietic Progenitor Cells (HPC) for allogeneic transplantation. HPC ex vivo expansion of a cord blood graft has been proposed as a way to increase the speed of engraftment and thus to reduce the occurrence of transplantation-related complications. This however necessitates the enrichment of HPC by for example immunoselection for CD34. To evaluate the accurate impact of CD34 selection on the frequency of engrafting cells compared to non-selection, we choose a limiting-dilution model where paired groups of either selected or non-selected CD34+ cord blood cells were transplanted into non-lethally irradiated NOD-SCID mice and the engraftment determined by FACS and quantitative PCR analysis. **Methods:** For each experiment, 9 to 10 cord blood buffy coat units were thawed using the modified Rubinstein thawing and washing protocol including DNAse. These cord blood units were pooled and the volume containing the required number of CD34+ cells for the non-selected arm was taken off. The remaining volume was processed with the CD34+ CliniMACSÒ kit and tubing set 150 devices according to the manufacturer's instructions. The cells were injected into non-lethally irradiated NOD-SCID mice adjusted to contain 1 × 105, 5 × 104, 1 × 104, 5 × 103, 1 × 103 CD34+ cells. After 6 weeks the animals were sacrificed and the levels of engraftment for each transplantation group determined in the bone marrow and peripheral blood by flow cytometry and a quantitative real time PCR. **Results:** Mice transplanted with non-selected UCB cells showed higher engraftment levels in the highest dose group than animals transplanted with selected cells quantified by both FACS and PCR. The precursor frequency calculated by using poisson statistic with the L-Calc software was 1 in 32,079 for bone marrow (BM) and 1 in 127,591 for peripheral blood (PB) in the non-selected group compared to 1 in 53,946 for BM and 1 in 169,594 for PB in the CD34+ group. **Conclusion:** We could show that closed system immunoselection for CD34 cells from cryopreserved cord blood units impaired the engraftment capacity compared to the non-manipulated counterpart resulting in a loss of 40% precursors in BM and 25% in PB. This initial precursor cell loss has to be taken into account when applying ex vivo expansion protocols, which so far even further seem to diminish the precursor cell frequency while enhancing their progeny.

P2.2

In vitro Modulation of NK Cells

C. Figueiredo, R. Blasczyk, A. Seltsam
Medizinische Hochschule Hannover, D

Purpose: Natural killer (NK) cells have the ability to mediate both bone marrow rejection and promote engraftment, as well as the ability to elicit potent anti-tumor effects. Ex vivo expansion is a critical issue that may influence the availability and cytolytic properties of NK cells. The modulation of activating and inhibitory receptors may hold the key to clinical success involving NK cells. In this study, we evaluated the effect of different cytokines on the expression of NK cell receptors and on the proliferative and cytolytic potential of NK cells. **Methods:** Primary NK cells or NK-92 cells were stimulated with a single or a combination of two cytokines. **Results:** Expression levels of the activating NK cell receptor NKG2D and the activating co-receptors NKp30, NKp44 and NKp46 were increased by up to two-fold when stimulated with IL-2, IL-4 and IL-1beta respectively. In contrast, cytokine stimulation resulted in a decrease of KIR3DS1 expression by up to 50% with IL-2 plus IL-1beta showing the greatest effect. Expression of the inhibitory NK cell receptors KIR2DL1 and KIR2DL2 was inhibited by up to 50% in the presence of IL-2, IL-8, IL-20 and IL-1beta. NKG2A expression was reduced by up to 10% after exposure to IL-8 and TNF-alpha and increased by 18% when treated with IL-12. Prestimulation of NK cells with IL-1beta and IL-4 increased cytotoxicity by up to 12%. NK cell proliferation was induced in the presence of IL-1beta, IL-2, IL-6, IL-8, IL-10, IL-12, IL-20, but not in the presence of IL-4. **Conclusions:** As it is known that activated NK cells are more effective at lysing targets that are resistant to nonactivated NK cells, the ability to manipulate the balance of activating and inhibitory receptors on NK cells may open new avenues in immunotherapy.

P2.3

Human Platelets Target Dendritic Cell Differentiation and Production of Proinflammatory Cytokines

K. Kissel, S. Berber, A. Nockher, S. Santoso, G. Bein, H. Hackstein
Justus Liebig Universität Giessen, D

Purpose: Dendritic cells (DCs) are the most potent antigen-presenting cells that initiate and regulate immune responses. They are unique in their feature to produce bioactive IL-12, a major pro-inflammatory cytokine connecting innate and adaptive immunity. Platelets (PLTs) are highly reactive components of the circulatory system with fundamental importance in hemostasis. Recently, immunomodulatory capacity of single specific human platelet-derived products on DC effector functions were identified. To improve the understanding of PLT-DC interactions, this study systematically investigates the influence of intact resting and activated PLTs on DC phenotype and key functions. **Methods:** Magnetic beads sorted CD14+ cells were expanded in the presence and absence of resting or activated PLTs. DC differentiation, maturation, allostimulatority capacity, antigen uptake and cytokine profile were estimated to control group. **Results:** Activated PLTs potently impaired DC differentiation according to CD1a expression (mean reduction, 62%, $p < 0.05$). Production of IL-12p70 and TNF-alpha was reduced in the presence of resting (mean reduction, 46% and 55%, respectively, $p < 0.05$) as well as activated PLTs (mean reduction, 63% and 49% respectively, $p < 0.05$). In contrast to the suppression of pro-inflammatory cytokines, activated PLTs increased production of the immunoregulatory cytokine IL-10 by DCs (mean increase, 52%; $p < 0.05$). In the presence of PLTs, DC allostimulatority capacity, antigen uptake and phenotypic maturation remained unaffected. **Conclusion:** It is proposed that intact PLTs connect immunity and hemostasis by interfering with DC differentiation and cytokine production. This interference might be of importance in different clinical settings, such as DC therapy and PLT transfusions.

P3: Regenerative Medicine

P3.1

Isolation Of Human Adipose Tissue-Derived Mesenchymal Stem Cells According to Good Manufacuring Practice Regulations for Clinical Use

A. Dada, A. Hoffmann, M. Marx-Müller, G. Schmitz
Klinikum der Universität Regensburg, D

Purpose: Tissue engineering offers considerable promise in the repair or replacement of diseased and/or damaged tissues. Recent reports have shown that mesenchymal stem cells (MSCs) can be implanted into tendon and ligament tissue in experimental animals. One source of MSCs has been bone marrow. These cells are, however, not easily harvested from human donors. Beside the side effects of G-CSF administration, collection may present risks to the donor. An alternative potential strategy to enhance ligament and tendon healing in humans is the transplantation of adipose tissue-derived MSCs (AT-MSCs). In this study we evaluate the generation of human AT-MSCs under GMP conditions for clinical use. **Methods:** Human adipose tissue was obtained by liposuction from 7 healthy donors undergoing abdominal or breast reductive surgery. AT-MSCs were isolated as described by Zuk et al. with minor modifications. Based on our established GMP protocols for other blood products, we elaborated a GMP-based standard operating procedure (SOP) for the isolation and propagation of AT-MSCs from Lipoaspirates obtained from reductive abdominal or breast surgery in cooperation with the Department of Hand- and Plastic Surgery of the Caritas Clinic St. Josef, Regensburg. According to this protocol only sterile instruments and one way materials were used for the preparation and isolation of AT-MSCs under clean room conditions. **Results:** A median of 63 g (35–100 g) adipose tissue was processed. The total number of extracted cells was 6.4 × 10 E5, Mononuclear cells were 6.5 × 10E4, cell viability 86%. A fibroblast-like population of cells was observed in all prepared tissues, that confirms the functional ability of the isolated cells. All preparation steps were free of microbial contamination after the preparation and isolation procedures. **Conclusions:** This study demonstrates the possibility of generation of human AT-MSCs under GMP-conditions for clinical use and therefore may represent a promising approach to adipose tissue engineering. The GMP-isolated AT-MSCs will play a key role to prepare the ground for the therapeutic use of human mesenchymal progenitors in many fields e.g. the field of tendon, cartilage and bone repair.

P4: Apheresis Therapeutic

P4.1

Low Density Lipoproteins Selections Aphereses with DALI for Child

A. Griskevicius, J. Audzijoniene, Z. Petrulioniene, A. Laucevicius, A. Baublys
Vilnius university hospital Santariskiu clinics, Vilnius (Lithuania)

Purpose: The lipid lowering is one of the main ways to achieve reduction of the atherosclerosis progress. In the rare patients with homozygous familial hypercholesterolemia low density lipoprotein cholesterol apheresis should be performed as these patients usually have extremely high low density lipoprotein cholesterol concentrations and these patients usually do not, or only insufficiently, respond to statin therapy. **Methods:** The most frequently used mechanical methods of cholesterol removal from blood include the procedure of extracorporeal apheresis. The case of rear complicated homozygous hypercholesterolemia treated by direct adsorbtion of lipoprotein (DALI) apheresis system (were performed using a hemoadsorbtion machine 4008 ADS and sterile disposable components manufactured by Fresenius Hemocare Adsorber Thechnology Division, Bad Homburg, Germany). All treatments were performed using a central or peripheral venous vascular approach. Blood was drawn via a 6.5 F or 18-gauge needle at a flow rate 30–50 ml/min. Total cholesterol, low density lipoprotein cholesterol and other lipids were measured enzymatically using a commercially available kit. **Results:** From 2004 June until 2006 April in total 22 sessions were performed on one patient 16 years old. First session we did when he was 14 years old. Lipids levels before and after lipids apheresis were measured during each session throughout the study period. He mean reduction of low density lipoprotein cholesterol was 34.3–58.0% compared to baseline, total cholesterol – 26.4–56.0%, lipoprotein (a) – 67.4–90.9%, apolipoprotein B – 26.4–58.0%. Clinically, 100% of the sessions were completely uneventful. **Conclusions:** Our results with whole blood direct adsorbtion of lipoprotein are very encouraging.

P4.2

The Effectiveness of Erythrapheresis Performed with Blood Separator MCS+ in Patients with Primary Polycythaemia

A. Uchimiak-Owieczko, B. Boczkowska-Radziwon, P. Radziwon
Regional Centre for Transfusion Medicine, Bialystok, PL

Introduction: Collective erythrapheresis performed with automated blood separator MCS+ (Haemonetics, USA) presents save and efficient procedure to the blood donor. The aim of our study was to assess the safety and effectiveness of automated apheresis performed with MCS+ in patients with primary polycythaemia. **Material and Methods:** Isovolemic erythrapheresis was performed in 44 patients, 26 women and 18 men. The blood volume proceed varied from 422 ml to 1268 ml. **Results:** The mean volume of red blood cells removed varied from 202 ml to 460 ml. The mean packed cell volume, mean hemoglobin concentration, mean number of erythrocytes decrease were of 14.1%, 13.83%, 15.8% in women and of 15.02%, 14.55%, 15.23% in men respectively. There were also observed changes in number of platelets and leukocytes. Leukocyte count was lower after every erythrapheresis. The mean drop was of 13.24% in women and of 17.05% in men. There was no clear tendency in platelet count after apheresis. **Discussion:** The therapeutic erythrapheresis prefomed with MCS+ was well tolerated by all patients and no complications occurred. It was also more efficient than previously applied phlebotomy in these patients.

P4.3

Rheopheresis for Dry Age Related Macular Degeneration: Preliminary Experience in 4 Patients

N. Worel[1], K. Schmid[2], G. Leitner[1], S. Binder[2], P. Höcker[1]
[1]Universitätsklinik Wien, A; [2]Dept. Ophtalmology Rudolfstiftung, Wien, A

Purpose: Age related macular degeneration (AMD) is the leading course of severe visual loss and blindness in the elderly. Two types of macular degeneration are defined: the nonexsudative form (dry AMD) and the exsudative form (wet AMD). Currently only a small group of patients with wet AMD is regarded as treatable by available therapeutic methods. In AMD protein and lipid deposits (drusen) in the retina impair retinal microcirculation and lead to progressive vision loss. Elimination of high molecular rheologically relevant plasma proteins by an extracorporeal plasmatherapy with rheopheresis, improves microcirculation. **Methods:** Four female patients with dry AMD on both eyes (71, 73, 80, 82 yrs old) underwent rheopheresis therapy at our institution. Plasma was separated from blood cells using the COBE Spectra device with an ACD-A ratio of 1:14 and prophylactic calcium infusion. Elimination of a defined spectrum of high molecular rheological relevant plasma proteins was achieved with subsequent plasma filtration using the rheofilter (ASAHI Kasei, Tokyo) and the plasma fractinator CF-100. Vascular access was established by puncture of peripheral veins and 80–100% of patient's plasma volume was treated per session. The treatment schedule was to perform 10 treatments over 20 weeks. **Results:** From December 2005 to June 2006, 34 rheopheresis treatments were performed. In 7/34 (21%) procedures mild citrate reactions were seen, responding to calcium administration. One 80 year old patient with atrioventricular block I, presented with hypotension and bradycardia at the 7th rheopheresis and was therefore excluded from further treatments. Ophtalmological data were analyzed in all patients after 6 rheopheresis treatments and showed an improvement of visual acuity (ETDRS) of >1 line <2 line in 2 eyes, <1 line in 1 eye and 2 eyes did not change. Three eyes showed a decrease in visual acuity. In all patients a decrease in expanse of soft drusen was seen. **Conclusion:** Rheopheresis is a safe treatment for elderly patients with dry AMD and is tolerated well in the majority of procedures. Citrate toxicity is a well known complication if ACD-A is used for anticoagulation, but side effects can easily be treated with Calcium administration. To evaluate if rheopheresis is the treatment of choice in patients with dry AMD a larger cohort of patients has to be studied.

P5: Apheresis Preparative

P5.1

Metabolic And Functional Parameters of Platelets Collected by Multicomponent Apheresis with Two Different Cell Separators

S. Macher, K. Schallmoser, S. Sipurzynski, K. Rosskopf, R. Gilli, E. Gruber, G. Lanzer
LKH Universitätsklinikum Graz – Univ. Klinik für Blutgruppenserologie und Transfusionsmedizin, Graz, A

Introduction: With multicomponent collection (MCC) it is possible to collect several standardized components during one blood donation session. We investigated platelet (plt) function and metabolic parameters in double plt concentrates (PC) collected by MCC additionally to a packed red blood cell (PRBC) concentrate by two devices with different collection modes. **Methods:** 15 donors were randomly allocated to either the TRIMA Access (Gambro BCT) or the AMICUS (Baxter) device and vice versa two months later. The separators collected 6 × 10E11 plts (2 units) and one unit of PRBC. We determined blood cell counts, metabolic markers, visual plt quality (swirling effect), activation of coagulation (on the ROTEM Coagulation Analyzer by standardized INTEG Assay and after addition of abciximab and cytochalasin D) and assays of hypotonic shock response (HSR) on day (d) 0 (donation day), d2 and d7.

Results: Plt yields on d0: 2.79 ± 0.23 (Trima-PC) and 2.70 ± 0.54 × 10E11/unit (Amicus-PC). Metabolic markers showed statistically significant ($p < 0.05$) lower values for A-PC concerning pH and glucose (d0, d2, d7), statistically significant higher values for A-PC concerning lactate and LDH (d0, d2, d7) and concerning potassium on d2. Bicarbonate values showed no statistically significant differences. Thrombelastography showed significant lower values for A-PC on d2, so did HSR on d0. Swirling effect was observed until d7 although 2 A-PC showed aggregates on d0. **Conclusion:** The mean plt yield on d0 showed no significant difference ($p = 0.59$). Metabolic markers were well maintained in both groups, although pH and glucose were partially significantly lower, lactate, potassium and LDH partially significantly higher in the A-PC. Thrombelastography of the T-PC showed significantly better in vitro function parameters on d2, so did the HSR results of T-PC on d0. If the partially improved in vitro metabolic and functional parameters of the T-PC are of in vivo relevance has to be evaluated in clinical trials.

P5.2

Function and Activation Markers of Platelets during Seven Days of Storage Collected by Multicomponent Apheresis with Two Different Devices

K. Schallmoser, S. Macher, S. Sipurzynski, K. Rosskopf, G. Lanzer
Medical University of Graz, A

Collection of RBC and platelets (plt) by multicomponent apheresis may reduce donor exposure of polytransfused patients. We compared plt activation and function in platelet concentrates (PC) collected by two different devices during 7 days storage to estimate an association between level of activation and collection modality as well as maintained plt function. Fifteen donors, each with two donations, were included in our study. For each donor we used the TRIMA Access (Gambro BCT) (T-PC) and AMICUS (Baxter) (A-PC) with an interval of at least two months in between. PC were tested on day 0, 2 and 7 for CD62P, CD63 and thrombospondin binding (TSP) by flow cytometry (FACSCalibur, BD). Aggregometry was performed (BCT, DB) and maximum aggregation (MA,%) was measured. Per apheresis a double PC and one unit of packed RBC (250 ml, hct 80%). were collected. Mean plt concentrations in T-PC and A-PC were comparable ($p = 0.09$). In A-PC we found statistically significant higher CD62P- (d0: A-PC 62.6 ± 18.5; T-PC 17.3 ± 6.1; and d2: A-PC 60.7 ± 23.6; T-PC 32.6 ± 12.6; $p < 0.01$) and CD63-expression (d0: A-PC 36.2 ± 16.5; T-PC 19.2 ± 9.4; d2: A-PC 62.1 ± 20.9; T-PC 34.9 ± 12.5; d7: A-PC 69.2 ± 19.2; T-PC 46.3 ± 8.8; $p < 0.01$) and TSP-binding (d0: A-PC 25.2 ± 7.1; T-PC 11.5 ± 5.1; $p < 0.01$; d2: A-PC 26.0 ± 9.2; T-PC 17.3 ± 6.1; d7: A-PC 28.9 ± 9.6; T-PC 21.4 ± 7.5; $p < 0.05$) compared to T-PC. In contrast, in aggregometry the disposition of plt to get activated was significantly lower in A-PC on d0 and d2 compared to T-PC. Standardised PC-collection in MCC is effective and well tolerated as expected and there are no differences in storage parameters in comparison to plt collection only. Preparation of plt by the AMICUS device leads to a higher activation level of plt and therefore to a reduced ability to be further activated in vitro. This fact may be due to the different plt collection modality. In the AMICUS device plt are centrifuged highly concentrated until the end of apheresis and resuspended in plasma afterwards contrary to the TRIMA Access, where plt rich plasma is collected outside the cell separator. However, the in vivo relevance of our findings has to be evaluated in clinical observations.

P5.3

Metabolic Differences between Full Citrate and Reduced Citrate Anticoagulation in Autologous Stem Cell Apheresis

A. Strate, J.-H. Maas, J. Riggert, T. Legler, M. Köhler
Georg-August-Universität Göttingen, D

Purpose: Administration of citrate during large volume stem cell apheresis can lead to considerable alteration of electrolyte metabolism. To reduce the amount of citrate returned to the patient, citrate infusion can be combined with heparin. We compared electrolyte and pH value changes in a randomized study with patients admitted to autologous stem cell apheresis who underwent either full citrate anticoagulation or reduced citrate anticoagulation combined with heparin. **Methods:** 42 patients were randomly allocated in two groups receiving either citrate anticoagulation with simultanous intravenous calcium substitution (group 1, 21 patients) or reduced citrate anticoagulation with heparin (group 2, 21 patients). Natrium (Na), potassium (K), ionized calcium (iCa) and total calcium (tCa) concentration as well as pH value and base excess (BE) were monitored before and after apheresis. **Results:** There was no difference between the two groups concerning any of the analyzed parameters before apheresis. iCa and K concentration decreased in both groups during apheresis (iCa median from 1.18 to 1.04 and 0.99 mmol/L, K median from 3.73 and 3.77 to 3.36 and 3.41 mmol/L in group 1 and 2, respectively; $p < 0.05$). The decrease of iCa was significantly stronger in patients with combined citrate/heparin anticoagulation than in patients with citrate anticoagulation and calcium substitution. BE and pH value increased in both groups (BE median from 3.1 and 3.6 to 7.9 and 7.1 mmol/L, pH median from 7.42 and 7.41 to 7.47 and 7.46 in group 1 and 2, respectively; $p < 0.05$), and the pH value at the end of apheresis was significantly higher in group 1 than in group 2. tCa clearly increased in group 1 (median from 2.29 to 2.45 mmol/L; $p < 0.05$) whereas it rather decreased in group 2. Na concentration was hardly affected by the apheresis procedure. **Conclusion:** In our study full citrate anticoagulation with simultanous calcium substitution and reduced citrate anticoagulation with heparin showed similar changes of electrolyte and acid base metabolism during apheresis. However, the metabolic alcalosis due to citrate can be better compensated with reduced citrate anticoagulation. Thus, patients with pathological acid base balance before apheresis should be anticoagulated citrate-reduced.

P5.4

Effectiveness of Different Thrombapheresis Procedures Performed on COM.TEC Blood Separator and Quality of Obtained Platelet Concentrates

B. Boczkowska-Radziwon, D. Sredzinski, P. Radziwon
Regional Centre for Transfusion Medicine, Bialystok, PL

Purpose: Thrombapheresis performed with automated blood separator COM.TEC (Fresenius HemoCare, Germany) may be performed with either one needle (intermittent flow) or two needle (semi continuous flow) techniques. The aim of our study was to compare the effectiveness of two different techniques of thrombapheresis and to compare the quality of collected platelet concentrates. **Methods:** 161 platelet donors have been divided into 3 groups. Group I of 60 donors donated one unit of platelets using one needle technique, group II of 41 donors donated one unit platelets using two needle technique and group III of 60 donors donated two units of platelets using two needle technique. The following parameters have been measured: platelet count in blood donors before and after apheresis, mean blood volume proceeded, time of apheresis, platelet count harvested from the donor, leukocyte count in platelet concentrate (Nageotte chamber). **Results:** The mean platelet counts in donors were: in group A 235 × 103/μl before and 171 × 103/μl after apheresis, in group B 219 × 103/μl before and 154 × 103/μl after apheresis, in group C 285 × 103/μl before and 184 × 103/μl after apheresis. Calculated platelet loose in donors was 23% (group A), 30% (group B), 35% (group C). The mean blood volume proceeded and the mean time of apheresis were: 2458 ml in 75 min (group A), 2825 ml in 53 min (group B) and 3572 ml in 61 min (group C). The mean amount of harvested platelets in group A (2.73 × 1011) was significantly ($p < 0.0001$) lower compare to groups B and C, and in group B (2.98 × 1011) was significantly lower than in group C (5.52 × 1011, $p < 0.0001$). The efficiency of the procedures were: A – 57%, B – 58%, C – 67%). Leukocyte number was controlled In each platelet concentrate using Nageotte chamber. In group A 96.7% and in groups B and C 100% platelet concentrates met criteria for leukodepleted (<106) however there were no significant differences between mean leukocyte number in concentrate in the groups (0.14 × 106, 0.08 × 106, 0.12 × 106 for groups A, B and C respectively). **Conclusions:** COM.TEC blood separator harvests high quality platelet concentrates. One needle technique offers more comfort for the donor however it takes more time and produces platelet concentrates of lower quality compare to two needle technique.

P5.5

Degranulation and Cytokine Release in Platelet Concentrates during Storage

C. Kneißler[1], A. Opitz[1], A. Kobsar[2], M. Böck[1], M. Eigenthaler[2]
[1]Universität Würzburg, Würzburg, D; [2]Institut für Klinische Biochemie und Pathobiochemie, Würzburg, D

Purpose: Non-hemolytic transfusion reactions frequently occur after platelet transfusions. Cytokines and chemokines generated in platelet concentrates during storage have been discussed as possible cause of such transfusion reactions. In leukocyte-depleted platelet concentrates, platelets themselves are the source of such cytokines. Therefore, we determined the time course of several cytokines released from platelets and correlated it to platelet aggregability and the appearance of platelet activation markers. Different cell collection devices were compared. **Methods:** Platelet concentrates were analyzed at days 1, 3, 6 and 8 for the plasma concentration of interleukin-6, interleukin-8, monocyte chemoattractant protein 1 (MCP-1), RANTES and fractalkine. At these time points, platelets were further analyzed for platelet surface expression of P-selektine and cytokine receptors, platelet cytokine content and collagen induced platelet aggregation. **Results:** During storage, platelets degranulated in a time-dependent manner as detected by increased P-selektin surface expression. In the same degree, platelets lost their aggregability from more than 90% at day 1 down to less than 22% and 10% at day 5 and day 8, respectively. At the same time course, cytokines continuously increased in the plasma. Interestingly, differences between various cell collection systems and citrate concentrations used were observed. **Conclusions:** Leukocyte-depleted platelet concentrates release large amounts of platelet-derived cytokines, thereby potentially contributing to leukocyte and monocyte activation in the recipient leading to non-hemolytic transfusion reactions. Certain cell collection procedures might provide advantages resulting in less platelet activation and cytokine release during the storage period.

P5.6

Optimisation of Collection Strategies Using Three Apheresis Platforms to Maximise Donor Eligibility and Platelet Supply

S. Lechner, R. Gassler, A. Sima
ÖRK Blutspendezentrale für Kärnten, Klagenfurt, A

Background: In order to decrease the incidence and risk of TRALI, we converted from 30% buffy coat platelet (PLT)/70% Single Donor Platelet (SDP) to 100% SDP collection. **Aims:** At the same time we moved to 100% SDP, we introduced double dose PLT collection to meet our demands and decrease the costs. In this evaluation, we report on the eligibility for double dose (DD) SDP collection of our donor base. **Methods:** From October 2005 until January 2006 a total of 320 SDP collections were performed in 134 male (M) and 185 female (F) donors with an average body weight (BW) and PLT pre-count of respectively 75 ± 15 kg and 261 ± 49 × 10^3/µl (range 158–400) ¡V using the following separators: 3 Amicus (A), 2 MCS+ and 1 Trima Accel (TA). **SDP Collection Strategy:** The target PLT yield for single dose (SD) and DD products was respectively 2.5 and 5.0 × 10^{11}. The DD target yield were programmed on A and TA if the predicted procedure time was < 90 minutes and the predicted post PLT count was > 150 × 10^3/µ. DD products were not targeted with MCS+ because the increased number of cycles caused more plasma loss for the donors, and did not meet our threshold for collection time. Donors with excellent venous access, high BW and PLT pre-count were preselected for donation on TA because missed pressure cuff requested good vein condition in order to achieve short donation time. Pre-selection criteria for donation on A were: donors who meet the acceptance criteria for SD as well as for DD products in general. **Results:** The overall PLT yield in 320 collections was 4.4 × 10^{11}. With the above described strategy, we collected 38% DD PLT products with an average PLT yield of 5.8 × 10^{11}. There was a significant difference in donor profile between A and TA with regard to the overall PLT pre-count and donor BW in DD PLT collection as confirmed by ANOVA ($p < 0.0001$). This explains the difference in % DDPLT products and the DD PLT procedure time (A: 79 ± 9 min, range 51–99; TA: 63 ± 11 min, range 46–95). Despite this fact, PLT collection efficiency was similar (A: 66 ± 8% and TA: 68 ± 6%. $p = 0.048$). **Conclusions:** We were able to convert to 100% SDP production and achieved a 38% split rate with the implementation of DD PLT collection. Both TA and A are capable of delivering DD PLT products within ~90 minutes. TA was preferably used for donors with high BW, high PLT count and excellent vein conditions, A for a broader donor population. Both devices showed similar collection efficiencies.

Table for Abstract P5.6

Results of 320 SDP collections						Donor profile DD PLT collections			
Device	n	M/F	Pre-PLT 10^3/µl	PLT yld ×10^{11}	DD PLT %	n	BW (kg)	Pre-PLT 10^3/µl	M/F
Amicus	157	71/86	263 ± 44* (170–386)	4.6 ± 1* (2.2–6.8)	36	57	68 ± 2* (51–110)	298 ± 29* (252–368)	18/39
MCS+	82	17/64	227 ± 27* (158–297)	3.4 ± 0.5* (2.3–4.9)	n.a.				
Trima Accel	81	46/35	303 ± 46* (201–400)	5.7 ± 0.8* (3.3–7.1)	80	65	82 ± 14* (54–116)	313 ± 43* (250–400)	34/31

*significant difference ($p < 0.05$) by ANOVA

P5.7

Hemolysis as a Complication in the Course of a Thrombapheresis – a Case Report

K. Wuttig, E. Becker, A. Parkner, E. Klatt, M. Koenigsmann, M.U. Heim
Otto-von-Guericke-Universität Magdeburg, D

Introduction: Blood donors voluntarily render an important service to the community. The caring for the health of the donor is one of the most important tasks of transfusion medicine. The preparative hemapheresis allows to separate blood into its different components, whereas the components that are not required will be given back to the donor immediately. For this purpose cell separators are used which are capable of building an extracorporal circulation. These machines must be under the regulation of the "law for medicine products" and are only to be used with disposable sets. The involved personnel must be able to recognize malfunctions immediately and react accordingly: so it is clear that a sound knowledge in emergency medical aid is necessary. **Case Report:** We report on a hemolytic complication during a thrombapheresis. Up to this point the donor mentioned has completed 50 thrombaphereses without any problems. The anamnesis and the blood cell count revealed no extraordinary results at the physical examination. The apheresis was performed with the Fresenius COM.TEC using the C5L-Set. In the course of 60 min separation time we observed a distinct red coloration of the collcection tube as well as the plasma tube. The separation was terminated. The centrifugation of blood samples that were drawn at the end of the separation showed a(n) haemolytic supernatant. Our donor reported noticeable dark urine. For this reason, he was sent to the hematologic department of the clinic of Internal medicine. Haptoglobin was depressed, while LDH was elevated. With the aid of a plentiful hydration the colour of the donor's urine turned clear and LDH and Creatinine normalized again. Hemoglobin remained normal. The coombs test showed a negative result before and after the separation. **Follow up:** We expected a mechanic hemolysis during the apheresis as the cause of these changes. After the event the manufacturer examined the apheresis set that was used. However, they could not find any technical failure. Their explanation was an erythrocyte overflow. But this would not explain to the dark urine of the donor. **Discussion:** In the end we could not find a final explanation for this incident. With regard to the safety of blood donors such events should be reported accordingly and the exchange of experiences with other apheresis centers is of great importance.

P6: Immunohematology of Red Cells, Granulocytes and Platelets

P6.1

Does a Negative Direct Antiglobulin Test Exclude Warm Autoimmune Hemolytic Anemia? A Prospective Study of 504 Cases

U. Sachs, S. Santoso, G. Bein
Justus Liebig-Universität Gießen, D

Introduction: Serological evidence of warm-type AIHA is generally obtained by a direct antiglobulin test (DAT). With few exceptions, a positive DAT is indicative for the presence of autoantibodies: However, DAT-negative AIHA is suspected to constitute up to 5% of all warm-type AIHAs. It can occur by several possible mechanisms, including sensitization by a small amount of IgG that falls below the detection threshold, and both IgA and IgM antibodies that remain undetected by polyspecific antiglobulin reagents. A highly sensitive gel technique has been introduced to overcome these problems. Accordingly, a negative DAT is now often interpreted as absence of autoantibodies and thus, as more or less preclusive for the diagnosis of AIHA. **Study Design:** We conducted a prospective study enrolling in- and outpatients in whom immune-mediated RBC destruction was to be excluded (n = 1388). An indirect antiglobulin test (IAT) and DAT including anti-IgG, -IgM, -IgA, -C3d, and -C3c specificities, respectively, were performed using gel technique. Acid elutions were subsequently performed on RBCs from all patients who were non-reactive in IAT and DAT (n = 504). **Results:** Out of the 504 eluates performed, 481 were non-reactive, but 23 (4.6%) contained RBC-specific antibodies. Two groups of patients were identified: patients with previously undiagnosed AIHA (15/23), and patients with allospecific antibodies (5/23). All AIHA patients were found to be anemic, with one exception in whom a haemoglobin concentration at the lower border of the normal range was observed. A secondary cause of AIHA was determined in 6 patients. One year after the initial diagnosis, 5 patients had responded to steroid treatment, and 7 displayed at least one positive DAT upon subsequent examinations (data on treatment not available). **Conclusions:** This, to our knowledge, is the first prospective study demonstrating that even with an improved, monospecific DAT, employing gel technique, a small, but not negligible amount of AIHA patients will remain undetected. The DAT must be interpreted in conjunction with clinical and other laboratory data to avoid erroneous conclusions; it can be expected to be false-negative in up to 3% of AIHA patients. Elution of RBC antibodies is a valid additional procedure to clarify whether autoantibodies are present in DAT negative patients.

P6.2

Flowcytometric Analysis of an Oxaliplatin-Induced Severe Thrombocytopenia

G. Bringmann[1], W. Lange[2], H. Ritter[1], H.-D. Eichler[1]
[1]DRK-Blutspendedienst West, Ratingen, D; [2]Johanniter-Krankenhaus Rheinhausen, Duisburg, D

Purpose: Oxaliplatin (OHP, Eloxatin®), a third-generation platinum compound, is frequently in use for the treatment of advanced colorectal cancer patients. Reports about OHP-induced thrombocytopenia are rare (Immunthrombozytopenie nach Gabe von Oxaliplatin. Dt. Ärzteblatt, 103, Ausgabe 12 vom 24.03.2006:A-806). None of the previously published cases includes a description of flow cytometric analysis. **Case Report:** We report the case of a 71-year-old female patient treated with OHP 85 mg/m^2, 5-fluorouracil 2,000 mg/m^2 and folinic acid 500 mg/m^2 for palliative chemotherapy. Several cycles have already been administered resulting in a partial tumor remission without severe side effects, and at the start of the described cycle patient's hematologic values were normal. However, within a few hours after drug infusion, platelet count decreased to <10 × 109/l followed by purpura and bleeding. Levels of WBC and RBC were found to be normal with negative DAT. Drug-dependent thrombocytopenia was suspected. **Methods:** OHP was diluted with saline solution to 1 mg/ml followed by testing for PLT-associated antibodies in the indirect MAIPA assay, Capture P immuno-assay, and by flow cytometry using the same protocol as for PLT crossmatching. PLTs of healthy donors were incubated with the patient's serum in the absence and presence of either OHP solution or patient's urine. Normal donor's serum was used as control. **Conclusions:** In all three test methods, patient's serum caused positive reactions in the presence of OHP but not in the presence of urine metabolites. MAIPA assay showed positive results against GPIIb/IIIa. Therefore, this report demonstrates that a quick and sensitive flow cytometric test procedure may be a useful tool to clarify cases of OHP-induced, drug-dependent thrombocytopenia.

P6.3

Severe Immune Haemolysis Due to Donor-Derived Anti-D Ten Weeks after Liver Transplantation

C. Weinstock[1], B. Bretz[2], F. Köster[1], W. Madla[1], C.B. Kölbel[2], A. Markovic[1]
[1]DRK-Blutspendedienst West, Bad Kreuznach, D; [2]Brüderkrankenhaus, Trier, D

Purpose: Immune hemolysis due to Rh-antibody producing donor lymphocytes is thought to be a rare complication of organ transplantation. Increasing data suggest that the true incidence might be significantly higher. Knowledge about incidence and the time course of antibody production will help to optimise monitoring in post-transplantation care. Early detection of hemolysis will improve the outcomes of patients and grafts. **History:** A 53-year-old patient was admitted to hospital with acute haemolytic anaemia. His haemoglobin was 6.4 g/dl, LDH was 633 U/L and bilirubin was 1.86 mg/dl in serum. The direct antiglobulin test was positive for IgG. When his serum was screened, antibodies reacting with Rh-D and Rh-C positive cells were found and, since the patient had the blood group A Rh positive (CcD.ee), were at first classified as autoantibodies with (mimicking) specificity for the Rh-D and Rh-C antigens. The eluate of the patient's red cells, however, contained an anti-D + anti-C with a clear allo-reactive pattern. Investigating the patient's history, it turned out that he was liver transplanted two months before haemolysis occurred, and that the donor of the allograft was A Rh D-negative and had had anti-D + anti-C antibodies. 70 mg prednisolone were started, and four units of red blood cells of group A Rh D-negative were crossmatched negative and transfused. The patient's hemoglobin increased to 9.6 g/dl, and the reticulocyte count decreased within a few days from 116 °/oo to 13 °/oo. (Please note: We will follow this patient during the next weeks and we also will show some data on further laboratory investigations.) **Conclusions:** Immune haemolysis due to Rh-D incompatibility may be an underestimated risk of organ transplantation. Hepatologists and primary care physicians should be aware of this complication in order to detect and successfully treat those patients at an early stage of the haemolysis.

P6.4

The Differential Antibody Absorption is a Useful Method to Identify Additional Alloantibodies in Patients with Complex Antibody Findings

F. Köster, C. Weinstock, K.-H. Schwenk, A. Markovic
DRK-Blutspendedienst West, Bad Kreuznach, D

Case Report: A seventy-year-old woman had to be operated on a fracture of the femoral neck. A transfusion of red blood cell concentrates became necessary. The caring hospital found positive antibody search tests, a positive direct Coombs test and positive cross matches. For further examination blood samples were sent to our immunohaematologic laboratory. The patient was known from recent examinations to have warm auto-antibodies and alloantibodies with the specifities anti-c, anti-S and anti-Jka. These alloantibodies had been differentiated by a differential absorption half a year ago. The now repeated differential absorption clearly showed a new fourth alloantibody which was anti-E. By means of this new finding the hospital could be supplied with safe products for this unusual case. The original examinations will be shown on the poster. **Conclusion:** The differential antibody absorption is as useful method to identify alloantibodies hidden by warm auto-antibodies. It is worth being repeated regularly because it can deliver new surprising findings.

P6.5

A New Mutation in Exon 14 of KEL Gene Found in a Patient with K Null Phenotype

A. Doescher[1], F.F Wagner[2], E.K Petershofen[1]

[1]BSD-NSTOB, Oldenburg-Bremen, D; [2]BSD-NSTOB, Springe, D

Introduction: A blood sample from a 70 year old patient with suspect for an antibody against high frequency antigens, was analyzed by extended serologic typing. Agglutionation tests with anti-K/-k monoclonal and polyclonal antibodies were negative. To further characterize these findings we extracted DNA from EDTA-anticoagulated blood of the patient and three sisters. **Methods:** Antibody differentiation has been done by IAT and rare frozen RBCs, antigen testing with monoclonal anti-K [MS-56 Optima, K1.1.21HM BAG] and polyclonal anti-k, Kpa, Kpb and Jsa IgG (Biolith, Optima, Biotest). DNAs were subject of multiplex PCR with 11 fluorescent primer pairs, including polymorphisms for Kell and other major antigens, e.g. Jk, Fy, S/s. Sequencing of KEL-specific DNA, including exons 1 to 19 and intron/exon borders, was performed by direct taq cycle-sequencing using bigdye-terminators v.1.1 in an ABI310. **Results:** see table 1. **Conclusion:** Patient and sister 1 were carrier of a mutation in KEL-specific exon 14, showing a polymorphism at position 1666 (C > T) which leads to a premature stop codon at amino acid 516 presenting a K null phenotype. Sister 2 has been shown to be heterozygous for this mutation, sister 3 carries the wildtype gene, both sisters express the k-antigen. Although the sisters were carrier of the heterozygous mutation/wildtype gene, a family tree could not be established since parental DNA was not available.

Table 1 for Abstract P6.5

Serology	patient	sister 1	sister 2	sister 3
anti-k	negative	negative	negative	negative
anti-k	negative	negative	positive	positive
crossmatch: samples of patient vs. sisters	/	negative	positive	positive
DNA				
multiplex-PCR	Kel 2/Kel 2	Kel 2/Kel 2	Kel 2/Kel 2	Kel 2/Kel 2
sequencing	1666 C > T	1666 C > T	1666 C + T	1666 T

P6.6

Significant Differences in the Sensitivity of Different Gel Centrifugation Techniques

V. Kretschmer, M. Bornmann, K. Schmidt, R. Karger

Uniklinikum Marburg, D

Objective: Gel centrifugation has proven to be a very sensitive and specific method for blood grouping, antibody screening and crossmatching since many years being clearly superior to tube tests. In the study presented two different test systems of gel centrifugation technique were compared. **Materials/ Methods:** 55 fresh and 130 stored frozen samples with known red cell antibodies (rbc-abs, n = 216) were investigated in parallel using two different test systems: the ID Micro Typing System = test system A with polyspecific LISS/AHG- and monospecific anti-IgG-cards, and ID DiaCell I,II,III test cells (= test system A), and the ScanGel System = test system B with polyspecific anti-IgG, -C3d- and monospecific anti-IgG-cards, and ScanCell I,II,III test cells. Two different test cell lots of both companies with almost identical expiration dates were used. Both test cell panels exhibited all the antigens necessary to detect the rbc-abs specificities present in our collection of samples. The methods were performed as prescribed by the manufacturers. In 23 fresh and 33 stored plasma antibody titers were determined diluting in fresh plasma of blood group AB. Thawed plasmas were carefully restored to pH 7.4 by adding 0.1N HCl. **Results:** In fresh plasmas three of the 63 (4.7%) rbc-abs (anti-E, -K, -M) could only be detected with test system B (polyspecific cards). When investigating stored plasma samples 11 (7.2%) rbc-abs were also only found with test system B: anti-C, -Cw (2), -E, -K, -Fya, -M (2), -P1, -Lea (2). Test system B demonstrated a significantly higher sensitivity (98.1 vs. 91.7%, $p < 0.01$) and the same specificity (99.7 vs. 100%, n. s.) compared to test system A. The titration results confirmed the higher sensitivity of test system B. Similar results were obtained with the monospecific anti-IgG cards. **Conclusion:** In the study presented, the ScanGel system was clearly more sensitive than the ID system for the detection of red cell antibodies. This was certainly not only due to the higher transparency of the plastic material of the ScanGel cards.

P6.7

CD47 Expression on Red Cells and Platelets in Patients with Autoimmune Hemolytic Anemia and/or Thrombocytopenia

N. Ahrens, C. Pagenkopf, H. Kiesewetter, A. Salama

Charité – Universitätsmedizin Berlin, D

Purpose: CD47 has been suggested to act as a "marker of self", since murine red blood cells (RBC) and platelets lacking this protein are rapidly eliminated by macrophages. Soluble CD47 has been shown to inhibit phagocytosis of colloidal drug carriers. In non-obese diabetic (NOD) mice, CD47 deficiency results in lethal autoimmune hemolytic anemia and mild thrombocytopenia. It is yet unknown whether CD47 has an impact on autoimmune hemolytic anemia (AIHA) or immune thrombocytopenia (ITP) in humans. Thus, we examined whether these patients show altered expression levels of CD47. **Methods:** Healthy blood donors (n = 11), patients with AIHA (n = 13) and patients with ITP (n = 18), and one patient with Rhnull phenotype were investigated. CD47 expression on RBC, platelets, lymphocytes, granulocytes and in plasma was determined by quantitative flow cytometry. **Results:** CD47 expression on RBCs, platelets, lymphocytes and granulocytes of patients with AIHA or ITP did not differ significantly from healthy blood donors. CD47 was also detectable in the plasma of all subjects with significantly higher levels in the plasma of patients with ITP. **Conclusions:** Since patients express normal CD47 levels, the evidence for a pathogenic role of CD47 in AIHA or ITP in humans could not be demonstrated. Nonetheless, a preventive contribution of CD47 cannot be completely excluded. Higher levels of soluble CD47 in patients with ITP may be consistent with increased concentrations of microparticles from shedding that are commonly found in these patients.

P6.8

Serological and Clinical Characteristics of Diclofenac-Dependent Red Cell Antibodies

N. Ahrens[1], R. Genth[1], T. Hoffmann[2], B. Mansouri[3], R. Offner[4], H. Kiesewetter[1], A. Salama[1]

[1]Charité – Universitätsmedizin Berlin, Berlin, D; [2]Universitätsklinik Düsseldorf, D; [3]Universität Bern, CH; [4]Institut für Transfusionsmedizin Bayreuth, D

Purpose: Diclofenac is a common over-the-counter NSAR that may lead to drug-dependent immune hemolytic anemia (IHA). We report 11 recent cases with di-clofenac-dependent antibodies and summarize all published cases (total n = 62). **Patient and Methods:** Tests for drug-dependent antibodies were performed in the presence and absence of the target drugs and their ex-vivo antigens (urine samples of patients treated with the drug). **Results:** Diclofenac- and/or ex-vivo antigen-dependent red cell antibodies were detected in all 11 cases. Two of the drug-dependent antibodies had partial C-specificity. From a clinical viewpoint, the patients were initially suspected to have an acute abdomen, stroke, and/or autoimmune hemolytic anemia of warm type. Acute renal failure was present in 5 of the 11 patients, and in 19 of 36 otherwise published cases. Four of the 11 patients and 4 of the 36 otherwise published patients died (total 17%). **Conclusion:** Diclofenac-dependent and/or ex-vivo antigens-dependent IHA should always be considered when a patient develops acute renal failure and/or IHA.

P6.9

Post-Transfusion Purpura in a Patient with HPA-1a and GPIa/IIa Antibodies

B. Flesch[1], C. Woelke[1], P. Eichler[2], G. Washington[1]
[1]University Hospital Schleswig-Holstein, Campus Kiel, D;
[2]Ernst-Moritz-Arndt-University, Greifswald, D

Purpose: Post-transfusion purpura (PTP) is a rare bleeding disorder characterized by severe and sudden thrombocytopenia within 3–12 days after blood transfusion. Typically, preformed antibodies directed against human platelet antigens, esp. HPA-1a, are associated with the clinical symptoms. A 46 year old female presenting to the hospital with acute progressive kidney insufficiency and anemia received two units of packed red blood cells (rbc) within two days. On day 7 platelet count felt from 414 to 189/nL and one day later dropped to 4/nL. Four platelet concentrates were applied without success. The reason of platelet refractoriness should be clarified for an optimized treatment and platelet supply of the patient. **Methods:** Platelet serology was performed by different ELISA-assays and indirect immunofluorescence. Additionally, DNA-typing was performed by PCR-SSP. **Results:** After serological confirmation of an HPA-1a antibody, the patient was treated with intravenous gamma immunoglobulin (ivIgG) and the platelet count increased to normal values on day 17. In addition to the persisting HPA-1a alloantibody, an antibody reactive with GPIa/IIa of HPA-5a and -5b positive platelets was detected during the acute phase of thrombocytopenia. After complete remission, the patient was transfused with four units of packed rbc from HPA-1a negative donors and platelet counts remained normal. **Conclusion:** Early recognition and clear differential diagnosis can prevent a harmful outcome of PTP. A second platelet antibody reacting with HPA-5a- and -5b-platelets in addition to the HPA-1a alloantibody could serve as an explanation for the pathophysiology of PTP.

P6.10

Comparison of the Isoagglutinin Titer and the Determination of Isohaemolysins in Sera of Blood Group O Donors

B. Flesch, I. Kunze, R. Kühl-Burmeister, G. Washington
Universitätsklinikum Schleswig-Holsten, Campus Kiel, D

Purpose: ABO minor incompatible transfusion of blood group (BG) O platelets can induce haemolytic transfusion reactions due to isoagglutinins and isohaemolysins in the donor plasma. To reduce this risk, we regularly test the serum of BG O platelet donors with respect to their ability to induce total haemolysis of BG A and BG B red blood cells in vitro. The question arose whether the results of total haemolysis correlated to those obtained by antibody titration in an isoagglutinin test. **Methods:** 41 sera from BG O platelet apheresis donors and from 13 whole blood donors were tested in parallel in the isohaemolysin test and in the isoagglutinin assay with titration of the sera in a gel card system (Liss/Coombs test). The serum and red blood cell volumes in the haemolysin test were adjusted to reach not more than about 20% of BG O samples with complete haemolysis. Only complete haemolysis was reported as positive. Results of both assays, including historic data of apheresis donors obtained with the isohaemolysin test, were compared. **Results:** With two exceptions, Anti-A and Anti-B isoagglutinin titers of 1:64 and lower went along with a negative haemolysin test. In addition, 15 out of 25 sera with Anti-A isoagglutinin titers of 1:128 and higher were associated with negative complete haemolysis as well as 9 out of 12 anti-B sera. With two exceptions the anamnestic data of the high titer isoagglutinin and negative haemolysin group showed at least one positive haemolysin test within the apheresis donors. Only 9 samples from apheresis donors were negative in both actual assays and had negative haemolysin results in each historic assay. **Conclusion:** Our strategy to transfuse ABO minor incompatible BG O platelets on the basis of a negative actual haemolysin assay will be reconsidered. In the future, platelets from donors with an anamnestic positive haemolysin test will be provided strictly for ABO compatible transfusions. The study will be extended to obtain additional data.

P6.11

Successful Small-Scale Extracorporeal Photochemotherapy without Need for Cellseparator-Devices in Critically Ill Children with Steroid-Refractory Graft-versus-Host Disease

J. Misterek[1], W. Wössmann[2], G. Bein[1], H. Hackstein[1]
[1]Institute for Clinical Immunology and Transfusion Medicine, Gießen, D;
[2]Justus-Liebig University of Giessen, D

Background: Extracorporeal photopheresis is an accepted method for the treatment of life-threatening steroid-refractory graft-versus-host disease (GVHD). However, the classical procedure requires collection of large numbers of leucocytes employing a cell separator device and subsequent UVA irradiation in the presence of 8-Methoxypsoralen (8-MOP). Since experimental animal models have showed that UVA irradiation of as few as 0.2% of the body's blood volume are sufficient to achieve an immune modulatory effect, we have developed a small scale extracorporeal photochemotherapy method that circumvents the use of a cell separator. This procedure allows extracorporeal photochemotherapy in critical ill patients with significant contraindications for apheresis. **Methods:** The mononuclear cells from 100 ml whole blood were collected with an umbilical cord blood sample bag and separated after centrifugation. Subsequently, the buffy coat fraction was diluted with sterile Saline in order to decrease the hematokrit <3%. After addition of 8-MOP the cells were irradiated with 2.5 J/cm^2 in a UVA chamber and reinfused to the patient. We treated two pediatric patients, age 2 and 5 years, with steroid-refractory skin GVHD twice weekly over an 6 week period with small-scale extracorporeal photochemotherapy. **Results and Conclusion:** Both critically ill patients showed no side effects after reinfusion of the irradiated leukocytes. The patients recovered promptly from steroid-refractory skin GVHD within 2 weeks after start of photochemotherapy. We propose that small-scale extracorporeal photochemotherapy is a simple and effective alternative to classical extracorporeal photochemotherapy that enables treatment of life threatening GVHD in critically ill children.

P6.12

GPIIb/IIIa Induced Amegacaryocytic Thrombocytopenia and Delayed Onset GPIIb/IIIa Inhibitor Induced Thrombocytopenia – Implications for Management

A. Greinacher[1], H. Zinke[2], B. Müllejans[2], W. Krüger[1], N. Lubenow[1], P. Eichler[1], W Motz[2]
[1]Ernst-Moritz-Arndt-Universität, Greifswald, D; [2]Klinikum Karslburg, D

Background: GPIIb/IIIa inhibitors reduce the incidence of complications after coronary angioplasty. We report atypical presentations of GPIIb/IIIa induced thrombocyto-penias (TP). **Materials and Methods:** Sera and platelets of patients with TP following treatment with GPIIb/IIIa inhibitors were assessed by whole platelet ELISA and by glycoprotein specific ELISA (MAIPA). **Results:** Of 24 patients with acute TP in conjunction with GPIIb/IIIa inhibitor treatment, we confirmed drug dependent antibodies in 13 patients, 8 abciximab, 4 tirofiban, 1 eptifibatide. In 3/6 evaluable patients, TP occurred within 24 hrs, 3 patients showed delayed onset of TP, after 5 and 9 days after cessation of abciximab and 8 days after cessation of tirofiban. The patient treated with eptifibatide had been preexposed to the drug 20 days before. He presented with an abrupt decrease of platelet counts from 400,000/µl to <5/µl after start of eptifibatide, complicated by pericardial hemorrhage. Transfusion of 2 platelet concentrates within the first 24 h was without any effect on platelet count. Despite its short half life of 2 h, after cessation of eptifibatide platelet counts remained <5/µl for 4 days associated with gastrointestinal and skin hemorrhage. ELISA and MAIPA showed eptifibatide dependent GPIIb/IIIa specific antibodies. Bone marrow on day 4 showed early stages of megakaryocyte development only. Platelet transfusion at day 4 resulted in a sharp increase in platelet counts and cessation of bleeding. Platelet counts then spontaneously rose to 150,000/µl on day 7. **Conclusion:** Delayed onset TP is not rare after GPIIb/IIIa inhibitor treatment and platelets should be monitored up to the second week after treatment. We also show the first case of aplastic TP induced by reexposure to eptifibatide. Other than in acute or delayed onset forms, bleeding in amegakaryocytic TP can and should be treated by platelet transfusion to prevent severe bleeding complications.

P6.13

Allocation of Transfusion Compatible Red Blood Cell Concentrates in the Presence of Warm-Reactive Antibodies – a Retrospective Comparison of Two Different Strategies

E. Matheis, B. Grossrieder, A.E. Böhlen-Bodmer, M. Furrer, B.M. Frey
Zürcher Blutspendedienst, Zürich, CH

Background: Allocation of tx compatible red blood cell concentrates (RBCC) in patients carrying warm-reactive autoantibodies (WRA) is often hampered by the WRA interfering x-match procedure. Therefore, simultaneously present alloreactive antibodies (ARA) may escape detection. Various strategies to uncover coexistent ARA or to overcome interfering WRA are in use, e.g. autologous/homologous serum adsorption of WRA (ASA and HAS resp), and others. However, these strategies have several drawbacks (technically demanding, must be repeated frequently, others). Molecular genotyping (MGT) of red cell antigens offers a new approach to allocate RBCCs. Retrospectively, we compared HAS vs MGT strategy for management of patients with WRA. **Methods:** From 1.5.2003 to 30.3.2006, 67 patients were managed (first by HAS exclusively, starting 11/2003 progressively by MGT). **Results:** see Table. Data on ARA specificities as well as genotype pecularities will be provided. **Conclusions:** 1. MGT based allocation strategies of RBCCs are safe, efficient and economic. 2. Commercial available genotyping kits need to be completed by in-house procedures. 3. After transfusion of cross-match positive RBCCs, search for newly induced ARA should be performed.

Table for Abstract P6.13

Number/Endpoint	HAS	MGT
Patients	30	37
Investigations	38	37
Repeated investigations	8	0
Allocated RBCCs	196	762
Work-up time/procedure (total, in h)	8 (296)	6 (222)
Preexisting ARA	13	45
Newly discovered ARA following Tx	3	0

P6.14

Antibodies against Abciximab-Coated Platelets Interfere with Platelet Autoantibody Detection and React with the Cleavage Site of Fab Fragments

V. Kiefel, S. von Stein, T. Müller, C. Nienaber
Universität Rostock, D

Immune-mediated acute thrombocytopenia is a well known side effect of abciximab occurring in about 0.7% of patients after first exposure and in about 5% after repeated administration. Antibodies reacting with platelets after exposure to abciximab have been observed in patients under laboratory investigation for AITP. **Purpose:** The incidence of glycoprotein (GP) IIb/IIIa specific IgG (GP PAIgG) on autologous platelets in patients treated with abciximab should be assessed and related to free antibody in serum samples obtained before abciximab treatment. **Methods:** In a prospective study, blood samples from cardiological patients were obtained prior to therapy with abciximab, 2–4 h and 24 h after initiation of therapy with abciximab. A serum sample was obtained before treatment. In all three samples, GP PAIgG was determined in the direct monoclonal immobilization of platelet antigens (MAIPA) assay using monoclonal antibodies (mabs) SZ21, Gi5. The serum sample was tested for antibody reacting with GP IIb/IIIa of abciximab coated test platelets. Positive sera were retested with abciximab-coated platelets after adsorption with Fab fragment of human IgG. **Results:** 28/52 patients presented with elevated GP PAIgG 2–4 h after begin of abciximab treatment and 36/50 patients 24 h following initiation of abciximab treatment. Thirteen of 52 sera contained antibodies reacting with abciximab-GP IIb/IIIa, signals correlated with GP PAIgG (Rs = 0.72, $p < 1 \times 10^{-6}$). Binding of these antibodies could be inhibited with human Fab fragments. In 5/52 patients, platelet counts fell below 50% of its initial value, in 2/52 below 25%. No significant correlation was found between change in platelet count and GP PAIgG (Rs = 0.26, p = 0.06). **Conclusion:** Therapy with abciximab enhances GP PAIgG in approximately 50–60% of patients, which may lead to false positive results in immunological tests for platelet autoantibodies. Thrombocytopenia develops only in a subset of patients with antibodies and therefore seems not to be exclusively related to these antibodies. Results of inhibition tests suggest that all antibodies identified in this study reacted with the cleavage site of the abciximab Fab fragment.

P6.15

Genotypic and Phenotypic Characterization of Dombrock (Do) Blood Group Antigens in Blood Donors

I. Hegemann, P. Jaquet, M. Furrer, B.M. Frey
Zürcher Blutspendedienst SRK, Zürich, CH

Purpose: Detection of antibodies to Do antigens (anti-Do) is difficult due to lack of both Do phenotyped reagent red cells (RRC) and lack of monospecific anti-Do antisera. Additionally, anti-Do usually are weakly reactive, deteriorate in vitro and are often present in antibody mixtures. Despite this, anti-Do are clinically significant and may cause severe hemolytic transfusion reactions as well as mild hemolytic disease of the newborn. We established methods to reliably identify Do genotype and phenotype of blood donors. Furthermore, we studied the respective allele frequencies, screened for Doa/b double-negative phenotypes (DoNull) and established red cell panels for anti-Do identification. **Methods:** Genomic DNA of consecutive blood donors (BD) were amplified for exon 2 of DO gene using formerly described primers DoF and DoR, which imply the 793A > G polymorphism responsible for Doa/b phenotype and being detected by BseRI mediated digestion of Dob amplicon (PCR-RFLP). Phenotyping of red blood cells (RBC) was performed by indirect immunofluorescence staining using rat monoclonal antibodies NONI-B4 and NONI-B63 (gift by F. Nolte, Hamburg), that recognize the ART4/Do protein (CD297). By FACS analysis, DoNull caused by various splice site mutations, which are missed by PCR-RFLP, were excluded. The impact of phospholipase C (PLC), DTT and ZZAP on ART4/Do protein structure was evaluated, aiming to confirm GPI anchoring of ART4/Do protein as well as structure dependent epitope expression. **Results:** PCR-RFLP analysis of 188 Swiss BD revealed the following genotype/gene frequencies: DoAA 17.6%, DoAB 50%, DoBB 32.4%, DOA 43.1%, DOB 56.9%. These data correspond to earlier findings of caucasian population. FACS of NONI-B4 and NONI-B63 binding, representing other sites on ART4/Do protein than Doa/b polymorphism, allowed to exclude DoNull phenotypes. Antibody binding is abrogated by PLC and DTT, simulating DoNull phenotypes. In contrast, ZZAP (papain) had only minor effect on antibody binding. **Conclusions:** The methods described permit adequate BD screening for Do phenotype/genotype, and also identify rare DoNull phenotypes. Thus characterized BD allow to establish selected RRC panels for anti-Do identification.

P6.16

Comparison of Two Immunohematological Assays

A. Mühlbacher[1], K. Göttfert[2]
[1]Paracelsusuniversität und Landeskrankenanstalten Salzburg, A;
[2]Diagast, Wien, A

Introduction: Our aim was to evaluate the performance of manual AB0 blood typing and the determination of Rhesus D phenotyps with GROUPA 2 LYS and the FREELYS Workstation (E.M. Technologie) in routine work. Besides this we tested selected samples of weak AB0 bloodgroups and some weak positive Rhesus D phenotypes in comparison to the Gel centrifugation test. Due to the magnetisation of the erythrocytes the E.M. (erythrocytes magnetising) Technology allows to perform immunohematology assays without centrifugation. **Material and Methods:** The samples were tested with GROUPA 2 LYS kit on the Freelys workstation and the Gel centrifugation test with its instrumentation for manual working. For the reverse testing we used premagnetized red blood cells HEMALYS. 56 patient samples collected on EDTA with clear result at AB0 D typing. 20 patient samples collected on EDTA with weak results at AB0 testing in the Gel centrifugation test and clear results in tube.

13 samples of patient serum samples which are showing clear results for isoagglutinins only at 4°C in tube and a negative or weak reaction in the Gel centrifugation test. 6 patient samples with weak D. Positive results obtained in tubes with IAT (Indirect Antihumanglobulin Test). **Results:** The analysis of the 56 patient samples with clear results showed no discrepancy between the two methods. All the weak AB0 samples (8 weak A, 8 weak B and 8 weak AB) showed crisp and clearer results with the E.M. Technology in comparison to the Gel centrifugation test. The detection of isoagglutinins which gives positive results only in tube at 4°C with HEMALYS test cells and GROUPA 2 LYS is equally less possible as with the Gel centrifugation test. Only one sample of 6 exclusivly in Indirect Antihumanglobulin Test positive weak D phenotypes showed a positive reaction with E.M. Technology. **Conclusion:** The determination of AB0 bloodgroups and D phenotypes with the GROUPA 2 LYS kit on the Freelys workstation is easy, fast and clear. The E.M. Technology seems to have some advantages in detecting weak bloodgroups. In comparison to the Gel centrifugation test the sensitivity in detecting weak D phenotypes is not equal.

P6.17

Detection and Clinical Relevance of Antibodies against Highly Frequent Antigens – a Case Report of Anti-LW(a) Needing Transfusions

H.-D. Barth, A.-M. Meißner
DRK BSD NSTOB, Gera, D

Purpose: Antibodies against highly frequent antigens usually require much effort regarding diagnosis and supply of compatible red cell concentrates. This applies especially to cases where additional serological problems are present; for example patients with rare rhesus antigens. **Case Report:** It is reported about a female patient in urgent need of transfusion: status after revision of a total-endoprothesis of the knee because of an infection with staphylococci; antibiotics therapy with Avalox after a change in medication because of anaphylaxis against Vancomycin; diabetes requiring insulin; Hb 4.2. The patient's sample had been sent to us because of indefinite antibody findings. Tests for irregular antibodies resulted, apart from a general reaction with all test-cells, in a semi-specificity (auto) anti-D with a mild reaction against own cells. Besides, a mild anti-E was verified. The presumption of an anti-c was traced by alloadsorption. The adsorption assay with ccddee cells did not confirm an anti-c. Instead after elution an astounding anti-D was to be found. All cross-matching responses reacted more or less positive with slight positive self-checking. dd-conserves showed distinctly weaker reactions. These results labelled "suspected of antibodies against highly frequent antigens" were sent to an external laboratory. Tests there found a specificity anti-LW(a) as well as anti-E and anti-Kell, which was not to be excluded. Based on the contradictory declarations about the relevance of anti-LW(a) in transfusions we decided to recommend 0 CCddee red cell concentrates. This was thought to be most compatible, so predictable problems in supplying were overlooked. As expected, cross-matching was less reactive then the CCD.ee samples. Transfusion of overall four units proceeded without any complications. **Conclusion:** In the case of anti-LW(a) antibodies matching dd-blood was chosen for cross-matching. Transfusions proceeded despite positive cross-matching successfully without complications. Due to the rare Rh-constellation CCee supplying blood required a lot of effort. But in the interest of minimizing risks in transfusion this should not be seen as a problem.

P6.18

Severe Hemolytic Disease of the Newborn due to Maternal Anti-K and Anti-E

A. Stenzel[1], G. Bringmann[1], U. Kreklau[1], E. Prüter[2], H. Eichler[1]
[1]DRK-Blutspendedienst West, Ratingen, D; [2]Städtisches Klinikum, Klinik für Kinder und Jugendliche, Solingen, D

Purpose: Maternal anti-K is known to cause severe anemia of the fetus by each shortened live time of DAT positive red blood cells (RBC) and by supression of fetal erythropoiesis. In addition, anti-K also inhibits fetal thrombopoiesis. We report the case of a newborn with severe HDN, hydrops fetalis and thrombocytopenia caused by maternal anti-K and aggravated by anti-E. **Case Report:** At the end of the first trimenon, the mother (2nd gravida) was routinely screened for the presence of irregular RBC antibodies (AB) by a clinical chemistry laboratory. Anti-E, anti-Jk(a), and anti-K were detected, but no information about AB titers or the potential harm of this AB constellation was transmitted to the gynecologist. Therefore, the pregnancy was not classified as potentially at 'high risk'. At 36 week of gestation, the fetus developed severe cardial arrhythmia, and the baby had to be delivered by urgent caesarean section (APGAR 1-4-6, Hb 4.6 g/dl, PLT 76/nl, LDH 3,307 U/L, bilirubine 6.7 mg/dl). **Materials:** Maternal anti-E, -Jk(a), and -K were confirmed by our laboratory (titers 64, 1, and 256, respectively). Fetal RBC tested strongly DAT positive with anti-IgG and -C3d. Anti-K and -E could be eluted. Surprisingly, serologic typing of native fetal RBC with anti-K test serum gave negative results, but molecular typing confirmed the newborn's Kk phenotype (father: Kk). Primary RBC exchange transfusion was performed. In the further clinical course also PLT transfusions were necessary over a period of weeks. **Conclusions:** Once irregular RBC AB are detected during pregnancy, the potential clinical significance has to be evaluated by a qualified physician. Moreover, the clinical course of risk pregnancies, e.g. defined by the presence of anti-K, must be closely observed. False negative serolgic typing of RBC coated with anti-K is possible.

P6.19

Hemolysis in a Liver Transplant Recipient by Donor Anti-Rh(D) and Anti-C

M. Kunz-Kostomanolakis, S. Runkel, W.E. Hitzler
Klinikum der Johannes Gutenberg, Mainz, D

Purpose: In recipients of AB0-mismatched grafts hemolytic reactions are well known. In the case we report here, AB0-compatible liver transplantation lead to hemolytic disease, caused by donor lymphocytes transferred with the graft, which produced antibodies against recipient's RBCs. **Patient and Methods:** A 56 year-old male patient with the blood group A Rh(D) positive, CcD.ee received a liver from a donor with the blood group A Rh(D) negative, ccddee. Antibody screening and DAT of the patient was negative before transplantation. The donor had antibodies with the specificity of anti-D and anti-C. All transfused units were leucodepleted and irradiated with 30 Gy. Two days after Transplantation, no antibody was detectable in the patient's serum and DAT was weakly positive. Hence passive transmission of antibody could be excluded. Another 5 days later anti-D and anti-C were detectable in the patient's Serum, leading to hemolysis and a decrease of Hb from 10.7 to 8.3 g/dL. DAT titer was 100 (IgG). The patient was transfused with Rh(D) negative packed red cells. 2.5 months later the patient was still anemic. **Conclusion:** In this case the transmission of donor lymphocytes with a liver graft lead to autoimmune hemolytic anemia in the recipient. Routine antibody screening of donors could help to reduce the risk of for hemolytic complications alter organ transplatation.

P6.20

Provision of HPA-1a-Negative Platelets for the Acute Treatment of Fetal and Neonatal Alloimmune Thrombocytopenia (FNAIT)

J.-P. Schmidt, S. Jorks, K. Winterstein, H. Kroll
Red Cross Blood Transfusion Service NSTOB, Dessau, D

Purpose: Fetal and neonatal alloimmune thrombocytopenia (FNAIT) is caused by maternal immunization against a human platelet alloantigen (HPA). About 75% of the cases are due to anti-HPA-1a and further 20% due to anti-HPA-5b (Kroll et al. 2005). The newborn is at high risk (10–20%) to develop intracranial hemorrhage. The usual clinical situation is unexpected thrombocytopenia of unknown origin in a newborn. Treatment is required without delay and before serologic analysis is available, since the bleeding risk is highest in the initial phase. Though recent observations indicate that incompatible platelet transfusion are helpful more frequently than previously expected (Kiefel et al. 2006), the optimal treatment to achieve a sustained raise of the platelet count is the transfusion of compatible platelets. Therefore, our aim was the regular availability of HPA-1a, 5b-negative platelets for immediate treatment of FNAIT. **Methods:** A pool of 450 donors from our institute with known HPA-type was reevaluated. In addition, 840 whole blood donors from donations in an area of 30 km around our centre were phenotyped for HPA-1a using an enzyme immunoassay (Diamed). Donors with HPA-1a-negative phenotype were genotyped for HPA-1-5 and 15 by PCR-SSP. Donors were contacted by phone call and/or ground mail to receive consent for platelet apheresis. **Results:** From the known donor pool, 14 individuals were HPA-1a-negative. Initially, only two of them were active donors. From 840 donors that were phenotyped, 11 turned out HPA-1a negative. Confirmatory genotyping showed perfect correlation between the results. Two donors dropped out of the program due to temporary or permanent deferral from donation, two others due to age above 60 years, two donors lived out of our area and one donor stopped blood donation completely due to unknown reasons. The blood group distribution reflected the donor population. All active donors were screened for anti-A and anti-B hemolysins. With the active donors, we were able establish a regular program in which HPA-1a-negative platelet apheresis donations are obtained twice weekly. **Conclusions:** The optimal treatment of unexpected FNAIT is the transfusion of HPA-1a-negative platelets. We established a program by which we are now able to provide a HPA-1a-negative platelet concentrate for the immediate use in thrombocytopenic newborns in our region.

P6.21

Heterogeneity of HPA-3 Alloantibodies: Consequences for the Diagnosis of Fetal and Neonatal Alloimmune Thrombocytopenia

I. Socher[1], C. Zwingel[1], K. Schallmoser[2], T. Hundhausen[3], S. Santoso[1], H. Kroll[4]

[1]Justus Liebig University, Institute for Clinical Immunology and Transfusion Medicine, Giessen, D; [2]University Clinic for Blood Group Serology and Transfusion Medicine, Graz, A; [3]German Red Cross Blood Service NSTOB, Oldenburg, D; [4]German Red Cross Blood Service NSTOB, Dessau, D

Purpose: Fetal and neonatal alloimmune thrombocytopenia (FNAIT) results from fetomaternal human platelet alloantigen (HPA)-incompatibility. Immunization against HPA-3a residing on the alphaIIbbeta3 integrin (glycoprotein IIb/IIIa) is responsible for at least 1–2% of the cases and can cause severe FNAIT. Recently, HPA-3a alloantibodies (alloabs) reacting only in whole platelet assays have been described. Since such antibodies could be overlooked by standard antigen capture assays the relevance of HPA-3 in FNAIT may be underestimated. **Methods:** Here, we investigated the reactivity of anti-HPA-3a (n = 11) and anti-HPA-3b (n = 1) using serological and immunochemical techniques. **Results:** Preliminary studies in the MAIPA assay with fresh homozygous and heterozygous HPA-3a platelets showed that 4/12 sera failed to react with heterozygous HPA-3a/b platelets. Therefore, only HPA-3a/a platelets were applied for further studies. The influence of the age of test platelets on alloab reactivity was analyzed. Whereas all sera reacted with alphaIIbbeta3 integrin from fresh platelets, a continuous reduction of reactivity was observed during a storage period of 14 days. We found 3 patterns of HPA-3a alloabs: a. complete loss of reactivity (n = 4), b. considerably weakened reaction (over 70% reduction; n = 4), and c. minor reduction of reactivity (less 40% decrease; n = 3). The HPA-3b alloab was non-reactive on day 14 (pattern a). Anti-HPA-1a used as control remained stably reactive. When kryopreserved platelets were used, 9/11 anti-HPA-3a and one HPA-3b alloabs reacted positive in MAIPA assay. There was no correlation between the reaction pattern and antibody titer. Next, we asked, if HPA-3 epitopes are heterogeneous. Interestingly, analysis of HPA-3 alloabs by immunoprecipitation revealed two different reaction patterns. Whilst, the majority of HPA-3 alloabs recognized alphaIIbbeta3 complex, two sera precipitated alphaIIb subunit. This finding could be confirmed by immunoblotting. Thus, HPA-3 alloabs are heterogeneous in respect to their alloantigenic determinants. This heterogeneity, however, did not correlate with the stability of HPA-3 reactivity during platelet storage. **Conclusion:** We provide evidence that a considerable heterogeneity of HPA-3 alloabs may hamper the serologic diagnosis of FNAIT. Fresh or nitrogen stored platelets should be used in antigen capture assays. Further studies addressing the molecular nature of HPA-3 epitopes are required to improve the laboratory diagnosis of FNAIT.

P6.22

O Blood Group, Where Art Thou?

A.Seltsam[1], C. Figueiredo[1], D. Grüger[1], C. DasGupta[2], O. Bock[1], R. Blasczyk[1]

[1]Hanover Medical School, Hanover, D; [2]Biotest AG, Dreieich, D

Purpose: Blood group O is thought to be based on C-terminally truncated, enzymatically inactive ABO transferases caused by a single nucleotide deletion at position 261 (261delG) in exon 6 of the ABO gene. However, so-called unusual ABO*O alleles with mutations also predicting premature truncation express weak blood group A phenotypes. The aim of the study was to investigate the crucial role of the 261delG mutation for a complete loss of enzymatic activity of the ABO transferase and to define the molecular mechanism responsible for A expression in the unusual ABO*O alleles. **Methods:** The ABO genotypes were determined by sequence-specific priming and sequencing. Expression studies in HeLa cells were performed using a panel of A- and O-specific ABO expression plasmids. Expression of recombinant ABO transferases was analyzed by immunoprecipitation and confocal laser microscopy using expression constructs encoding for V5/His- or GFP-ABO transferase fusion proteins. Transcription levels of ABO transferases were measured using real time RT-PCR. **Results:** Red blood cells from donors genotyped to have unusual ABO*O alleles expressed weak blood group A phenotypes. Accordingly, HeLa cells transfected with expression constructs encoding for the unusual ABO*O alleles showed weak A antigen expression. In contrast, transfectants treated with constructs encoding for the common 261delG-ABO*O alleles retained a blood group O phenotype. Interestingly, N-terminally truncated A transferases were detectable in HeLa cells transfected with expression constructs encoding for the unusual ABO*O alleles. Using A-specific expression constructs in which the Met1 start codon and 9 potential alternative start sites had successively been interrupted, A antigen activity was measurable on HeLa cells until the Met189 codon was affected. No difference in ABO transcription levels was observed in the peripheral blood samples and bone marrow between blood group A and O individuals. **Conclusion:** The real O blood group seems to be based on 261delG. N-terminally truncated A transferases driven by alternative initiation sites are responsible for weak blood group A phenotypes in non-261delG ABO*O alleles. This finding may have a great impact on future ABO genotyping strategies suitable for clinical purposes.

P6.23

Variable Expression of the Neonatal Fc Receptor Alpha-Chain Promotor May Influence Fetal and Neonatal Platelet Counts in Alloimmune Thrombocytopenia

I. Socher[1], R. Bald[2], U.JH Sachs[1], G. Giers[3], S. Santoso[1], H. Kroll[4]

[1]Institut für Klinische Immunologie und Transfusionsmedizin, Gießen, D; [2]Clinics for Obstetrics and Gynecology, Leverkusen, D; [3]Heinrich Heine University, Düsseldorf, D; [4]German Red Cross Blood Service NSTOB, Dessau, D

Purpose: The neonatal Fc receptor (FcRn) plays an important role as IgG transporter across placental barriers and mediator in IgG metabolism. Recently, a variable number of tandem repeats region (VNTR) within the FcRn promoter has been described (VNTR1–VNTR5). In Caucasians, the two most frequent alleles (VNTR2, VNTR3) are associated with variable expression of FcRn on the monocyte surface: VNTR2 carriers express less FcRn than VNTR3 homozygotes. Given that these differences are also relevant on the syncytiotrophoblast, FcRn density could influence the effectiveness of diaplacental IgG transfer in fetal/neonatal alloimmune thrombocytopenia (FNAIT) and have, thereby, an impact on the clinical severity. **Methods:** Here, we analyzed the FcRn VNTR alleles from 104 FNAIT cases due to anti-HPA-1a by PCR. 54 samples were obtained antenatally during intrauterine platelet transfusion and 50 samples were from newborns with FNAIT. Genotypes were related to fetal or neonatal platelet counts, respectively. Statistical analysis was performed using the SPSS 12.0 and SigmaStat 3.1 software. **Results:** Genotyping revealed similar VNTR3:VNTR2 gene frequencies as found in a large cohort of 420 unrelated healthy individuals (92.0:7.5). The frequencies were 94.4:5.6 (antenatal) and 92.0:8.0 (postnatal). We asked if there was a relationship between severity of thrombocytopenia and the VNTR genotype

(VNTR 3/3, VNTR 2/3). The intrauterine pre-treatment fetal platelet counts did not show an association with VNTR genotype. Interestingly, VNTR 3 homozygotes displayed a tendency (p = 0.364) to lower nadir platelet counts than VNTR2 carriers (median 18/nl vs. 33/nl). Similarly, neonates with VNTR 3/3 genotype had lower median platelet counts compared to VNTR 2/3 genotype (21/nl vs. 34/nl, p = 0.267). **Conclusions:** In this study, we observed a trend to lower platelet counts in FNAIT patients with higher FcRn density. Thus, high expression of FcRn may result in an increased transport rate of pathogenic antibodies. However, due the low frequency of the VNTR 2 allele other mechanisms besides VNTR alleles must contribute to clinical heterogeneity. Further studies will have to confirm our observations.

P6.24

PECAM-1 on Human Platelets Expresses ABH Antigenic Determinant: Application in Platelet Crossmatching

S. Santoso, S. Santoso
Clinical Immunology and Transfusion Medicine, Giessen, D

Transfusion of ABH-incompatible platelets can be associated with decreased recovery, shortened survival and an increased incidence of HLA-immune refractoriness. Although ABH incompatibility can adversely affect platelet recovery, the clinical outcome is highly variable between transfusion and individual patients. In this study, we analyzed the expression of ABH antigen on platelet glycoproteins (GPs) by the use of sera derived from polytransfused patients who developed refractoriness to blood group A1 platelet transfusions. When labelled platelets of blood group A1 were analyzed by immunoprecipitation, a major band migrating with an apparent molecular weight of ~120 kDa was observed. Further analysis by two dimensional gel electrophoresis indicated that two GPs, PECAM-1 (CD31) and GPIIa (beta1 integrin) may superimpose in this band. Therefore, we performed preclearing experiments to differentiate both GPs. After successive preclearing with anti-GPIIa, a strong 120 kDa band still could be precipitated with patient's sera. Absorption with anti-PECAM-1 specific mab Gi18 showed that this remaining band corresponds to PECAM-1. These results were supported by data obtained with the glycoprotein specific immunoassay (MAIPA). When platelets of blood group A1 were analyzed with patient's serum, positive reaction was detectable using anti-PECAM-1. In contrast, no reaction was observed with platelets of blood group O or blood group A2. Comparison with other mabs (anti-GPIIa, -GPIIb/IIIa and -GPIb/IX) showed that PECAM-1 specific mabs gave a higher signal. These data suggest that PECAM-1 is the major GP on platelets carrying the A1 blood group determinants. To examine the clinical impact of this finding we analyzed retrospectively different samples of patient's serum by crossmatching analysis in the MAIPA assay. Interestingly, direct association of low platelet increment with the presence of immune anti-A was detectable when anti-PECAM-1 was applied. Thus, platelet crossmatching using PECAM-1 specific mab may be useful to identify high level of immune anti-A or anti-B.

P6.25

Gel Antigen Specific Assay (GASA) for the Detection of Platelet Alloantibodies

T. Bakchoul[1], S. Santoso[1], T. Bakchoul[1], A. Agaylan[2], O. Meyer[2], G. Bein[1], S. Bombard[3], A. Salama[2]
[1]Clinical Immunology and Transfusion Medicine, Giessen, D; [2]Charite; Berlin, D; [3]Diamed, Cressier, CH

The identification of platelet alloantibodies is indispensable for the diagnostics of alloimmune mediated thrombocytopenia. Currently, antigen capture assay (MAIPA) based on immobilization of platelet antigens by monoclonal antibodies is the most common used technique for alloantibodies detection. This technique, however, is time consuming and is limited by different factors. Here, we develop a rapid gel particle assay by the use of purified antigens (termed Gel Antigen Specific Assay; GASA). Glycoprotein IIb-IIIa derived from homozygous HPA-1aa or HPA-1bb phenotyped platelets were purified by affinity column using mab Gi5 and were proved by silverstaining and immunoblotting. To determine the activity of the purified antigens, real-time analysis of antigen-antibody binding by surface plasmon resonance technology (SPR) was performed using monoclonal antibody specific for HPA-1a. Purified antigens were then coated onto red-dye beads. Coated beads were incubated with patient's sera and were applied onto microtyping system containing anti-human IgG. Positive antigen-antibody reactions could be observed as a layer of particles on the top of the gel tube after centrifugation. Different HPA-1a sera (n = 10) and HPA-1b (n = 2) antibodies derived from mothers with NAIT and polytransfused patients were tested to evaluate this technique. In the control experiments, AB-sera, HPA-5b and HLA class I alloantibodies were tested in parallel. In all HPA-1a sera specific agglutination was detected in GASA using purified HPA-1a protein, whereas no specific reaction was observed with HPA-1b antigen. Vice versa, HPA-1b antibody was selectively reacted with HPA-1b antigen, but not with HPA-1a. As expected, no agglutination was found with all control sera. These results showed good correlation with the MAIPA assay. In the future, other platelet reactive antibodies (autoantibodies, drug-dependent antibodies) should be tested to determine the value of GASA for platelet antibody detection.

P6.26

Retrospective, Comparative Typing of Rh(D) Negative and Weak D Blood Donors with Serological and Genotyping Methods

J. Thierbach, A. Jung, W.E. Hitzler
Klinikum der Johannes Gutenberg Universität, Mainz, D

Purpose: The aim of this study was a retrospective, internal quality control to detect, if there could be found any difference using serological and genotyping methods in typing Rh(D) negative blood donors. **Material and Methods:** For serological testing we combined three tube tests with a positive, and a negative control and an autoagglutination test. One test includes monoclonal anti-D, that cannot detect DVI und two anti-D blend IgG and IgM tests, that can discriminate all known categories of the D-antigens partly also some D-variants. In addition a gel-matrix-test with human anti-D and an indirect antiglobulin test for differentiation of weak D was added. For genotyping the BAGene partial D-type and the BAGene weak-D-type PCR-SSP were used. **Results:** In this study 950 donors were tested retrospectively. 17 of these donors had already been tested serologically as weak D. All other 923 donors were serologically typed as Rh(D) negative. Only in one case genotyping could find a DEL. **Discussion:** RHD-blood group alleles with reduced or absent antigen expression, are a clinically significant and heterogeneous group of utmost clinical importance, that requires reliable test methods without causing enormous costs. The aim of this Study was to estimate retrospectively, if the combination of serologically methods with the PCR-SSP in special cases, will detect the most common, relevant and known RHD-blood group alleles.

P6.27

Performance Evaluation of a Novel Lateral Flow Device for Rapid Multi-Parameter Blood Grouping without Centrifugation

C. Geisen[1], P. Schwind[2], E. Seifried[1]
[1]DRK-Blutspendedienst BW-Hessen, Frankfurt, D; [2]Medion Diagnostics AG, Düdingen, CH

Background: A novel lateral flow assay ("MDmulticard") allows for simultaneous multi-parameter testing in a single assay, providing a stable end-point without centrifugation. The aim of this study is to evaluate the performance of MDmulticard in routine testing on statistically significant donor and patient populations as opposed to state-of-the-art methods. **Methods:** 4276 blood samples, comprising 3550 samples of blood donors and 726 authentic clinical samples of hospitalized patients were tested for ABO, D, K and Rhesus subgroups. Challenging samples i.e. neonatal samples (n = 86), samples with weak antigen expression (n = 88) (weak D, partial D, weak A, Ax, Ael, weak B) as well as samples with mixed field reactions were included. The lateral flow based assay (MDmulticard, Medion Diagnostics) was compared with established methods: a microtiter plate agglutination assay (Olympus PK-7200) in blood donors and a gel agglutination assay (ID-System, DiaMed) in clinical samples. Briefly, in the lateral flow method 100 µl of diluted blood or erythrocyte sediment are pipetted into the application zone of the MDmulticard, followed by 300 µl of a rinsing buffer. Results can be read after 5 minutes. Positive results are recognized as distinct red bands, negative results are recognized by the absence of the respective band. **Results:** In 4271 samples ABO, D, K and Rhesus subgroup typing concurred. 5 samples showed discrepant results. In one sample Rhesus e-antigen was typed negative in the lateral flow assay while different monoclonal antibodies gave variable results in the gel agglutination assay suggesting a partial e-antigen. In two samples false positive results were observed initially, which were most likely due to excessive hyperlipaemia and high titer IgG-autoantibodies, respectively. After washing red blood cells regular results in the lateral flow assay could be obtained in both samples. In one sample with high cold agglutinin titer due to complete auto agglutination in the application zone of the lateral flow device no band could be observed. After preincubation of the sample at 37°C the lateral flow assay gave concurring results. In one weak A sample a positive result with Anti-A could only be observed with MDmulticard but not with the gel agglutination test. **Conclusions:** The lateral flow assay "MDmulticard" represents a highly sensitive and specific method for ABO, D, K and Rhesus subgroup antigen typing within 5 minutes without a centrifugation step. Therefore MDmulticard is highly suitable for emergency diagnostics.

P6.28

Frequency of Irregular Antibodies during Pregnancy and Comparison of Antibody-Titers Using Two Different Techniques

B. Mansouri Taleghani[1], P. Thalmann-Zingg[2], H. Hustinx[3], S. Fontana[3]

[1]Klinik und Poliklinik für Hämatologie und Hämatologisches Zentrallabor, Bern, CH; [2]Kantonsspital Winterthur, Winterthur, CH; [3]Blutspendedienst SRK Bern, Bern, CH

Background: Pregnancies may be complicated by clinical significant alloimmunization to fetal red-cell antigens. Different methods are used for screening and titration of corresponding antibodies. We assessed the frequency of antibody specificities in a major Swiss region and compared titers being determined by means of the classical tube technique or gel microcolumns, respectively. **Study Design and Methods:** All maternal irregular antibodies (n = 376), which were identified or confirmed at our Swiss reference laboratory for immuno-haematology between June 2003 and December 2005, were retrospectively evaluated. For the initial antibody screen an indirect antiglobulin test (IAT) was performed using commercially available gel cards (Diamed, Cressier, Switzerland). Samples showing a positive result were further analyzed including an antibody identification test (gel cards, IAT) and the determination of their titers, simultaneously using the tube and the gel IAT. **Results:** The specificities of identified antibodies and their frequencies were (n/%): E (80/21.8), D (64/17.4), K (53/14.4), c (45/12.3), M (32/8.7), Kpa (18/4.9), Fya (13/3.5), Cw (12/3.3), Lua (11/3), C (9/2.5), Jka (9/2.5), S (9/2.5), Lub (3/0.8), Coa (1/0.3), e (1/0.3), G (2/0.5), Ge (1/0.3), Jra (1/0.3), s (1/0.3), Vw (1/0.3), Wra (1/0.3), Yta (1/0.3). Linear regression analysis showed a very good correlation of the titers determined with the tube and the gel IAT, respectively (r = 0.96), but with consistently higher titers using the gel cards (y = 1.01x + 1.74). **Discussion:** Our outlined spectrum of pregnancy induced irregular antibodies shows some peculiarities which may be ascribed to our position being the corresponding national reference laboratory. For assessment of the course of an antibody titer during pregnancy it seems reasonable to convert the results of the tube and gel IAT to each other by means of a statistically verified formula.

P6.29

A Case of Severe Fetal Anemia Caused by Maternal Anti-K and Complicated by Maternal Anti-Fya due to Immunization by Serial Intrauterine Transfusions

C. Brockmann, H. Hennig, M. Ziemann, T. Schulze, S. Sharifzadeh, P. Schlenke, S. Görg

UK S-H, Campus Lübeck, Lübeck, D

Background: Maternal anti-Kell (K) alloantibodies in pregnancies with a K positive fetus can cause severe haemolytic disease of the newborn. Rare cases of fatal anaemia are due to hemolysis and impaired red blood cell production, as the K antigen appears early in erythropoiesis. Anti-Fya is the relevant alloantibody in about 5% of fetal or neonatal haemolytic disease. **Case Report:** We report a case of severe fetal anemia caused by maternal anti-K with development of a second maternal alloantibody due to multiple intrauterine transfusions. Doppler studies in the middle cerebral artery (MCA) and ultrasound scans were performed with a GE Voluson-730 Expert, fetal blood sampling and intrauterine transfusion conducted with a 22G needle. A 34 year old woman presented at 29 weeks of gestation with an anti-K (titer 1024) and fetal hydrops. Doppler studies showed a MCA peak velocity of 85 cm/s. The Hb in the fetal blood sample was 29 g/L. Fetal cells showed a strongly positive direct Coombs test (C3d and IgG). The antigen K was not detectable on fetal erythrocytes, while polymerase chain reaction (PCR) studies showed a Kell-positive result. Immediate intrauterine transfusion (IUT) of 50 ml was performed with a K-negative unit of packed red cells. Two days later a second IUT of 60 ml was performed, increasing the Hb level from 58 to 82 g/L. A third IUT was carried out after an interval of 3 days. Eleven days later an additional alloantibody with the specificity anti-Fya was detected. Retrospectively, two of the three transfused red cell units were tested positive for Fya while the fetus was tested negative for Fya by PCR. Further units were selected both Fya- and Kell negative. **Conclusions:** As shown in this case, intrauterine transfusions hold the risk of additional maternal allo-immunizations against transfused blood and therefore the risk of aggravated hemolysis in the fetus. This might result in a higher frequency of necessary IUTs and, postpartum, in a delayed transfusion reaction of the newborn which may aggravate the underlying hemolytic disease. Therefore, regular antibody screening and identification is essential for early detection of additional alloantibodies. To prevent further alloimmunizations by IUTs even Duffy- and the Kidd-antigens should be considered in the selection of compatible units for intrauterine transfusions.

P6.30

Weak RhC Expression in a Patient with a Mutation in Exon 3 of the RhCE Gene

P. Hoyer[1], A. Döscher[2], I. Wojtzyk[1], E.K. Petershofen[2], H. Kroll[1]

[1]DRK Blutspendedienst NSTOB, Dessau, D; [2]DRK Blutspendedienst NSTOB, Oldenburg, D

Purpose: Several single point mutations of the RHD gene have been described in relation with altered expression of the RhD protein (weak D). The mechanism by which these mutations impair antigen density on the cell surface is not fully understood. Variants of the RhC, Rhc, RhE and Rhe antigen expression have been observed, suggesting that molecular variations comparable to RHD are responsible. We report on a patient who presented with weak RhC. **Methods:** The 62-year-old Caucasoid woman was admitted to hospital for suspected thrombosis. Clinical and laboratory investigation did not reveal signs of hematological or infectious disease. Blood groups of the patient were typed by serological tube agglutination method using IgM monoclonal antibody clones: anti-C (MS273, MS24, Immucor), anti-Cw (MS110, Immucor), anti-c (MS33, MS35, Immucor), anti-E (MS258-MS906, MS12-MS260, Immucor), anti-e (MS16-MS2, MS62-MS6, Immucor) and anti-D (RUM1 and MS 201, Biolith). In addition, polyclonal anti-Cw was used in indirect antiglobulin technique (Ch204s, Biolith). RHD and RHCE genotyping was performed by multiplex-PCR with 24 fluorescent primer pairs. Sequencing of exons 1 to 10 of the RHCE gene including intron/exon borders was performed from genomic DNA by Taq cycle-sequencing using Bigdye-terminators v.1.1 in an ABI310 (Applied Biosystems). **Results:** Phenotyping of the RhC antigen with two monoclonal antibodies showed clearly weakend reactions (2+). In contrast, anti-Rhc, anti-Rhe, and anti-RhD antigens showed strong agglutinations (4+) with the patient's red blood cells. The RhE and RhCw antigens were not detectable. Upon genotyping positive results were obtained for RHD-exons 2–7, 9, 10 and polymorphisms associated with antigens RhC, Rhc, and Rhe. Sequencing of the RHCE gene showed a single C340T point mutation in exon 3 in comparison to the consensus sequence. **Conclusion:** In our patient, the weak RhC was induced by an amino acid substitution R114W which is located in the transmembranous part of the RhCE protein. The mutation has formerly been described as RhCeMA. Interestingly, a R114W amino acid substitution has already been observed in the RHD gene in association with weak D type 17. One may speculate if mutation has independently occurred in the RHCE gene or if it has been arisen from by crossing over between the two RH genes. Further studies on the antigen density will help to elucidate similarities and discrepancies between expression mechanisms of RhD and RhCE.

P6.31

Anti-G Alloimmunisation in Combination with Anti-C in a Patient with Rh(D+) Phenotype

P. Hoyer[1], *A. Döscher*[2], *H. Kroll*[1], *E.K. Petershofen*[2], *I. Wojtzyk*[1], *B. Müller*[1]
[1]DRK Blutspendedienst NSTOB, Dessau, D; [2]DRK Blutspendedienst NSTOB, Oldenburg, D

Purpose: The antigen G is characterized by serine in amino acid position 103 of the Rh(D) polypeptide and is usually associated with D+ and C+ phenotype. G(−) is characterized by proline 103 and is usually associated with Rh(D−) phenotype. Anti-G is commonly found as a component of anti-D and/or anti-C in Rh(D−) individuals. Here we report a case of anti-G that mimicked anti-D in an Rh(D+) individual. **Methods:** The 75-year-old female patient required red cell transfusions due to intracerebral hemorrhage. Blood group typing was performed with monoclonal antibodies against RhD, RhC, Rhc, RhE and Rhe in standard tube agglutination assay. Pretransfusion antibody screening was performed in indirect antiglobulin test and enzyme test by gel column agglutination method. For genotyping of RHD and RHCE genes polymerase chain reaction with sequence-specific primers (PCR-SSP) was used (Innotrain). Sequence analysis of the RHD gene was performed by Taq cycle sequencing of exons 1–10 including intron/exon borders. **Results:** The red cells of the patient were serologically typed Rh(D+, C−, C+, E+, E+), K(−). No common variant D, weak D or altered RHCE gene were detected by commercial PCR-SSP. The serum showed reactivity with all Rh(C+), Rh(D+), and K+ test cells indicating anti-C, anti-D, anti-K. The direct antiglobulin test with anti-IgG and anti-C3d was negative as well as acid elution from autologous red cells. We then searched for anti-G in a sequential adsorption elution procedure. First, the serum was absorbed twice with ccD.ee, K(−) red cells. The remaining supernatant still showed anti-C and anti-K. Interestingly, an acid eluate obtained from the cells that had been used for adsorption still showed reactivity with Rh(C+) and Rh(D+) cells. When the serum was absorbed with CCddee, K(−) red cells only anti-K remained in the supernatant. The eluate again showed reactivity with Rh(C+) and Rh(D+) indicating that the antibody reacted with a common epitope on both Rh proteins, i.e. G. Thus, the serum contained anti-C, anti-G and anti-K. Sequence analysis revealed the G-specific single nucleotide mutation (T307C) of the RHD gene which is responsible for a S103P amino acid exchange in the second exofacial loop of the RhD protein. **Conclusions:** This case of anti-G in a Rh(D+) individual underlines the necessity to carefully distinguish between anti-C, auto-anti-D and anti-G in persons with strong antigen RhD expression. Patients with anti-G require G-negative blood. Thus, Rh(D−) blood may be required in patients with Rh(D+) phenotype.

P6.32

Clinical Relevance of Serum Autoabsorption in 73 Patients with Warm Type Red Cell Autoantibodies

K. Winterstein, I. Wojtzyk, B. Müller, H. Kroll
Red Cross Blood Transfusion Service NSTOB, Dessau, D

Purpose: Autoabsorption of serum with autologous red cells is used for the detection of alloantibodies coexisting with unbound serum autoantibodies. However, its worth and necessity is sometimes questioned, particularly in patients with acute warm type autoimmune haemolytic anaemia. We were interested in clinically relevant alloantibodies that could only be detected after serum autoabsorption. **Methods:** All autoabsorption procedures that were performed in our institute during the year 2005 were evaluated. Autoabsorption was performed when the patient showed warm type autoantibodies in indirect antiglobulin test (IAT) and a positive direct antiglobulin test. The autologous red cells were washed and an acid-elution of cell-bound autoantibodies was performed. Subsequently, the cells were treated with papain. Equal amounts of patient serum and pretreated packed red cells were incubated for 60 minutes by 37°C. If the serum was still reactive in IAT, a second autoabsorption step with another aliquot of eluted red cells was performed. Antibody identification was then performed by IAT. **Results:** Sera from 73 patients with warm type red cell autoantibodies were analysed. In five patients, new alloantibodies were suspected by analysis of the serum in IAT [anti-C (1), anti-E (1), anti-E + anti-K (1), anti-E + anti-c (1), anti-Kp(a) (1)]. After autoabsorption, the alloantibodies in the first three sera were clearly visible. In four further patients, alloantibodies [anti-Jk(b) (1), anti-E (1), anti-Cw (1), anti-c + anti-Kp(a) (1)] could be identified only after autoabsorption of the sera. Interestingly, all these antibodies were detectable after the first autoabsorption, whereas subsequent absorption steps did not reveal further alloantibodies. In 35 patients (48%) the autoabsorbate reacted negative in IAT. In 30 further patients (41.1%) the autoantibodies could not be completely eliminated by autoabsorption, most probably due to low avidity of the antibodies. In 20 patients (27.4%) the "least incompatible" red cells were transfused. One patient with Non-Hodgkin's lymphoma and secondary autoimmune hemolytic anemia showed worsened hemolysis after transfusion. Autoadsorption had been performed months before without alloantibody detection and not repeated before the actual transfusion. Upon reanalysis, anti-Jk(a) was identified. **Conclusions:** Autoabsorption revealed otherwise undetectable clinically relevant antibodies in 5.5% of our patients with warm type red cell autoantibodies and should, therefore, be performed regularly. Furthermore, a hemolytic transfusion reaction due to anti-Jk(a) could have been prevented by consequent autoabsorption.

P6.33

Molecular Genetic RHCE Characterization of 99 Cases with Problems in Automated RH Determination

F. Wagner[1], *A. Döscher*[2], *P. Niggemeier*[1], *E.K Petershofen*[2]
[1]DRK Blutspendedienst NSTOB, Springe, D; [2]DRK Blutspendedienst NSTOB, Oldenburg, D

Introduction: Discrepant results for RHCE in automated blood donor typing may be due to RHCE allele variants. The alleles underlying such problems in Northern Germany have not been extensively studied. **Methods:** Samples with discrepant results in RH phenotype determination using two sets of anti-C, c, E and e antibodies on a PK 7200 automated blood group analyzer were further analyzed by manual serology and DNA typing. Manual serologic investigations were performed using column and tube techniques and commercial antisera. RHD/RHCE typing was performed by multiplex-PCR with 24 fluorescent primer pairs. Positive results were obtained for RHD-exons 2–7, 9, 10 and polymorphisms associated with antigens C, c, Cw, E and e. Sequencing of RHCE-sequences, including exons 1 to 10 and intron/exon borders, were done by direct taq cycle-sequencing using bigdye-terminators v.1.1 in an ABI310. **Results:** 99 samples were analysed by serology and molecular genetics. The antigen causing typing problems were most frequently C (n = 43), followed by E (n = 43), e (n = 23), c (n = 6). Problems in C and e often occurred together (n = 11). Genotyping results are given in table 1.

Table 1

	n	allele		n	allele
RhC	3	G96S	RHC, -e	1	G96S
	3	L115R		1	L297P
	1	S122L		3	RHCE-D-CE
	3	*RHCE-D-CE*		7	No change detected *
	1	408 stop codon > Tyr	Rhc	1	G96S
	20	No change detected *		1	exon1:RHc; exon 2:RHCc
				2	No change detected *
Rhe	1	W16C; G163R; R114Q	Rhc, -E	2	M167K
	1	V223F			
	1	H171R		35	M167K
			RhE		
	1	S230T		1	M155R; N159K
	1	Q233E; M238V; L245V; R263G		1	RHCE-D-CE
	6	No change detected*		4	No change detected*

*no polymorphisms in RHCE exons 1–10 (± 10nt intron sequence)

Conclusion: The allele most frequently involved was E variant type I, which caused typing problems for E as well as c. The remaining problems were caused by 13 different alleles. No change could be detected in 39 samples, suggesting that some frequent mechanism of antigen alteration, possibly hybrid allele masked by a normal RHCE allele in trans, cannot be detected by our current analysis strategy.

P6.34

Suspected RHD-Allo-Antibodies in RHD Positive Patients – Report of Three Cases

E. Förstemann, K. Feldmann, E. Thomas, C. Huebler
DRK Blutspendedienst Sachsen, Dresden, D

Purpose: To date, more than 70 different partial-D alleles and more than 53 weak-D types have been described. This high RhD variety and the high sensivity and specifity of available serological test kits may cause problems when routine matching tests are performed in serological laboratories prior to blood transfusions. Sometimes it may be difficult to decide if the testing should focus on auto- or alloantibody search. **Case Reports: Case 1:** A 56-year old male with RhD positive blood type and known warm autoantibodies had been formerly received RhD positive blood. In a first step, his RhD positive blood type was confirmed using pre-transfusional serologic routine blood tests with two different monoclonal antisera. Positive results in direct antiglobulin test (DAT) were followed by an antibody search that yielded anti-D. Allo- or auto-anti-D in association with the known warm autoantibodies were differentiated using PCR-SSP. A weak D type 11 was found, which is capable to form alloantibodies. **Case 2:** An 84-year old female with RhD positive blood type and known warm autoantibodies had a history of multiple transfusions with RhD positive blood, all performed recently. The case was referred to confirm or exclude possible alloantibodies before further transfusions. DAT and search for antibodies were both positive. Due to the short period between transfusions, no identification of the antibody was possible. However, following a period of five weeks without further transfusions, we were able to identify anti-D similar to case one: PCR-SSP yielded again weak D type 11. **Case 3:** An 80 year old female with RhD positive blood type had a history of transfusions with RhD blood. Antibody search was negative at the time of these transfusions. The case was now referred to identify/differentiate antibodies following positive testing. The tests we performed yielded anti-D. PCR-SSP found D Cat. IIIb, which is also known to act as alloantibody. **Results:** Testing with two different monoclonal antisera yielded anti-D in multiple identification panels and thus confirmed the serological RhD positive blood samples. DNA-SSP found alterations in RhD locus of all patients. These alterations are known for their ability to form antibodies. **Conclusions:** During pre-transfusional routine testing divergent results of RhD-tests are common problems. Clinically important is the distinction between allo- and autoantibodies because RhD negative donors are less numerous. In our cases we strongly suspect boostering of anti-D during former transfusions. The signs of immunisation in Patient 3 were obvious only after several transfusions over many years. The history of case 2 is more clouded because of interfering warm autoantibodies and the short gap between transfusions. A clear detection and identification of the alleged allo-anti-D was only possible with some delay. Future studies should investigate if RhD positive patients with anti-D should be tested for alterations in their D locus.

P6.35

Severe IgA-Mediated Auto-Immune Haemolytic Anaemia (AIHA) in a Paediatric Patient

S. Wienzek[1], D. Schranz[2], H. Hackstein[1], G. Bein[1]
[1]Universitätsklinikum Giessen-Marburg, Giessen, D; [2]Zentrum für Kinderheilkunde und Jugendmedizin, Giessen, D

Auto-immune haemolytic anaemia (AIHA) is characterised by haemolysis associated with the presence of the immunoglobulins IgG, IgM or IgA, and/or components of the complement system on the autologous red cell membrane. Cases of IgA-only warm-type AIHA are exceedingly rare. Here we demonstrate the case of a 3.5 year-old boy. He developed severe IgA-mediated autoimmune haemolytic anaemia under immunosuppressive therapy (Sandimmun/Imurek) due to orthotopic cardiac transplantation 3 years before. He suffered from dyspnea and the blood analysis revealed a haemoglobin concentration of 5.5 g/l, elevated LDH (2396 U/l) and elevated total bilirubin (4.0 mg/dl) levels. Haptoglobin was not detectable (<0.07 g/l). Performing direct antiglobulin tests with monospecific anti-globulin, we found a very strong positive reaction with IgA antiglobulin. The eluted auto-antibodies reacted predominantly with Rhesus C-positive test cells (blood group of patient: 0 Rh pos, CcDee). Direct antiglobulin tests with monospecific anti-globulin sera anti-IgG, anti-IgM, anti-C3d, and anti-C3c were doubtful positive. After treatment with glucocorticosteroids the haemo-globin concentration increased and a control investigation 6 months later showed a weakly positive direct antiglobulin test with IgA antiglobulin. This case emphasized that in any patient with suspicion of AIHA, the anti-globulin test should include anti-IgA antibodies.

P6.36

Cellbind Screen Micro Column Affinity Test: Results of a Multi Center Trial

E. Van der Donk, De Jong, Visser, Melsert, Engelfriet
Sanquin Blood Supply, Amsterdam, NL

Purpose: To evaluate the micro column affinity test Cellbind Screen, an international study was performed in five transfusion laboratories in Italy, Germany, Sweden, the Czech Republic and the Netherlands, comparing Cellbind to the ID-Gel test. **Methods:** Serum and EDTA plasma samples from 400 patients per laboratory were tested for the presence of red cell alloantibodies. For antibody screening the Sanquin 3-cell panel was used, for antibody identification the Sanquin 16-cell panel and for the auto control the patient's own red cells. LISS diluents from both manufacturers were used to prepare 0.5% and 0.8% cell suspensions. The titer of detected alloantibodies was determined using the corresponding LISS as diluent. **Results:** Antibody screening 2000 patient samples were screened in the two techniques. With 53 samples a positive reaction was obtained in both techniques and the specificity of the antibodies could be determined. Eight samples gave discordant reactions in the two techniques, five of them only reacting in the Cellbind technique and two only reacting in the ID-Gel test. Cross-matches. A total of 417 cross-matches were performed, 42 of them being positive in both techniques with the reaction strength being more or less equal. However, in two cross-matches with blood group B serum and A2B red cells, the reactions in Cellbind were stronger, which was considered to be important. Identification and titration of "known antibodies" Sera known to contain red cell alloantibodies of defined specificity were titrated. The titer and/or score of several sera was clearly (sometimes considerably) higher in Cellbind than in the ID-Gel test. Direct antiglobulin test (DAT). The DAT was performed on the red cells from 74 patients, yielding 40 patient samples positive for IgG and/or C3d. The reactions with IgG-DAT samples were stronger in the ID-Gel test than in Cellbind whereas the reactions with C3d-DAT samples were generally stronger in Cellbind. **Conclusions:** For screening of patient sera for the presence of red cell alloantibodies, the Cellbind technique and ID-Gel test seem to perform equally well. There is no explanation for the few discrepancies found, but technical mistakes have not been excluded. Also in the cross-match the results with the two techniques were similar. It appeared that in the DAT the reactions with red cells from patients with a positive IgG-DAT were weaker in Cellbind than in the ID-Gel test but none were missed. Finally, the higher titer in Cellbind of known alloantibodies, most of which must be IgG antibodies, might be due to a strongly increased reactivity caused by the LISS for the Cellbind technique.

P7: Histocompatibility and Immunogenetics

P7.1

A New and simple Particleagglutination Assay for HLA-B27 Typing

O. Meyer[1], Z. Abdallah[1], C. Schönemann[1], F. Hugo[2], A. Agaylan[1], H. Kiesewetter[1], A. Salama[1]
[1]Charité, Universitätsmedizin Berlin, D; [2]Institut für Medizinische Diagnostik, Berlin, D

Purpose: The human leukocyte antigen (HLA) B27 is associated with spondyloarthropathies. The strongest association exists with ankylosing spondylitis.

Therefore, HLA-B27 is the most frequently typed single antigen. Here, we describe a simple and rapid particle agglutination assay (PaGIA) for HLA-B27 typing. **Methods:** Superparamagnetic particles with carboxylic acid groups were coated with a monoclonal antibody to HLA-B27 (clone HLA-ABC-m3, Serotec, Düsseldorf, Germany), and subsequently used for testing. Anticoagulated whole blood samples were from healthy blood donors (n = 194) with known HLA patterns, and from patients (n = 51) who had been typed positive for HLA-B27 by flow cytometry. The agglutination reaction was visualized using the ID-microtyping system (DiaMed AG, Cressier s/Morat, Switzerland). **Results:** The particles agglutinated only after incubation with HLA-27 positive blood samples. Positive reactions were clearly distinguishable from negative reactions in all cases tested. Twenty-one (10.8%) of the 194 samples from healthy blood donors were found to be positive for HLA-B27 by the particle agglutination assay. These results were in complete concordance to the known HLA-pattern. No false positive results were obtained from HLA-B7, -B13, -B40, -B47, and -B73 positive samples. Furthermore, 50 samples from patients that had been previously typed positive for HLA-B27 by flow cytometry were also positive by the particle agglutination assay. In one another case, the result of the flow cytometric typing was indeterminate, but the PaGIA was negative, and the patient was also found to be HLA-27 negative using PCR-SSO. **Conclusion:** The new HLA-B27-PaGIA is suitable for rapid HLA-B27 typing. The assay is simple, easy to perform, and can be implemented in any routine laboratory.

P7.2

High Resolution HLA-A, -B and -Cw Typing with an Allele Group-Specific Sequencing Approach in Hematopoietic Stem Cell Transplant Patients and Their Unrelated Donors

K. Hirv, A. Merz, H. Schrezenmeier, J. Mytilineos
Institute for Clinical Transfusion Medicine and Immunogenetics, Ulm, D

The major histocompatibility complex is one of the most polymorphic human gene regions. Over 1200 HLA-A, -B, -Cw alleles are known, and the number of new alleles, submitted to the WHO have reached more than 200 submissions per year. Sophisticated strategies are needed for accurate and efficient HLA typing. HLA sequencing (SBT) is the most informative HLA typing method, and allows an unambiguous identification of all known as well as new alleles. High resolution HLA-A, -B and -Cw typing for patients and their unrelated hematopoietic stem cell donors is required for donor search and matching. We have developed a reliable and cost-effective in-house HLA class I typing strategy for high sample throughput. A generic amplification does in most cases not allow an unambiguous typing of HLA alleles because of the enormous diversity of the HLA system and because of the inability to define the cis/trans linkages of sequence motifs. By splitting the alleles in multiple groups, the proportion of homozygous sequences can be increased and leads to a lower number of ambiguities. Our approach utilises 3 group-specific primer pairs for HLA-A (generic, A2 and A24), 4 for HLA-B (BCG, BTA, B7 and B44) and 1 for HLA-Cw amplification. Furthermore, in selected cases HLA-A3, -B18 or -B51 group specific primers are used. Our assay allows the simultaneous processing of up to 12 samples on one 96-well plate in a mean time of 4.7 calendar days. Ambiguities were analysed in a representative pool of 274 samples. Unambiguous HLA-A, -B and -Cw typings are achieved in 97%, 95% and 68% of the cases, respectively. The most common ambiguities were A*0101,2902/2903,3604 and B*0801,3901/0812,3903. The proportion of unambiguous HLA-Cw typing results can be increased to the 89% of samples, if additional group-specific amplifications with Cw6 and Cw7 specific primers are included in the assay. With our allele group-specific amplification approach of only 8–9 primer pairs for the HLA-A, -B and -Cw loci, unambiguous SBT results are achieved in 97% and 95% of samples for HLA-A and -B, respectively. A generic amplification for HLA-Cw is not sufficient for unambiguous SBT.

P7.3

A PCR-SSP Method for NOD2/CARD15 Gene 3 SNP Analysis

A. Merz, A. Skambraks, H. Schrezenmeier, J. Mytilineos
Institute for Clinical Transfusion Medicine and Immunogenetics Ulm, D

Single Nucleotide Polymorphisms (SNPs) within the NOD2/CARD15 gene (SNP8, 12, 13) have been associated with an increased incidence of Crohn's disease and an higher transplant related mortality (TRM) after hematopoietic stem cell transplantation. Ligation of muramyl-dipeptide (MDP) to NOD2/CARD15 induces a signal transduction cascade finally leading to activation of the transcription factor NF-kB, and subsequent inflammatory response in epithelial cells of the ileum as well as in monocyte/macrophage derived cells. NOD2/CARD15 variants may affect this interaction thus leading to a dysregulated macrophage/monocyte or epithelial response to microbial challenges. We developed a PCR-SSP method for the detection of the 3 well characterized NOD2/CARD15 SNPs (SNP8, 12, 13). For each polymorphism we designed primers which allowed a discrimination of single base exchanges. The design of the primers allows PCR conditions which are identical to those for HLA-typing by most of the commercial PCR-SSP reagents. A total of 6 PCR mixes was used for the detection of all wild types and variants. A 440 bp fragment of the CRP gene was co-amplified in each PCR tube as an internal amplification control. PCR-products of all SNP's were confirmed by sequencing. 98 healthy Caucasian individuals were tested. The frequency of mutated NOD2/CARD15 alleles occured as follows: NOD8 7%, NOD12 2.5% and NOD13 5.1%. 27.5% of the individuals tested had at least one mutation. Only one individual had two mutations (NOD8 & 12). The genotype frequencies of all SNP were in Hardy-Weinberg equilibrium. There was no significant difference in the distribution of genotypes when compared with other published Caucasian populations. The described method can easily be used in routine transplant immunology laboratories which perform studies on the effect of NOD2/CARD15 in stem cell transplantation as well as in other inflammatory or autoimmune diseases. In order to asses the role of NOD2/CARD15 variants on the long term outcome of allogeneic stem cell transplantation a retroperspective analysis of 340 recipients and their unrelated stem cell donors is planned.

P7.4

Ranking of Mismatches within the B*41 Group by Peptide Motif Characteristics

C. Bade-Doeding, A. Seltsam, R. Blasczyk, B. Eiz-Vesper
Hanover Medical School, Hanover, D

Purpose: For a variety of alleles, peptide motifs have been described, but few studies have addressed the question to which extent variants of the same allelic group differ in their peptide motifs. However, this information is of great importance to describe functional similarities between alleles for mismatching purposes. **Methods:** Peptide binding motifs of B*4101, *4102, *4103, *4104, *4105 and *4106 were investigated because all of their polymorphic differences affect their peptide binding groove. To obtain peptides, recombinant B41 molecules were expressed in HEK293 cells and their eluted ligands were determined by mass spectrometry. **Results:** Sequence analysis of eluted peptides revealed that all B*41 alleles have an identical P2 (E) but different PÙ anchors. For the ligands from B*4101 and *4106 P and V were detected at PÙ. B*4102, *4103 and *4104 strictly present L at PÙ. B*4105 presents a L, P and V motif at PÙ. **Conclusions:** In B*4105 Lys at position 80 and Trp at position 95 are apparently responsible for this broadening of the peptide binding spectrum. The complete motif overlap in B*4102, *4103 and *4104 suggests that they are permissive in both transplant directions. Because of the absence of an overlap between B*4101, *4106 and B*4102, *4103 or *4104 no permissivity can be expected. Additionally, the B*4105 shaped T-cell receptor (TCR) repertoire should be more permissive for *4101, *4102, *4103, *4104 or *4106 recipients, because of a larger TCR gap. Inversely, a B*4101, *4102, *4103, *4104 and *4106 shaped TCR repertoire should be less permissive for B*4105 recipients, because of a smaller TCR gap. This peptide motif based ranking of allelic mismatches can contribute to the donor selection process when no HLA-identical donor is available to prevent mismatching being a matter of chance.

P7.5

The Problem of Positive Major Cross-Matches Caused by Anti-HLA Antibodies

M. Mosebach
Institut für Transfusionsmedizin und Immunhämatologie, Magdeburg, D

Background: HLA class I molecules are expressed more or less strongly on mature red-blood-cells (RBCs) and well known as Bennett-Goodspeed (Bg) antigens. Bg antibodies are directed against specific HLA-antigens like HLA-B7, HLA-B17 and HLA-A2 and usually have no clinical relevance in transfusion practice. Nevertheless in three published cases red-cell reactive HLA-antibodies were accused of delayed and acute hemolytic transfusion reactions. **Case Report:** Major cross-matches, using EDTA-treated-plasma from a 52 year-old women, were performed with column agglutination technology (Ortho-Clinical Diagnostics GmbH, Neckargemuend, Germany). One out of twelve major cross-matches showed incompatibility at AHG phase. RBC antibody screens for the patient were negative (4°C, RT, 37°C with LISS and AHG phase). The direct antiglobulin test (DAT) for the RBC unit also was negative. A rare RBC antibody could not be approved and Anti-Bg-antibody testings also were negative. We assumed the possibility of HLA-antibodies not specific for HLA-B7, HLA-B17 and HLA-A2 antigens in the patient plasma. The HLA antibody screen and identification by ELISA (Biotest, Dreieich, Germany) and the complement-dependent-cytotoxicity (CDC) based assay (One Lambda, Meerbusch, Germany) for the patient detected HLA-alloantibodies against HLA-Bw6 molecules. For further information the following major cross-matches were done: Twelve with homozygote HLA-Bw6 antigen positive tested RBC units, seven with HLA-Bw4/Bw6 antigen positive tested RBC units and four with homozygote HLA-Bw4 antigen positive tested RBC units. Positive cross-matches could only be found in three out of twelve homozygote HLA-Bw6 antigen positive tested units. **Discussion:** HLA-molecules are present on mature RBCs and differ in their expression. This could be an explanation for the reported observations. 16% of the HLA-Bw6 antigen positive tested RBCs showed positive cross-matches with the patient sera, containing Anti-HLA-Bw6 antibodies. HLA-antibodies seem to be usually clinically insignificant in transfusion practice of RBC units, but considerable workload is expended in their identification. Conventional RBC antibody screens could not detect HLA-antibodies other than anti-Bg-antibodies. The suspense of a potentially rare RBC antibody with clinical significance persists and complicates the transfusion procedure, even if positive major cross-matches are found and the RBC antibody screens remain negative. In this case an investigation for HLA-antibodies could be done for transfused or multiparous patients, when isolated positive major cross-matches are found.

P7.6

Immuntherapie mit paternalen Lymphozyten bei wiederholtem Abort und erfolgloser IVF-Behandlung

S. Wegener[1], K. Schnurstein[1], S. Hansch[2], M. Bolz[2], R. Sudik[3], V. Briese[2], R. Wegener[1], A. Busecke[4], H. Müller[4]

[1]Institut für Transfusionsmedizin, Rostock, D; [2]Klinik für Gynäkologie und Geburtshilfe Universität Rostock, D; [3]Klinik für Gynäkologie und Geburtshilfe Neubrandenburg, D; [4]Praxiszentrum Frauenheilkunde Rostock, D

Einleitung: Für ungeklärte wiederholte Aborte (WA) wird ursächlich eine verminderte Immunantwort des mütterlichen Immunsystems auf den Feten mit ausbleibender mütterlich-fetaler Toleranz diskutiert. Daraus ergibt sich ein Behandlungsansatz der Immunisierung mit paternalen Lymphozyten, über den von verschiedenen Autoren mit z.T. widersprüchlichen Ergebnissen berichtet wird. Wir stellen unsere fünfzehnjährige Erfahrung mit der aktiven Immuntherapie (AI) bei WA und erste Ergebnisse bei erfolgloser IVF-Behandlung vor. **Patienten und Methoden:** 1990 bis 2004 wurden 202 Frauen mit WA und 47 Patientinnen mit erfolgloser IVF-Therapie mit 3–5 $\times$ 107 paternalen Lymphozyten aus 50 ml Vollblut i.c. immunisiert. Die Infektionsdiagnostik vor AI wurde entspr. den Hämotherapie-Richtlinien durchgeführt. Zusätzlich erfolgten HLA-Typisierung der Paare und HLA-Antikörpertestung der Patientin im CDC. **Ergebnisse:** Die Erfolgsrate (Geburten in gesamter Patientinnengruppe) betrug bei den Frauen mit WA 75% (132/177); einen erfolgreichen Schwangerschaftsverlauf gab es bei 87% (132/152). Von den 47 Patientinnen mit erfolgloser IVF-Behandlung wurden nach AI und Embryotransfer 34% (16/47) schwanger, davon bekamen 75% (12/16) ein gesundes Kind. Außer vorübergehenden entzündlichen Reaktionen an den Injektionsstellen wurden keine schweren Nebenwirkungen registriert. **Schlussfolgerungen:** Die Immuntherapie mit paternalen Lymphozyten ist eine therapeutische Option für Patienten mit WA mit einer Erfolgsrate von 75% und einer erfolgreichen Schwangerschaftsrate von 87%. Bei Patientinnen mit erfolglosem IVF-Programm kann die Erfolgsrate durch die AI erhöht werden. Die HLA-Antikörpertestung dient dabei als Auswahlkriterium für den immunlogisch bedingten Abort, als Entscheidungsfindung für die Wiederholungsimmunisierung und bei positivem Befund als prädiktiver Test für einen erfolgreichen Schwangerschaftsverlauf.

P8: Hemostaseology

P8.1

No Evidence for Involvement of Thrombophilic Mutations in the Genes of Factor V, Prothrombin, and the Methylenetetrahydrofolate Reductase in the Pathogenesis of Thrombotic Microangiopathies.

C. Sucker, F. Farokhzad, F. Dahhan, B. Grabensee, R. Loncar, R.B. Zotz, R.E. Scharf

Heinrich-Heine-Universität Düsseldorf, D

Introduction: Determinants contributing to the onset and modulating the severity of thrombotic microangiopathies are largely unknown, although recent research has elucidated the pathogenesis of these rare thrombotic disorders to some extent. **Methods:** In the present study, we used a case-control and a case-only design, enrolling 35 patients (mean age [$\pm$SD] 38 $\pm$ 11 years) with a history of thrombotic microangiopathy and 728 control subjects to assess the G1691A mutation in the factor V gene (factor V Leiden), the G20210A mutation in the prothrombin gene, and the C677T mutation in the methylentetrahydrofolate reductase (MTHFR) gene as risk factors for the manifestation of thrombotic microangiopathies, and as determinants of the clinical course. The severity of thrombotic microangiopathies was graded according to a clinical score, including degree of thrombocytopenia and anemia, and extent of neurological or renal involvement. Genotyping for respective mutations was performed according to standard procedures. **Results:** The prevalences of factor V Leiden (8.6% vs. 7.7%, odds ratio 1.12, 95% CI 0.3 – 3.8, $p = 0.74$), G20210A prothrombin gene mutation (2.9% vs. 2.9%, odds ratio 1, 95% CI 0.1–7.6, $p = 1$), and MTHFR 677 TT genotype (17.1% vs. 10%, odds ratio 1.9, 95% CI 0.7–4.6, $p = 0.16$) did not differ significantly between patients with thrombotic microangiopathies and healthy control subjects. In addition, the presence of these mutations did not predict a more severe clinical course of thrombotic microangiopathies. **Discussion:** Our findings argue against a role of thrombophilic mutations in the pathogenesis of thrombotic microangiopathies. Thus, screening for these mutations does not allow the identification of individuals at increased risk or the prediction of the clinical course of these rare thrombotic disorders.

P8.2

Heat Shock Inhibits Lipopolysacharide-Induced Tissue-Factor Expression in Whole Blood Samples: Evidence from an In-Vitro Sepsis Model of Gramnegative Sepsis Based on Coagulometry

C. Sucker[1], R. Berkels[2], K. Zacharowski[2], Matthias Hartmann[3]

[1]Heinrich-Heine-Universität Düsseldorf, D; [2]Department of Anesthesiology, Düsseldorf, D; [3]Department of Anesthesiology and Intensice Care Medicine, Essen, D

Background: In gramnegative sepsis, tissue-factor is expressed on peripheral blood monocytes, consequently leading to activation of hemostasis. Recently, we demonstrated that thrombelastography provides a suitable tool to assess lipopolysaccharide (LPS-) -induced activation of hemostasis in vitro. Since inhibition of tissue-factor expression by heat-shock has recently been demonstrated in HUVEC cells, we used thrombelastography to evaluate the effect of heat-shock on LPS-induced activation of hemostasis in human whole blood and isolated leucocytes. **Methods:** After adding of LPS, human whole blood obtained from healthy volunteers was incubated at 37°C for 5 hours or at 43°C for 2 hours followed by an incubation at 37°C for 3 hours. After incubation, clotting time (CT) was determined using a coagulometer (Amelung KC4). The experiments were also performed with leucocyte suspensions isolated from citrate-anticoagulated human whole blood. Activation of hemostasis by LPS was further evaluated by use of ASIS, a tissue-factor antagonist, and cycloheximide, an inhibitor of protein synthesis. **Results:** Incubation of whole blood with LPS (100 μg/ml) at 37°C for 5 h led to significant shortening of CT from 357 $\pm$ 108 sec to 82 $\pm$ 8 sec ($n = 12$; $p < 0.05$). The shortening of CT was completely inhibited by heat-shock (incubation at 43°C for 2 hours, followed by 37°C for 3 hours; CT 312 ± 66 sec vs. 277 ± 65 sec). Further experiments employing ASIS and cycloheximide demonstrated that LPS-induced activation of hemostasis is mediated by tissue-factor and requires protein synthesis. The inhibitory effect of heat shock on hemostasis was also observed in leucocyte suspensions, although cell integrity of leukocytes was not affected as judged by FACS analysis. **Conclusions:** Hyperthermic conditions ("heat shock") inhibit LPS-induced tissue-factor expression in human whole blood and leucocyte suspensions. The clinical relevance of this finding requires further evaluation.

P8.3

Evaluation of a New Assay for Measuring ADAMTS-13 Activity and Antigen from the Same Sample (TECHNOZYM® ADAMTS-13)

S. Colle[1], S. Geiter[1], H. Vetr[1], M. Dockal[2], F. Scheiflinger[2], P.A. Kyrle[3], B.R. Binder[4]

[1]Technoclone GmbH, Wien, A; [2]Baxter Bioscience, Wien, A; [3]Dept.Internal Medicine, Medical University Vienna, Wien, A; [4]Dept. Vasc.Biol. and Thromb.Res., Medical University Vienna, Wien, A

Purpose: The aim of this study is to evaluate a new assay for quantification of ADAMTS-13 activity and antigen levels in the same sample allowing determination of specific activities. Defects in the activity of ADAMTS-13, the von Willebrand Factor (vWF) cleaving protease, is the major cause for TTP, a microvascular thrombotic disorder, which is inevitably fatal if not treated immediately by plasma exchange. **Methods:** The method is based on the Actibindechnology®, using a catching monoclonal antibody not interfering with ADAMTS-13 activity, assaying activity by a fluorogenic substrate and bound antigen thereafter by a peroxidase labelled polyclonal antibody. ADAMTS-13 autoantibodies were measured by TECHNOZYM® ADAMTS-13 INH. **Results:** Samples from TTP patients (n = 43) had significantly lower levels of ADAMTS-13 activity and antigen than those from normal donors (n = 38; $p < 0.05$). The majority of TTP samples (37 out of 43) had ADAMTS-13 activities below 50%. These low activities correlated with high levels of anti-ADAMTS-13 antibodies. Moreover, the TTP samples had significantly higher levels of vWF:CBA activity ($p < 0.05$) consistent with the presence of high molecular weight vWF. **Conclusion/Results:** obtained with the new assay for measuring ADAMTS-13 activity/antigen (TECHNOZYM® ADAMTS-13) correlate with the clinical picture and the decreased functional activity of ADAMTS-13 leading to increased levels of vWF multimers and in turn platelet consumption. Thus this new assay clearly adds to differentiate patients with TTP.

P8.4

Risk for Thromboembolic Disease in Lupus Anticoagulant Patients Due to Pathways Involving P-Selectin and CD154

K. Stamer[1], I. Pabinger[2], B. Eichelberger[2], D. Koren[2], H. Klüter[1], S. Panzer[2], P. Bugert[1]

[1]Institut für Transfusionsmedizin und Immunologie, Mannheim, D; [2]Klinik für Blutgruppenserologie, Wien, A

Objective: Individuals with Lupus anticoagulant (LA) are at risk for thromboembolism (TE). Because platelets play a key role in inflammation and TE we investigated whether gene polymorphisms as well as plasma levels of platelet receptors are associated with the development of TE and are therefore useful predictors of TE in LA patients. **Methods:** LA was diagnosed in 109 patients according to international criteria and 68% of the patients had a history of thromboembolic disease (LA/TE+; n = 74), 62 with venous thrombosis (VT), 18 with arterial thrombosis (AT), 6 of the latter had both, VT and AT. The remaining 35 LA patients had no previous thrombosis (LA/TE−). Genotyping for P-selectin, PSGL-1, and CD154 polymorphisms was performed using PCR methods. Plasma levels of soluble P-selectin and CD154 were determined by ELISA. **Results:** None of the gene polymorphisms proved to be a predictor for the general risk of TE in LA patients. Interestingly, the P-selectin Pro715 allele was slightly more frequent in VT (logistic regression adjusted for age and sex: p = 0.0594; OR = 3.167, 95% CI [0.955–10.503]) but no patient with AT had this allele (p = 0.0238; OR = 0.099, 95% CI [0.001–0.790]). Thus, the Pro715 allele may protect from the development of AT. Plasma levels of soluble P-selectin were significantly higher in LA/TE+ patients (ANOVA adjusted for age and sex: p = 0.0205) and were associated with VT (p = 0.0388) but not AT (p = 0.4713). The CA repeat polymorphism in the 3′-noncoding region of the CD154 was significantly associated with the development of AT (p = 0.0138; OR = 4.035, 95% CI [1.329–12.249] after logistic regression adjusted for age and sex). Plasma levels of sCD154 were not different among the various groups. **Conclusion:** Gene polymorphism of P-selectin (Thr715Pro) and CD154 (CA repeats) are presumably modulating the risk for VT and AT. Further, plasma levels of soluble P-selectin and CD154 are elevated in LA patients, but their role to predict TE needs to be evaluated in a prospective study.

P8.5

Dopamine is a Coactivator for Platelet Adhesion to Collagen and Acts via D2-Like Receptors

A. Schedel[1], P. Schloss[2], H. Klüter[1], P. Bugert[1]

[1]DRK-Blutspendedienst Baden-Württemberg – Hessen, Mannheim, D; [2]Central Institute of Mental Health, Mannheim, D

Background: Monoamines such as serotonin and epinephrine are known to be involved in platelet activation and aggregation. The effect of dopamine is barely understood so far. Different dopamine receptors, such as D2R, D3R and D5R, have been described on human platelets and recently, we could also demonstrate a functional dopamine transporter (DAT) on platelets. We now investigated the role of dopamine in platelet activation and adhesion and defined the receptors involved in this pathways. **Methods:** Platelet-rich plasma (PRP) was isolated from citrated blood samples of 12 healthy individuals. PRP was treated with different agonists (ADP, epinephrine, dopamine) and combinations of them. Platelet activation markers (CD62P and CD63) were measured by flow cytometry. Platelet adhesion to collagen was investigated in a flow chamber system and quantified by using an image analysis software. Different dopamine receptor and DAT antagonists were applied in order to identify the molecules involved in the dopaminergic system of platelets. **Results:** ADP, epinephrine and ADP/epinephrine treatment but not dopamine or ADP/dopamine treatment lead to platelet activation measured by CD62P and CD63 expression. Platelet adhesion to collagen under flow was remarkably increased after ADP (3.8 ± 2.2 times), ADP/epinephrine (9.2 ± 2.2 times) and also ADP/dopamine (5.5 ± 2.7 times) treatment compared to untreated platelets. Pre-incubation of platelets with D2-like receptor antagonists prior to the incubation with ADP/dopamine deminished the dopamine effect on platelet adhesion to collagen. D1-like receptor antagonists as well as DAT antagonists did not affect the dopamine-induced platelet adhesion. **Conclusions:** ADP/dopamine co-activation does not cause release of alpha and dense granules, but leads to a significant increase of platelet adhesion to collagen. The dopaminergic system of platelets includes D2-like receptors for outside-in signalling. The dopamine-induced platelet adhesion to collagen may put further link to clinical data about increased risk for thromboembolic complications in patients with mental disorders amongst others caused by dopamine imbalance.

P8.6

The Marburg I Polymorphism of Factor VII-Activating Protease Is Not Associated with Deep Venous Thrombosis

V. Weisbach, R. Ruppel, J. Ringwald, R. Eckstein

Universitätsklinikum Erlangen, D

Purpose: The role of the factor VII-activating protease (FSAP) variant Marburg I in the occurrence of venous thromboembolism (VTE) is controversial. **Methods:** We determined the Marburg I 1601G > A polymorphism using PCR amplification with specific primers and the Light Cycler device (Roche, Germany) in 241 patients with confirmed VTE who were admitted to our institution for thrombophilia work-up and 241 sex- and age-matched healthy controls. Patients with axillary, mesenteric or cerebral vein thrombosis were excluded. Controls were recruited from our blood donors and from patients who were attended at our hospital without having thrombosis. Statistical analysis was done by means of Fisher's exact test. **Results:** In the whole study population, the prevalence of the Marburg I polymorphism was similar in patients and controls (N = 18; 7.5% versus N = 15; 6.2%; p = 0.36; OR = 0.9; 95% CI 0.7–1.3). In the subgroup of 58 patients who had a first and idiopathic incident of VTE the incidence of the Marburg I polymorphism was higher (p = 0.20) in the patients compared to the controls (N = 6; 10.3% versus N = 15; 6.2%; OR = 1.1; 95% CI 0.9–1.5). **Conclusions:** The results of the present study rule out a strong association between the FSAP variant Marburg I and unselected VTE. This result is in line with all three previous reports on this subject which were published since 2005. We could not confirm an association of the Marburg I variant with idiopathic VTE, which was described in one of these previous reports. Whether there is a weak effect of the Marburg I polymorphism on thrombotic risk, especially in idiopathic VTE, remains to be determined by the observation of very large study populations. The present and future studies may contribute to the generation of such a database.

P8.7

Importance of Platelet Count in Intensive Care Patients with HIT II

K. Erdlenbruch, B. Stephan, J. Schenk, G. Pindur
Universitätsklinik des Saarlandes, Homburg-Saar, D

Introduction: Heparin induced thrombocytopenia Type II (HIT II) is one of the most serious complications for patients treated with heparin. Heparin induces platelet aggregation which can lead to thrombosis which can result in organ failure or limbthreatening complications. Regular control of platelet count especially during the first days of treatment with heparin is important to give a hint for the development of a HIT by drop of platelet count. In intensive care patients it can be difficult to distinguish between HIT II and other causes for low platelet count. In HIT II treatment of choice is danaparoid or lepirudin. Platelet count should increase after switch from heparin to alternative treatment except in case of crossreactivity of HIT II antibodies to the alternative anticoagulant. In such a case severe clinical complications can occur. We report the clinical course of a patient with HIT II which highlights the importance for regular labcontrol even after switch of therapy. **Clinical Course:** 56 year old female patient with polytrauma, impaired renal function and massive transfusion received UFH iv. for primary prophylaxis. Though massive bleeding could be controlled and all parameters normalized the platelet count remained at 62.000/µl. In parallel D-Dimers increased continuously up to 3.3 mg/l, normal range 0–0.2 mg/l. There was no clinical sign of thrombosis. A screening test for HIT II was performed by gelcard assay, Diamed, and confirmed by ELISA technique with positive result. Therefore treatment was switched from Heparin to danaparoid. Danaparoid was chosen due to reduced renal function. During the next 3 days under danaparoid platelet count fell continously to 37.000/µl. D-Dimers remained increasing, too. This was a hint for a suspected crossreactivity of HIT II antibodies with danaparoid. Due to these results of platelet count monitoring a crossreactivity of danaparoid with hit antibodies was considered. Treatment was switched from danaparoid to lepirudin. After switch to lepirudin platelet count increased pretty fast from 37.000/µl to 66.000/µl in 5 h and to 113.00/µl in 24 h. Also D-Dimers begun to decrease. During the next days under treatment with lepirudin platelet count and D-Dimers fully normalized. **Discussion:** This case shows the importance of regular platelet count monitoring – not only during treatment with heparin. Even in case of confirmed HIT II close monitoring is important to detect crossreactivity to alternative anticoagulants.

P8.8

Do Patients in Major Liver Resections Benefit from Anti-Fibrinolytic Drugs?

B. Stephan, M. Weinrich, K. Erdlenbruch, C. Justinger, K. Benesch, J.L. Borchers, V.M. Petrescu-Jipa, S. Windischmann, J.F. Schenk, M.K. Schilling, G. Pindur
University Hospital of the Saarland, Homburg-Saar, D

Purpose: Central molecules in fibrinolysis and its inhibition are plasminogen and alpha-2-antiplasmin (alpha-plasmin inhibitor). Decreased levels of plasminogen and alpha-2-antiplasmin can be found in liver diseases, hyperfibrinolysis and blood loss. A lack of alpha-2-antiplasmin may result in a bleeding disorder. Anti-fibrinolytic drugs like tranexam acid inhibit directly the plasmin effect. Activated coagulation with increased thrombin generation can be described with the plasma concentration of the thrombin-antithrombin complex (TAT). Increased TAT is often seen in DIC, thromboembolism, polytrauma, shock, severe liver or heart failure, anticoagulant or thrombolytic therapy and patients with fresh wounds. TAT determination is very sensitive to pre-analytic influences. Surgical bleeding control in typical or atypical major liver resection can be performed by selective vascular clamping (SVC) or Pringle manoeuvre which cause a short-time circulatory stasis. **Methods:** Five female and four male patients (53.6 years in average, 31 to 71 years) underwent elective major liver resection. Samples for the determination of plasminogen, alpha-2-antiplasmin and TAT were taken from peripheral veins before and after operation. **Results:** The preoperative samples showed normal values for alpha-2-antiplasmin (0.7–1.2 U/ml) and plasminogen (0.7–1.4 U/ml) in all patients. Preoperative TAT (normal <5 µg/l) levels were found normal in only three patients, six patients had increased levels. Postoperative alpha-2-antiplasmin activity was decreased in five patients (normal in four patients), postoperative plasminogen activity was normal in six patients and below normal in three patients. Alpha-2-antiplasmin decreased from an average of 0.9 to 0.63 U/ml and plasminogen from an average of 0.9 to 0.72 U/ml. Postoperative TAT was increased in all patients from a preoperative average concentration of 12.1 to to a postoperative average concentration of 19.7 µg/l. Komolgoroff-Smirnoff statistic assay detected a significant pre- to postoperative difference in all three parameters. **Conclusion:** Fibrinolysis, its inhibition and thrombin generation are significantly altered in major liver resection as the decrease of plasminogen and alpha-2-antiplasmin and the increase of TAT show. Anti-fibrinolytic drugs could partially stabilise fibrinolysis. Further investigations should aim on the clinical effect of anti-fibrinolytic drugs in major liver operations.

P8.9

Reducing Blood Component Transfusion Therapy by Thrombelastography in a Case of Severe Bleeding Episode after Hip Revision Surgery

S.J. Hopp, B. Stephan, H. Rensing, T. Pohlemann, J. Schenk
University of Saarland, Homburg-Saar, D

Purpose: Severe bleeding complications require adequate hemostatic balance besides restrictive transfusion policy. We aimed to find out if thrombelastography (TEG) as a viscoelastic monitoring device is appropriate for managing patients efficiently and cost-effectively. **Methods:** A 74 year old female patient suffering from a chronic multiresistent inflammation of the right hip joint after implantation of hip prosthesis and a "girdlestone situation" at present underwent multiple revision surgeries leading to polytransfusion therapy. No signs/symptoms for hemostatic abnormalities existed. Thus severe bleeding led to transferral to ICU. Besides global coagulation assays and blood cells, PLT counts and function, F XIII activity, v.Willebrand specific parameters (Rcof). In addition the fibrinolytic system was controlled (reptilase time, d-dimers) and dysfibrinogenmemia excluded. Coagulation time (CT), clot forming time (CFT) and the maximum clot firmness (MCF) were evaluated by a computerized TEG (ROTEM®, Pentapharm, Munich) in citrated whole blood. Extrinsic and intrinsic pathways were analyzed using "ExTEM", and "InTEM", as well as a specific reagent (FibTEM) including GpIIb/IIIa inhibitor was used to exclude PLT interferences. Fibrinolysis was verified by ApTEM. **Results:** After transfusion of 9 RBC, 6 FFP and 2 PLT concentrates abnormal blood coagulation parameters (PT 63%, PTT 63′, fibrinogen 82 mg/dl, AT III 34%) could be normalized as well as blood cell and PLT count improved while PLT function remained abnormal. Rcof, d-dimers, and TEG using ApTEM to exclude fibrinolytic activity were found to be normal. TEG measurements implicated F XIII deficiency and/or severe reduction of fibrinogen leading to F XIII activity measurements. MCF-FibTEM demonstrated zero-line before BW adapted supplementation of 2500 U F XIII within 12 hrs. CT and MCF-FibTEM normalized to 74′, and 11 mm respectively. F XIII increased from 23 to 102%. As a consequence CFT changes representing the improvement of the dynamic coagulation process became evident. Serosanguinous drain secretion was markedly reduced (from 5500 ml to 660 ml per day). Substitution for 3 days led to uneventful revision surgery. Hypothermia and acidosis could be excluded (36.6°C, pH 7.46). **Conclusion:** In our case, adjustment of TEG (ROTEM) has proofed to be very effective in detecting coagulation disorders by reducing necessity for blood products and minimizing transfusion risks, respectively.

P8.10

Von Willebrand Syndrome Type San Diego – Step Wise Approach of a Rare Case of Combined Hemostatic Abnormality

V.-M. Petrescu-Jipa, M. Mennicke, C. Benesch, G. Pindur, J. Schenk
University of Saarland, Homburg-Saar, D

Introduction: A 38 years old female patient with moderate signs/symptoms of bleeding diathesis but extremely prolonged aPTT values (>160″), became suspicious by routine lab controls. No drug interference existed. At least the reason of this phenomenon remained unclear as well as the history/family history did not help to elucidate any hypothetic underlying disease. **Methods:** Global coagulation assays (PT, aPTT, TT, fibrinogen – immunologically based method and according to Clauss) were measured using platelet poor plasma besides d-dimers, reptilase-time, and antithrombin activity/concentration. To exclude acute phase reactions e.g. C-reactive protein was determined. Special assays were performed to complete step-wise procedure: lupus anticoagulant (ratio), phospholipid antibodies, alpha 2-antiplasmin, plasminogen-activity and a plasma mixing assay. Platelet counts were controlled using citrated and EDTA whole blood. Bleeding time (acc. to Duke) and platelet aggregation (acc. to Born) were controlled. VWF activity (Rcof)/concentration (vWF:Ag) as well as vWF multimers were analysed and the endogenous coagulation system (factor XII, XI, IX, and VIII activity) was controlled besides factor XIII activity. **Results:** Platelet count (217000/µl-EDTA whole blood; 204000/µl – citrated whole blood), bleeding time acc. to Duke (1′55″; n: < 4′), and platelet aggregation were found to be normal. Abnormal laboratory results were registered as follows: aPTT >140″ (n: <34′), Rcof activity 35% and vWF related antigen 39% (n: >60% (Rcof); >70% (vWF:Ag)). Factor VIII activity 44% (n: >70%). Multimer analysis demonstrated the presence of all molecular classes of proteins, and normal structured oligomers. Furthermore collagen binding capacity (n: >50%) was also found to be pathologic (43%; ratio: vWF:CB/vWF Ag: 0.87 (n: 0.8–2.0)). F XII activity was severely reduced (<1.6%; n: >70%). Inhibitor of the endogenous system could not be verified. **Conclusions:** A rare case of mild vWJ-syndrome, type San Diego was diagnosed. Bleeding In the context of the patient's bleeding history vWJ-S seem to be of predominant importance. We therefore suggest weight adapted application of DDAVP/Minirin since necessary also reflecting the thrombophilic risk related with factor XII deficiency by the critical use of anticoagulants.

P8.11

Clinical Impact of the C677T Methylentetrahydrofolate Reductase and Association with Homocysteine in Serum

A. Ihle, M. Ames, B. Stephan, J. Schenk
University of Saarland, Homburg-Saar, D

Purpose: The gene variant of C677T MTHFR may be associated with hyperhomocysteinemia. Its clinical relevance is meanwhile controversially discussed. We therefore aimed to get insights by the following questions: Does the function loss of the enzyme "MTHFR" at patients with thrombotic complications (group I) and asymtomatic mutant carriers (group II) necessarily associated with hyperhomocysteinemia? Does the kind and/or severity of the underlying thrombotic complication play any role and do homcysteine values age related differ between both groups? **Patients and Methods:** Group I: 65 more or less severe (venous/arterial) thrombotic patients and proved homozygous (n = 18), and heterozygous (n = 47) MTHFR defect. Group II: 35 asymptomatic mutant carriers for MTHFR (homozygous: n = 13; heterozygous: n = 22). Homocysteine in serum (n: <15 µmol/l) was measured by HPLC in EDTA whole blood. DNA analysis was performed by agarose gel electrophoresis (acc. to Schröder & Herrmann/Greifswald). Means and SD was calculated and the chi square assay was used to. **Results:** Group I: In 27/65 patients (42%) hyperhomocysteinemia (16.2 ± 8.0 µmol/l) was diagnosed. The measurements of patient with recurrent events did not differ from single thrombotic complications (15.1 ± 6.0 µmol/l vs. 16.1 ± 4.5 µmol/l) as well as in comparison with group II. In some single arterial thrombotic patients (n = 12) homocysteine serum levels were more elevated than in venous patients (n = 51) (19.6 ± 13.7 µmol/l vs. 15.6 ± 6.6 µmol/l). In most thrombotic patients (group I) normal homocysteine concentrations were measured in serum (11.1 ± 2.4 µmol/l). In asymptomatic mutant carriers (group II) slightly higher homocysteine values (16.0 ± 6.5 µmol/l) were found compared with group II. Furthermore neither in group I/II homozygous mutant carriers did demonstrate higher serum levels for homocysteine than heterozygous MTHFR gene defects (16.9 ± 7.4 µmol/l vs. 15.8 ± 7.4 µmol/l). After randomization to age-related groups (<30 J./30–59 J./>59 J). No significantly higher homocysteine values in group I compared with group II became obvious. **Conclusion:** The gene defect encoding the C677T variants of MTHFR does not necessarily correlate with hyperhomocysteinemia and is of no clinical significance as risk variable in thrombotic patients. Hyperhomocysteinemia seem to be more attributable with arterial than venous thrombotic patients but has to be critically reviewed as a thrombophilic risk factor.

P8.12

Is Point-of Care Testing via Thrombelastography an Approach for Monitoring Oral Anticoagulants?

S.J. Hopp, A. Nemeh, B. Stephan, T. Pohlemann, J. Schenk
University of Saarland, Homburg-Saar, D

Purpose: The evaluation of coagulation abnormalities as well as its monitoring may become obvious by thrombelastography (TEG). We aimed to clarify if patients on VKA treatment can be monitored using the ROTEM Coagulation Analyzer (Pentapharm, Munich, Germany). **Methods:** Citrated whole blood samples from 27 patients (17 males and 10 females), 18–81 years of age (average 52 years) with an acquired extrinsic coagulation disorder caused by VKA treatment comprised the experimental study material. The average prothrombin (PT)-value – performed with the coagulometer according to Schnitger and Gross – was 27.84 percent, the average INR at the time of blood withdrawal as 2.28 (1.27–3.53). Thrombelastographic profiles were produced by incubating 0.3 ml of at least 30-min-rested, prewarmed (37 degrees C) whole blood with defined amounts of activating reagent. Blood coagulation was induced by the activation of the extrinsic (ExTEM), and intrinsic (InTEM) pathways, as well as by a specific reagent (ReoPro) including small amounts of a GpIIb/IIIa inhibitor (FibTEM) and CaCl2. Traditional thrombelastographic parameters like Coagulation Time (CT), Clot forming time (CFT), and Maximum Clot Firmness (MCF) were recorded. The reference levels of the ROTEM in our laboratory were established by using citrated whole blood from 70 healthy blood donors of both genders in our department. **Results:** The clotting profiles of the 27 patients receiving VKA treatment demonstrated a significantly prolonged initiation of whole blood clot formation as expressed in the CT-ExTEM (VKA group, 36.63 ± 6.88 sec. vs. reference group, 31.79 ± 5.77 sec.; $p < 0.01$) and correlated significantly with increasing INR in a dose-related manner ($r = 0.664$, $p < 0.001$). Nevertheless, the CT-ExTEM values of the VKA patients surprisingly remained within normal ranges which has been confirmed by a ROC calculation (AUC: 0.704, $p < 0.01$, sensitivity: 3.7%, specifity: ~ 93%). Additionally the CT-FibTEM was significantly prolonged in cases of higher INR values ($r = 0.502$, $p < 0.05$). Besides a week but not significant correlation between INR and CT-InTEG ($r = 0.392$, $p = 0.053$) no other significant correlation was found. **Conclusion:** Our present findings demonstrate that ROTEM and especially the strongest parameter CT-ExTEM in this issue neither is a useful tool for detecting sensitively patients with hemorrhagic diatheses due to oral anticoagulation nor an application to patients′ self-management of monitoring VKA treatment.

P8.13

Effects of Soluble CD40L on Platelet Thrombus Formation under Arterial Flow Conditions

R.E. Scharf, E. Reiff, E. Atunlu, V.R. Stoldt
Heinrich Heine University Medical Center, Düsseldorf, D

Introduction: CD40 ligand (CD40L) is a transmembrane protein belonging to the tumor necrosis factor family. Recent studies have demonstrated that CD40L stabilizes arterial thrombi by a beta3 integrin–dependent mechanism and, thus, can contribute to arterial thrombogenesis. We have now explored the effects of soluble CD40L (sCD40L) on thrombus formation and progression under arterial flow conditions using an established in vitro model. **Material and Methods:** Citrate-anticoagulated blood was obtained from healthy donors (n = 8) and perfused at an initial wall shear rate of 1,000 sec-1 through a rectangular flow chamber coated with type I collagen. Prior to perfusion, blood samples were incubated with recombinant sCD40L at concentrations of 1, 5, 10, or 100 ng/ml. Thrombus formation was quantified 3-dimensionally by mepacrine-prelabelled platelets using confocal laser scanning microscopy and a voxel-based software (ECCET http://eccet.acs.uni-duesseldorf.de/index.html#top) for analysis. **Results:** Under control conditions (no sCD40L added), thrombus volume (mean ± SD) was 8,412 ± 1,472 μm^3 after 5 min and 34,022 ± 4,776 μm^3 after 10 min (n = 8, $p < 0.05$). Clinically relevant sCD40L concentrations of 1 ng/ml or 5 ng/ml caused a significant increase in thrombus volume of 20,641 ± 6,604 μm^3 (5 min) and 64,131 ± 13,840 μm^3 (10 min, sCD40L 1 ng/ml) or of 31,091 ± 15,740 μm^3 (5 min) and 69,707 ± 35,373 μm^3 (10 min, sCD40L 5 ng/ml), respectively (p each < 0.05, as compared to corresponding control values). Immunolabelling of formed thrombi with monoclonal antibodies against P-selectin and bound sCDL demonstrated colocalization of both antigens on the thrombus surface. At sCD4L concentrations of 10 or 100 ng/ml, no additional effect on thrombus growth was detected. Moreover, exposure of platelet thrombi to continously increasing wall shear rates (>1,500 sec-1) revealed that preincubation with sCD40L at concentrations of 1 or 5 ng/ml resulted in significantly more stable platelet thrombi, as compared to thrombi without preincubation of whole blood with sCD40L ($p < 0.05$). Again, higher concentrations of sCD40L had no additional effect on thrombus resistance to increasing wall shear rates, as shown in this setting of displacement experiments (n = 3). **Conclusion:** Our findings demonstrate that soluble CD40L at clinically relevant concentrations does indeed promote thrombus formation and stability under arterial flow conditions. These in vitro observations are in accordance with the contention that soluble CD40L can display prothrombotic effects and thereby increase arterial thrombus formation in vivo leading to acute vascular occlusion and ischemic syndromes.

P8.14

Clinical Impact of PLT and Blood Cell Activation by Shear Stress: Microscopic Evaluation Using the Retention Test of Homburg-II (RTH-II)

M.A. Nemeh, P. Mestres, E. Morgenstern, J. Schenk
University of Saarland, Homburg-Saar, D

Purpose: Clinical impact of platelet (PLT) and blood cell activation in-vitro (coincidence of PLT adhesion and aggregation) is rather unclear. To match biological conditions, PLT, leucocytes (WBC) and erythrocytes (RBC) response to activation was evaluated by investigating their interactions with the athrombogenic filter of RTH-II forced by shear stress. **Methods:** 500 μL isotonic citrated whole blood (1:10) obtained from healthy individuals (n = 70) was added to Eppendorf retention tubes and forced through RTH filter by centrifugation (110 g/5 min) within 30 min. after blood withdrawal. The percentage of the difference between CBC measurements before (b.F) and after (a.F) the passage of the filter represented the retention index (RI) of PLT (PLT-RI), WBC (WBC-RI), and RBC (RBC-RI). Phase-contrast microscopy was done on b.F and a.F blood after fixation. For characterizing the interactions of PLT, WBC and RBC with the filter, scanning and transmission electron microscopy was used. Wilcoxon and Kolmogorov-Smirnov (KS) tests were 2SD; KS: applied for statistics. **Results:** Based on normal theory (mean $p < 0.005$), the reference ranges of RBC-RI levels were significantly lower than 8.2%; p 8.3% vs. −3.3 WBC-RI (4.2 < 0.0005), while PLT-RI revealed much higher 12.5%; p values (PLT-RI: 25.2 < 0.0005). Phase-contrast and electron microscopy proved these phenomena. PLT adhered and spread relevantly on the filter forming aggregates bridging the opposite surfaces of its pores with mild degranulation. WBC and RBC showed evident signs of activation e.g., direct adherence to the filter substantially less than PLT, leukocyte degranulation and erythrocyte coin-rolls and agglutinations. **Conclusion:** PLT multiple responses to activation by shear stress were reflected by high retention despite their smaller size than WBC, RBC and the filter interconnected pores (16–22 μm). The substantially lower retention of WBC and RBC seems to be mainly proportional to their sizes. The evident activation of WBC and RBC and their direct adherence on the filter underline the specific interactions with the filter. This is further supported by their reliable and reproducible RI levels and their ability to pass through the filter besides constant correlations of WBC-RI (r = 0.183) and RBC-RI (r = 0.129) with PLT-RI. These conclusions confirm the reliability and significance of RTH-II as a simple assay for screening PLT function and urge to study the impact of blood cell activation in future clinical studies.

P8.15

Is thrombelastography an Useful Tool for Monitoring Hemophilic Patients?

S.J. Hopp, A. Nemeh, B. Stephan, T. Pohlemann, J. Schenk
University of Saarland, Homburg, D

Purpose: In our study we aimed to evaluate the influence of hemostatic changes and drug influence on thrombelastographic measurements in hemophilic patients. **Methods:** 11 adult and pediatric patients, 4–40 years of age (average 17.64 years) suffering from hereditary factor VIII deficiency (9 severe, 1 moderate, 1 mild hemophilia) were substituted with BW adapted factor VIII concentrates. Recovery measurements of factor VIII activity and PTT were performed in our coagulation laboratory before and 15 min. after the replacement of factor VIII. Coagulation Time (CT, reflecting time for initiation of fibrin formation), Clot forming time (CFT, reflecting the dynamics and speed of clot formation) and Maximum Clot Firmness (MCF, reflecting the maximal clot strength) were evaluated by a computerized TEG (ROTEM®) in citrated whole blood. Blood coagulation was induced via the activation of the extrinsic (ExTEM) and intrinsic (InTEM) pathways and CaCl2. Prior to the factor VIII administration the average PTT value was 62.25 sec. and factor VIII activity 2.38%, respectively. Blood cell and platelet counts were measured by an automatic blood cell counting system ("M-2000" Sysmex-Analyzer). The reference levels of the ROTEM in our laboratory were established by using citrated whole blood from 70 healthy blood donors of both genders in our department. **Results:** In hemophilia A patients the BW adapted supplementation of factor VIII concentrates resulted in a significant decrease of PTT (62.25 to 34.13 sec, $p < 0.01$) and an increase of the FVIII:C (2.38 to 46.25%, $p < 0.01$), as well as a significant normalization of the CT-InTEM (326 to 160.56 sec, $p < 0.01$). The coagulation response to factor VIII supplementation varied amongst patients. Only a slight tendency but no significant correlation between the CT-InTEM and the PTT (r = 0.551, $p > 0.05$), as well as the FVIII:C (r = 0.616, $p > 0.05$) was objected. Regarding the selectivity of this test system there might be no superiority of the PTT compared to the CT-InTEM (AUC: 1.00, $p < 0.001$, sensitivity: 100%, specifity: 98.5–100%) for diagnosing disturbances of the intrinsic system. **Conclusion:** Our data implicate that ROTEM and in paticular CT-InTEM can be used as a rough indicator of adequate therapy in hemophilic patients. The missing correlation of PTT and CT-InTEM probably is caused by the different sensitivity of the thromboplastin reagents.

P8.16

Fibrinogen Gene Mutations in Relation to the Clinical Manifestations of Dysfibrinogenemia

W. Miesbach[1], V. Catania[1], C. von Auer[2], D.K. Galanakis[3], I. Scharrer[2]
[1]Universitätsklinik Frankfurt, D; [2]Universitätsklinik Mainz, D; [3]State University of New York, USA

The congenital dysfibrinogenemia is a rare clotting disorder which is based on a structural defect in the fibrinogen molecule. Approximately 350 cases of unrelated families with dysfibrinogenemia have been reported. Of these, the structural defects have been determined in nearly 170 families. **Patients and Methods:** We describe the clinical manifestations in 50 patients from 19 families from Frankfurt. Up to now the underlying structural defect could be found in 43/50 (86%) of the patients and 14/19 (74%) of the families (Galanakis, New York, von Depka, Hannover). **Results:** In 19 families, 50 patients were found with dysfibrinogenemia (52% female, age median: 52 years-old, 9–89 years old). The fibrinogen level, according to Clauss decreased in median with 51 mg% (15–86 mg/dl, norm: 150–450 mg/dl). The determination of the other fibrinogen levels resulted in the normal range. Fibrinogen according to Schulz: 240 mg/dl, immunological fibrinogen: 244 mg/dl. The Reptilase time was prolonged to 55 sec (median, norm: – 20 sec). 50% of the patients stated a distinct bleeding tendency and mostly a tendency for haematoma (59%) and secondary haemorrhaging (45%). 13 patients had a thrombotic disease, of which 80% were arterially caused. 12% of the patients stated a tendency for bleeding as well as for thrombosis. 19% of the patients had miscarriages, partly recurrent and 18/50 (36%) of the patients were asymptomatic. Furthermore, it was observed that the clinical symptoms are often similar in the affected families. In 11 of the families, an Aalpha 16 Arg-Cys mutation was found. In the other three families there were found gamma mutations, e.g., gamma 356 Ala-Thr, gamma 318–319 del and gamma 318 Ap-Gly. The clinical manifestations in the families with Aalpha 16 Arg-Cys mutation were bleeding (65%), thrombosis (22%) and abortions (16%). 25% were asymptomatic and 12% of the patients experienced both, bleeding and thrombosis. **Conclusion:** The investigations of the Frankfurt patient group with dysfibrinogenemia showed a high rate of clinical manifestations, mostly the tendency for haematoma and secondary haemorrhaging. The tendency for thrombosis is concerned rather with the arterial vessels. The high tendency for miscarriage is striking, which makes the administration of fibrinogen concentrate during pregnancy necessary. The most common found fibrinogen mutation was at the Alpha chain in position 16. In patients with this mutation mostly both, bleeding and thrombosis occurred. Thus, management of patients with this mutation may be complicated by the variablility of clinical manifestations of congenital dysfibrinogenemia.

P8.17

Establishment of an International Registry of Patients with Congenital FXIII Deficiency

V. Ivaskevicius[1], R. Seitz[2], H.P. Kohler[3], L. Muszbek[4], R.AS Ariens[5], E. Seifried[6], J. Oldenburg[1]

[1]Institute of Experimental Haematology and Transfusion Medicine, Bonn, D; [2]Paul-Ehrlich-Institute, Erlangen, D; [3]University Clinic of Bern, CH; [4]University of Debrecen, HU; [5]University of Leeds, UK; [6]Institute of Transfusion Medicine, Frankfurt, D

Introduction: FXIII deficiency is a rare autosomal recessive disorder affecting approximatly 1 out of 1–3 million inhabitans. The disease is characterized by bleeding, impaired wound repair and spontanious abortions in females. Extracellular FXIII molecule has a tetramer structure composing of two catalytic A-subunits and two B-subunits that act as a carrier molecules. Based on genotype there are two types of FXIII deficiency: A-subunit deficiency when mutation affects F13A gene and much rarely B-subunit deficiency when mutation affects F13B gene. In 1993, the ETRO Working Party on factor XIII initiated a Europe-wide questionnaire on congenital FXIII deficiency with several aims: (1) establish a patient registry (2) join a study group (3) accumulate and exchange informations on symptoms, diagnostic approach, and treatment; (4) stimulate reseach on protein and gene defects and their relation to clinical symptoms. **Results:** We followed this registry and so far included 104 questionnaire patients (QP) out of 88 families representing 24 nations. Fifty-six were females and 48 were males. Before the introduction of treatment severe bleeding symptoms were recognized in 55 (53%) QP, moderate bleeding in 36 (34.6%) QP, mild bleeding in 10 (9.6%) QP and non-bleeding in 3 (2.9%) QP. Muscle bleeding was occured in 51 (49%)/104 patients, joint bleeding in 37 (35.6%)/104 patients, intracranial haemorrhage in 35 (33.7%)/104 patients, umbilical cord bleeding in 58 (55.8%)/104. Impaired wound healing was seen in 30 (28.8%)/104 cases. Prophylactic treatment was initiated in 72 (69.2%). No treatment was required in 21 patients: 16 with mild deficiency, 3 with severe deficiency, 1 with B-subunit deficiency, 1 with FXIII inhibitors. So far the molecular defects have been detected in 50 (48.1%)/104 patients. Point mutations (predominantly missens) were found to be the most common type of mutations due to the higher proportion of hot-spot mutations at CpG dinucleotides. The most frequent mutation affecting F13A gene was a splice site mutation in intron 5 (IVS5–1G > A). This type of mutation in homozygous or heterozygous status was elucidated in 10 out of 50 analyzed individuals originating from 8 european countries. In year 2005, the ISTH FXIII and Fibrinogen subcommittee supported our initiative to enlarge the data of ETRO Working Party aiming the development of an international registry including clinical, phenotypic and genotypic data.

P8.18

Gene Polymorphisms Implicated in Influencing Susceptibility to Venous Thromboembolism: Association with Other Diseases?

B. Hoppe, T. Dörner, H. Kiesewetter, A. Salama

Charité – Universitätsmedizin Berlin, D

Perturbation of the hemostatic system is central to the pathogenesis of thrombosis affecting the venous system. In addition to environmental factors, which are well known to influence the risk of cardiovascular diseases (CVD), a multitude of hereditary factors have been implicated in influencing susceptibility to venous thromboembolism (VTE). The influence of these hereditary factors on other diseases was analyzed in the present study.

P8.19

HIT-II-Diagnostic

H. Alber, B. Schnabel, E. Förstemann

DRK-BSD Sachsen, Dresden, D

Antibodies against platelets. Evidence of high and low molecular heparines in lab testing. **Purpose:** Apart from the drop of platelets of up to 50% and/or new thromboembolic complications in heparine induced drop of platelets (HIT II) the unwanted side effect dreaded most is the building of heparine induced platelet antibodies. So tests to detect and specify those antibodies are an important tool in the different diagnosis. Over a period of five years probes of patients (hospital as well as out-patient-clinic) treated with heparine and suspected HIT II were tested. Included were patients with low platelet counts but missing symptoms. **Methods:** Tests used to detect and specify platelet antibodies

Particle Gel Immuno Assay
"Heparin/PF4 antibody test"
Aggregation test (HIPA) from A. Greinacher
Heparine derivates used for anticoagulation in the study
Heparin-Natrium (Heparin-Natrium)
Clexane* (Enoxaparin – Natrium)
Mono-Embolex* (Certoparin – Natrium)
Fraxiparin* (Nadroparin – Calcium)
Liquemin* (Heparin – Natrium)
Fragmin P* (Dalteparin – Natrium)

Results: In the study significant differences between the above mentioned heparine derivates could neither be found in relation towards the development of antibodies nor in their expression.

P9: Hemovigilance and Materiovigilance

P9.1

A Ten Years Experience of the Evaluation of Adverse Transfusion Reactions

E. Strobel

Klinikum Schwabing, München, D

Background: The evaluation of an adverse transfusion reaction is important for the further treatment of the involved patient, i.e. to prevent the patient from being exposed to the same offending agent in subsequent transfusions. On the other hand, reporting and analyzing transfusion complications is a preliminary condition for the risk management in transfusion medicine, especially for describing and assessing existing risks, communicating them and developing and performing measures to prevent them. **Materials and Methods:** As the basis for risk assessment of blood transfusion in a municipal hospital with more than 1000 beds we have analyzed all non-infectious transfusion complications that had been reported from 1996 to 2005 to our immunohaematological laboratory. If possible, the adverse transfusion reactions were evaluated for red blood cell incompatibility, sterility of the blood product, IgA deficiency of the recipient and – beginning from 1997 – for HLA-antibodies. **Results:** From 1996 to 2005 a total of 237 cases of suspected adverse transfusion reactions had been reported. In about 51% of the cases red blood cell concentrates were involved, in 40% platelet concentrates, in 4% fresh frozen plasma and in 4% more than one kind of blood product. The relative incidence of suspected adverse reactions was 0.24% for all blood products, 0.13% for red blood cell concentrates, 0.90% for platelet concentrates and 0.07% for FFP. The incidence of reports of adverse reactions in platelet transfusions showed a marked increase in the last two years, whereas the incidence in RBC transfusions was not significantly different. The symptoms were (on average of 10 years) febrile in about 27%, allergic in 40%, unspecific in 26% and in 4% a combination of symptoms was reported. Only the number of suspected cases of allergic reactions showed an obvious increase in the last year. In altogether 11 cases (2 of them in combination with other symptoms) a haemolytic transfusion complication was suspected, but in none of them a RBC incompatibility was found. **Conclusions:** General introduction of leukocyte depletion of blood products in 2001 had no obvious positive influence on the number of reports of adverse transfusion reactions in our hospital so far. The increased incidence of reported adverse reactions in platelet transfusions in the last 2 years may probably be due to a more sensitive reporting behaviour of the physicians as there had been no change in the kind of platelet concentrates (all from apheresis) used for transfusion in our hospital since 1996.

P9.2

Safety of Haemotherapy – Evaluation of the Haemovigilance Data 1999 – 2005 of the University of Muenster

C. Baumann, J. Recke, D. Stahl, W. Sibrowski
Institute of Transfusion Medicine, Münster, D

Background: The reporting of serious transfusion reactions (TR) has become mandatory since the new EU Blood Directive is implemented in November 2005. We here review transfusion-related events recorded in the University Clinic of Münster between 1999 and 2005. Since October 2001, only leucocyte-reduced ($<1 \times 10^6$ leucocytes per unit) blood components have been distributed. To study the role of leucoreduction we compared the transfusion related events before and afterwards introducing leucoreduction procedures. **Material and Methods:** 343,244 blood products, 177,380 packed red cells, 64,466 platelet concentrates (apheresis) and 101,398 fresh-frozen plasma (predominantly single donor plasma) were transfused (01.01.1999–01.06.2005). A transfusion reaction was identified when a clinical complication occurred in relation to a determined blood product according to a modified classification of Bux et al. (7TM European Haemovigilance Seminar London 2005): Definitions of transfusion-related events (TRE): ICT = immunological complication of transfusion; ICT,a = acute non haemolytic transfusion reaction, non febril; ICT,b = acute non haemolytic transfusion reaction, febril; ICT,c = acute haemolytic transfusion reaction; ICT,d = delayed transfusion reaction; ICT, V.a. TRALI = transfusion-related acute lung injury; CC/MC: with cardial component or metabolic component; TTI = transfusion transmitted infection; PUCT = previously unknown complication of transfusion. The severity of reactions was graded according to a score system: Slight, moderate, severe or most severe. **Results:** The incidence of transfusion reactions (n = 591) was 2.9 per 1000 blood products delivered to patients. Transfusion errors and near miss events were analysed separately. Platelet concentrates gave rise to a significantly greater number (n = 256, 4 per 1000) of adverse events than packed red cells (n = 234, 1.32 per 1000) or fresh-frozen plasma (n = 69, 0.7 per 1000). 27 cases could not finally be classified because of incomplete documentation.

TRE	RBC 177,380	TR	+CC/MC	Plt 64,466	TR	+CC/MC	FFP 101,398	TR	+CC/MC
ICT,a		155	68		216	44		56	18
ICT,b		71	18		38	13		10	4
ICT,c		4	2						
ICT,d									
ICT, V.a. TRALI		2	2		1	1			
TTI		2	1		1			3	2
PUCT									
Transfusion errors		4						1	

	Slight	Moderate	Severe	Most severe
RBC	80 (34%)	119 (51%)	16 (7%)	19 (8%)
Plt	147 (58%)	88 (34%)	14 (5%)	7 (3%)
FFP	37 (54%)	21 (30%)	6 (9%)	5 (7%)

Conclusions: 1. Most reactions were benigne and without long-term side-effects. 2. The incidence and the type of transfusion reactions was different with the blood product distributed. 3. Non febrile acute non haemolytic transfusion reactions were the most frequent observed transfusion-related events. 4. Allergic reactions were observed more frequently with platelet concentrates than with red packed cells or FFP. 5. No significant difference in the profile of adverse transfusion reactions were observed after implementation of general leucoreduction procedures of blood components. There is a need to classify and report more precisely and uniform transfusion reactions and transfusion-related events in order to obtain an internationally comprehensive haemovigilance system. Certain adverse transfusion reactions like the delayed transfusion reaction or TRALI may be underestimated by the clinicians in this study.

P9.3

Epidemiology of HIV, HCV and HBV Infections in about 1.4 Million Voluntary, Non-Remunerated Blood Donations of the German Red Cross Blood Donor Service Baden-Wuerttemberg-Hessen in the Year 2005

E. Schellenberg[1], S. Findhammer[1], K. Frank[2], M. Loehr[3], G. Geusendam[4], T. Dengler[5], U. Mayr-Wohlfahrt[6], M. Schmidt[1], E. Seifried[1], W. Sireis[1]
[1]DRK Blutspendedienst Baden-Württemberg, Frankfurt, D; [2]DRK Blutspendedienst Sachsen, Plauen, D; [3]DRK Blutspendedienst Berlin und Brandenburg, Cottbus, D; [4]DRK Blutspendedienst Schleswig-Holstein, Luetjensee, D; [5]DRK Blutspendedienst Baden-Württemberg-Hessen, Baden-Baden, D; [6]DRK Blutspendedienst Baden-Württemberg-Hessen, Ulm, D

Background and Objective: Surveillance of infectious disease markers in the blood donor population is of high value to estimate the prevalence and incidence of transfusion relevant infections. Here we estimate the prevalence and incidence of HIV, HBV and HCV among non-remunerated voluntary blood donors of the German Red Cross Blood Donor Service Baden-Wuerttemberg-Hessen in 2005. **Study Design and Methods:** Laboratory testing of 1,361,481 blood and plasma donations for anti-HIV 1,2, anti-HCV, HBsAg and HIV 1, HCV, HBV Pool-NAT, were evaluated with regard to the prevalence of the respective infection. Repeat reactive samples were additionally confirmed by HIV-, HCV-Immunoblot, HBsAg-Neutralization test and ID-NAT. To calculate the prevalence, reactive donors were estimated within different age groups related to all blood donations within this group. The incidence was calculated from the reactive donations from repeat donors only. **Results:** Within 1.4 million voluntary, non-remunerated blood donations, 15 donations were confirmed reactive for HIV, 119 for HCV and 218 for HBV, respectively. Among these 5 first time donors were positive for HIV, 103 for HCV and 207 for HBV. In contrast, 10 repeat donors seroconverted for HIV, 16 for HCV and 11 for HBV. The calculated prevalence per 10E5 donations was 4.42 for HIV, 91.99 for HCV and 183.10 for HBV. The incidence per 10E5 donations was 0.88 for HIV, 1.40 for HCV and 0.97 for HBV. As expected, there was a higher prevalence of HCV and HBV in older donors and males. In contrast, young males appeared to have the highest incidence for HIV with 4.7/10E5 among 18–24 year old donors and 2.9/10E5 in 35–44 year old donors, respectively. **Conclusion:** The prevalence and incidence of the transfusion relevant viruses HCV, HIV and HBV is considerable low in the population of non-remunerated voluntary german blood donors. Confirmed positive blood donations due to seroconversion were 66-times lower for HCV and 188-times lower for HBV compared to the prevalence in first time donors per 10E5 donations, supporting the view that a selected and large population of repeat blood donors contributes to a safe blood supply.

P10: Quality Management and Regulatory Affairs

P10.1

Whole Blood Donation without Prior Hemoglobin Testing – a Comfortable Alternative for Donors with Sufficient Historical Hemoglobin Values?

M. Ziemann, D. Steppat, C. Brockmann, H. Kirchner, G. Washington, P. Schlenke
Universitätsklinikum Schleswig-Holstein, Lübeck, D

Purpose: Prior to whole blood donation, hemoglobin (Hb) measurement is required. Selecting donors for prephlebotomy Hb testing according to their last predonation Hb could avoid unnecessary finger pricks or additional venous punctures. Especially after prolonged interdonation intervals the usefulness of this strategy is unknown. **Methods:** Predonation Hb levels were measured in 81913 consecutive donors using diversion samples. As these results were not available in time to defer donors with low Hb, donor admission was based on historical Hb values. Only donors with historical Hb values below 129 g/L or 139 g/L for females and males, respectively, underwent additional venous Hb measurement prior to donation using an automated hematology analyzer. All other donations were collected without prephlebotomy Hb testing. Hb values from diversion samples were analyzed grouping donors according to interdonation intervals of less than 6 months, 6 months to 1 year, 1 to 2 years and 2 years or more. **Results:** Independently of interdonation intervals, the screening resulted in an excellent accuracy of 95 to 96%. Sensitivities for detecting donors with Hb levels below the limits of 125 g/L and 135 g/L for female and male donors, respectively, were 56% after interdonation intervals of less than 6 months, 59% after 6 to 11 months and 67% after 12 to 23 months and 24 or more months. Donors with Hb levels below 110 g/L were detected with sensitivities of 86%, 82%, 88% and 80%, respectively. All sensitivities were at least comparable with results reported for capillary Hb screening. Selecting donors spared 77.7% from additional venous punctures or finger pricks and showed a specificity of 29%. Only 13 donors (0.016%) were bled despite Hb levels below 110 g/L. **Conclusions:** Donors with sufficient historical Hb levels can safely be admitted to whole blood donation without prior Hb measurement even after prolonged interdonation intervals. As only 126 donors in our study had interdonation intervals beyond 40 months, predonation Hb testing of this subgroup seems prudent.

P10.2

Qualification of Olympus PK7300 Automated Blood Type Analyser

F. Reinhardt[1], G. Galle[2], B. Siebert[3], G. Geusendam[3]
[1]DRK-Blutspendedienst Sachsen, Plauen, D; [2]DRK-Blutspendedienst Sachsen, Chemnitz, D; [3]DRK-Blutspendedienst Nord, Lütjensee, D

Background: Proof of correct blood typing as well as qualification of a complex analysis system require the use of predefined guidelines for performing a design, installation, functional and performance qualification of the device in the framework of a method validation. **Material and Methodology:** With the introduction of the new Olympus PK7300 automated blood type analyser by the DRK (German Red Cross) Blood Donation Service in Saxony and the North, comprehensive qualification documentation needed to be created in order to prove the functional capability of the analyser and the correct blood typing. A requirement specification was created by the users in the course of the design qualification on the basis of which key functionalities for automated blood typing were defined. Practically all requirements were already considered by the device manufacturer in the enhanced development of the device and were also already included in the specification. Using the procedure defined in the quality management system, the qualification focused on technical features rather than validation of the methodology, as this is already applied successfully worldwide in the previous model, the Olympus PK7200. **Result:** In the framework of the installation, function and performance qualification, important system modules were assessed in accordance with the requirements of the Common Technical Specification. Following the successful device qualification, the methodology for automated blood typing was validated on the basis of a comparative investigation of over 3,000 samples. The blood typing performed in parallel on the PK7200 compared with the PK7300 in the period between November 25 2004 and March 03 2005 at the DRK Blood Donation Service in the North (Lütjensee Institute) and between September 21 2005 and September 28 2005 at the DRK Blood Donation Service in Saxony (Chemnitz Institute) found no deviations in the typing of AB0-, D, C, c, E, e and Kell features. **Conclusion:** The use of the algorithm for device qualification, which is prescribed in the quality management system of the DRK Blood Donation Service of Baden-Württemberg and Hessen as well as the DRK Blood Donation Services of Saxony and the North as its subsidiaries, allows the successful qualification of the Olympus PK7300 automated blood type analyser. The requisite organisation and coordination of activities from a number of areas can only take place in the framework of a validation team, in which employees responsible for quality management, Data Processing and lab departments cooperate together with key personnel according to the principles of AMG (Medical Preparations Act).

P10.3

Interference of PLT Activation in-vitro on the Reliability of Measuring PLT Count and Function: Insights by the Retention Test of Homburg-II (RTH-II)

M.A. Nemeh, P. Mestres, E. Morgenstern, J. Schenk
University of Saarland, Homburg-Saar, D

Purpose: Reliable measurements of PLT count (PC) and function are essential to control the hemostatic system and to optimize a restrictive transfusion policy. PLT response to activation was assessed by RTH-II. The retention index (RI) of PLT (PLT-RI) indicates the percentage of PC decrease in the a.F blood (after passing an athrombogenic filter forced by shear stress). **Methods:** Serial precision and variability of PC and PLT-RI were evaluated by reflecting their interactions with the RIs of leucocytes (WBC-RI) and erythrocytes (RBC-RI). 10 mL isotonic citrated whole blood (1:10) prepared from healthy individuals was distributed into a series of 10 Eppendorf retention tubes (0.5 mL each), then centrifuged simultaneously (110 g/5 min). CBC and phase-contrast microscopy were performed before (b.F) and after passing the filter. Increasing time intervals were used for a.F measurements of each series. a.F blood was mixed by vortex: (a) 1–3 min as in previous RTH procedures, (b) <3 sec slight vortex as standardized in RTH-II. Wilcoxon and spearman tests were used for statistical analysis. **Results:** All b.F measurements showed acceptable PC variations ($CV < 1.4\%$). Vortex (a) was applied on 7 series and (b) on 3 ones. Means and variations were substantially higher in series (a) vs. (b) (mean = 62.5% vs. 27.9%, SD = 14.8 vs. 3.7; $p < 0.0005$). PLT-RI values in series (a) correlated negatively with WBC-RI ($r = -0.82$; $p < 0.0005$) and increased by a.F time (30–180 min; $r = 0.717$; $p < 0.0005$). Compared with series (a), series (b) revealed significantly higher WBC-RI levels (a: −19.5% vs. b: +5.9%; $p < 0.0005$) positively correlated with PLT-RI ($r = 0.3$) with no increase by time. Similar but less pronounced effect revealed by RBC-RI (a: −6.2% vs. b: −3.7%; $p < 0.0005$). Phase-contrast microscopy of series (a) compared with (b) showed excessive a.F increases of stimulated PLT and PLT aggregates proportional to PLT-RI increases. The sizes of aggregates corresponded with WBC-RI and RBC-RI decreases. **Conclusion:** Aggressive mixing of PLT pre-stimulated by shear stress can lead to PLT hyperactivation demonstrated by PLT aggregates and false PLT-RI increases. This effect amplifies by time and associated with WBC-RI and RBC-RI decreases related to the sizes of aggregates and inversely to cell concentrations. These phenomena are eliminated by applying slight vortex mode implicating the improved reliability of RTH-II vs. RTH. Convenient blood handling is essential for reliable CBC and PLT function measurements.

P10.4

Development of Platelet Standard: New Perspectives on the Effect of the Platelet Medium by Using RTH-II Assay and Morphological Control

M.A. Nemeh, P. Mestres, E. Morgenstern, J. Schenk
University of Saarland, Homburg-Saar, D

Purpose: Commercial PLT preparations used to control PLT count (PC) are not useful as reference control for PLT function. We try to bridge this gap by developing PLT standard using RTH-II and morphological control for validating PC and PLT function. We focus herein on difficulties triggered by variant PLT mediums which may have also interest for transfusion of PLT preparations. **Methods:** PLT standard was prepared by 2 approaches. (A) Unstimulated fresh PLT: Citrated whole blood (cWB) was drawn from 15 healthy individuals, 10 mL each, and cPRP was prepared (110 g/30 min), filtered by gel chromatography (Sepharose 2B) to obtain isolated PLT (iPLT), then rested at 37°C/30 min. (B) Fixed PLT: cPRP was prepared from 15 healthy individuals, fixed, then washed by centrifugation (220 g/20 min) and resuspension. RTH-II was applied on cWB, iPLT unwashed (Suw) and washed (Sw) standards; 500 μL tested material was forced to pass an "athrombogenic" filter by centrifugation (110 g/5 min). PC and morphological control were done before and after passing the filter. Percentage of PC decrease (PLT-RI; PLT retention index) reflects PLT response to activation by shear stress while passing the filter. Significance was tested by spearman and paired sample t tests. **Results:** PLT-RI values of iPLT vs. cWB increased substantially (>95.7%; $p < 0.0005$) in samples 1–7 (60.6% vs. 32.1%) and similarly in samples 8–15 (93.3%, $p < 0.0005$; iPLT vs. cWB: 53.1% vs. 28.1%) despite applying longer resting periods (30–120 min) before performing RTH-II. PLT spreading proved these effects: iPLT were intact, unstimulated, well spread, and compared with cWB, more activated mainly after passing RTH filter. Washing fixed cPRP revealed sharply higher PLT-RI increases (489.3%: $p < 0.0005$; Suw: 5.8% vs. Sw: 34.2%) which was reflected by increased PLT stickiness and agglutinates, as proved by phase-contrast microscopy. **Conclusion:** PLT predisposition to activation seems to increase by partial absence of normal blood medium. Compared with sustained PLT, Potency of fixed PLT to compensate such effect is basically less and associated with extensive increase in stickiness and agglutination. Dynamic functional balance in hemostasis seems to be preserved by PLT interactions within normal blood medium. Further studies are required to set practical solutions for preparing PLT standard as well as to consider these phenomena in the clinical evaluation of PLT mediums to e.g. optimize the quality assurance of PLT concentrates.

P10.5

Transport of Blood Products in a New Unique System

D. Nehring[1], K. Bienert[1], D. Radke[2], R. Linke[3], J. Neuhaus[3], R. Knels[3]

[1]delta T, Giessen, D; [2]Transmed Medizintechnik, Bad Wünnenberg, D; [3]German Red Cross Blood Donation Service Saxony, Dresden, D

Purpose: At the moment the German Red Cross Blood Donation Service in Saxony (BSD) uses for the transport of blood products insulated boxes in conjunction with compressor cold vans. This solution is expensive and requires car modifications for the car room cooling. Moreover, it is harmful for the environment, due to the start of the motor 1/2 h before transport in order to pre-cool. To change the situation the BSD searched for boxes, which give adequate conditions to transport the several types of blood products in conjunction with commercial thermal stabilizing elements. **Methods:** To find an appropriate box the BSD defined the following conditions: thermal stability by one till max. quantity in conjunction with the elements, robust, washable, lightweight, RFID labels can be read trough the box material. All conditions we found by a commercial foam box (delta T, Giessen, Germany). This box was designed for whole blood, red blood cell, platelets and fresh frozen plasma transport. To validate the conditions we washed the box 100-times, tested the robustness and measured the temperature with several quantities of the different blood products at several places in the box under several temperature conditions and with calibrated sensors. **Results:** By testing the machine-washing procedure and the sturdiness the material stayed stable and clean. The test of the BSD gave input for redesign of the box in relation of the practicability. Furthermore, throughout the foam RFID-labels can be read. By the temperature tests for the different types of blood products we used different precooled thermal stabilizing elements (plasma: −30°C, red cells: 2 to 6°C, whole blood and platelets 22°C). First we found, that the wall thickness of the foam bottom of the box was not enough to conserve the temperature in some of the tested conditions. Another problem was the temperature stability by a small (1–4) number of red cell products and a maximum number (12) of whole bloods. After re-design with a thicker bottom, 4 instead of 2 levels for the cooling elements and a new top and grip the BSD tested the new prototypes again and found acceptable results for the red cells for 12 h, the whole blood for 6 h with one cooling plate. **Conclusion:** With this system it is possible to meet the quality requirements for the transport of blood products. Since there is only one size of insulated container for all blood products the system is very simple to use and parameters such as temperature stability, weight, filling capacity for blood products, volume of the box, stability of the box, the possibility of washing and the use of RFID tags inside make this system suitable for middle long transport in transfusion medicine.

P10.6

Free Haemoglobin (Free-Hb) – Validation of 2 Photometric Kits and New Reference Materials

T. Ristau, H. Nader

RECIPE Chemicals + Instruments Labortechnik, München, D

Purpose: Since the "Guide to the prevention, use and quality assurance of blood components" has been introduced by the Council of Europe (6th edition (2001)) the determination of free haemoglobin is recommended to blood donation centres as a marker for the quality of donated blood. The haemolysis rate should be lower than 0.8% of the erythrocytes. Additional free haemoglobin is determinated in medical laboritories in suspicion of haemolysis. The results of the INSTAND e. V. EQA-surveys have shown that more than 40% of the participants use the 3-wavelength method originally descibed by Harboe. Users of the cyanmethaemoglobin method are at the same share. **Methods:** Since around 3 years we offer control material for these methods and due to discussions with our customers we learnt that there is a need of commercial available validated kits for the determination of free haemoglobin. Therefore we decided to develop a ready to use kit for the two most used methods 3-wavelength and cyanmethaemoglobin method. Tested reference materials for clinical and blood donation purposes in independend available control ranges (3 levels clinical: around 50 mg/l and 3 levels blood donation: around 1,500 mg/l) will be intruded. **Results:** A easy sample preperation is the main characteristic of both commercial available ready to use kits (3-wavelength and cyanmethaemoglobin method). Methodical differences with view of application will be dicussed. Data like linearity, inter- and intraassay precision will be given and compared with each other in the poster. **Conclusions:** We had evalutated two easy to handle and full validated ready to use kits based on 3-wavelength and cyanmethaemoglobin method with a variety of reference materials. The disposable reference materials in 6 different concentration levels have a prominent long time stability. All materials comply with the determination of the IVD-directive and are labeled with CE sign.

P11: Virus and Bacterial Testing and Inactivation

P11.1

The Inactivation of Pathogens in Platelet Concentrates by UVB Is Strongly Improved in Unfixed Irradiation Bags

H. Mohr[1], A. Bayer[1], F. Tolksdorf[2], W.H. Walker[2], T.H. Müller[1]

[1]DRK-Blutspendedienst NSTOB, Springe, D; [2]MacoPharma, Langen, D

Background: A two-step procedure for the inactivation of pathogens in plasma-reduced platelet concentrates (PCs) was worked out, consisting of photodynamic treatment with thionine (Th)/light followed by irradiation with ultraviolet B light (UVB, wavelength range: 280–315 nm). Th/light is intended to inactivate viruses, UVB to inactivate bacteria and leukocytes. The efficacy of either treatment is mutually increased. That of UVB is, however, strongly reduced by the low UVB-permeability of PC suspensions. The aim of this study was to improve the efficacy of UVB irradiation, especially to inactivate bacteria. **Methods:** PCs in storage medium SSP+ (MacoPharma) containing approx. 30% plasma were prepared from pools of 5 buffy coats. PC-aliquots or complete PCs (volume approx. 330 mL) were spiked with up to 105 CFU/mL of bacteria or up to 107 TCID50/mL of viruses. Other samples were treated without spiking. Irradiation with UVB light was from both sides of the bags. In addition they were agitated at different speeds using different types of agitators. Before and after irradiation bacteria or virus titers or platelet parameters were measured. Sterility was tested by the BacT/Alert method. **Results:** PCs were spiked with S. epidermidis and irradiated with UVB at doses between 0.8 and 1.2 J/cm^2. Titer reduction in samples clamped between quartz plates during agitation was not more than approx. 1.5 log10 at all UV doses applied. In contrast in loose PCs the bacteria titers were reduced by 3 log10 at 0.8 and by 4–4.5 log10 at 1 and 1.2 J/cm². The inactivation of other bacteria and of viruses was also enhanced when the agitated samples remained unfixed during agitation. The efficacy of the improved procedure was tested in experiments in which PCs were prepared from blood units spiked with 10–25 CFU/mL of S. aureus. The fixed PCs could not be sterilized at UVB doses up to 1.5 J/cm², at which platelet functions were strongly impaired. In contrast 0.6 J/cm² were sufficient to sterilize those PCs which were loosely placed during irradiation. At this dose platelet functions were only moderately influenced, and the storage stability of the treated products for up to 6 days after treatment (8 days after blood donation) was maintained. **Conclusions:** Pathogen inactivation of PCs by UVB light is considerably improved when the PCs are not fixed and in addition agitated during irradiation. The UVB dose can be reduced to such an extent that platelet damage becomes marginal.

P11.2

Introducing Anti-HBC Screening in Germany – Possible Implications for the Blood Donation Service

T. Zeiler, R. Karger, J. Slonka, K. Radsak, V. Kretschmer
Universitätsklinikum Giessen und Marburg, Marburg, D

Background: The German "National advisory committee" (AK-Blut), recently recommended testing of blood and plasma donations for antibodies against the hepatitis B core antigen (anti-HBc). We assessed possible effects of this intended measure on donor deferral rate and look back procedures. **Study design and Methods:** 3,964 consecutive blood donors were tested for anti-HBc for the first time. Anti-HBc positive samples were further investigated employing an alternative anti-HBc test, quantitative determination of anti-HBs and HBV-NAT. **Results:** 46 (1.16%) of the samples were tested specifically anti-HBc positive. Following the recommendations of the "AK-Blut", 9 (0.23% of all) donors had to be permanently deferred. 8 of these were repeat donors and had already donated 353 blood components which had been transfused to 285 recipients during the past 17 years. **Conclusions:** Implementation of anti-HBc testing in Germany will result in an acceptable loss of blood donors. However, the realization of look back procedures is problematic due to the huge number of transfused blood components, the long period of time those donors gave blood, and particularly the impossibility to precisely determine the time of seroconversion.

P11.3

Photodynamic Inactivation of Human Hepatitis B Virus in Plasma-Reduced Platelet Concentrates as Revealed by Long-Range Real-Time PCR

J. Knüver-Hopf, U. Gravemann, H. Mohr, T.H. Müller
DRK-Blutspendedienst NSTOB, Springe, D

Purpose: There is no infectivity assay available to investigate whether human hepatitis B virus (HBV) is susceptible to virus inactivation procedures. One of the target structures of photodynamic treatment in the presence of photosensitizers like methylene blue (MB) or thionine (Th) is the viral nucleic acid. Inactivation of viruses therefore might be determined by PCR. Standard PCR (whose amplicon is 130 base pairs long), however detects no influence on the genome of HBV after treatment. We investigated whether HBV-DNA degradation is observed when a long-range real-time PCR (LR-PCR) is used in which the amplicon covers 1090 base pairs, i.e. approx. 1/3 of the HBV genome. For this approach we tested HBV-infected plasma-reduced platelet concentrates (PC) before and after Th/light/UVB treatment, and Th- or UVB-treatment alone. **Material and Methods:** PC in storage medium SSP+ (MacoPharma, Langen, Germany) containing approx. 30% plasma were prepared from pools of 4 buffy coats. Photodynamic treatment with Th/light was performed on a MacoTronic illumination device (MacoPharma, Langen, Germany). Th concentration was 1 μM, the light dose was 94 J/cm². Irradiation with UVB was carried out on a BioGenic irradiator (Vilber Lourmat, Marne La Vallee, France) emitting broad band UVB light (wavelength range 280–320 nm). UVB dose was 1.2 J/cm². The QIAamp Blood Mini Kit (QIAGEN, Hilden, Germany) was used for isolation of DNA from all samples. For LR-PCR the LightCycler was used (Roche, Mannheim, Germany). Primers and hybridization probes were synthesized by TIB MOLBIOL (Berlin, Germany). Primers were selected for the nucleotide positions 44–2187 of the circular HBV genome. **Results:** The copy numbers of HBV genome were lowered from approx. 10 × E6 /ml to approx. 10 × E4 /ml by treatment with Th/light/UVB, i.e. by 99%. By treatment with Th alone the copy numbers were still lowered by 79%. In contrast, HBV nucleic acid was much more resistent to UVB alone. **Conclusion:** The results of the LR-PCR assay demonstrate HBV nucleic acid destruction after photodynamic treatment with Th/light in combination with UVB irradiation. This suggests that hepatitis B virus in plasma-reduced platelet concentrates can be inactivated by this procedure.

P11.4

Performance of Real-Time RT-PCR in Routine Sterility Testing of Platelet Concentrates

M. Störmer, K. Kleesiek, J. Dreier
Herz- und Diabeteszentrum Nordrhein-Westfalen, D

Purpose: The risk of bacterial contamination of platelet concentrates (PCs) remains and is now the most frequent transfusion-related infectious adverse event. Therefore, a screening method allowing the early detection of very low levels of bacteria in PCs would improve transfusion safety. The aim of this study was to evaluate the applicability of our previous described real-time RT-PCR method as a routine screening system in blood banks. **Methods:** Based on spiking and growth studies, we implemented a detection strategy and instituted the bacterial screening into our routine diagnostic scope of duties. Since then, 540 apheresis-derived single donor platelets were tested by real-time RT-PCR while the BacT/Alert automated culturing system served as reference method served as the reference method. After standard processing of PCs and storage of up to 20 hours at 22°C with agitation, samples were taken under aseptic conditions and used for microbial and molecular sterility testing. Nucleic acids were extracted using an automated high-volume extraction method based on magnetic separation technology and real-time RT-PCR was performed using the "locked nucleic acid" (LNA) technology. To make the assay appropiate as a routine screening method, an internal control and run controls with low bacterial titers were implemented. **Results:** Of all 540 tested PCs, one was detected positive in culture (18 hours after sampling) and RT-PCR (4 hours after sampling) and documented as Staphylococcus warneri. All remainding specimens were tested negative. **Conclusions:** The PCR has a much shorter turnaround time than culture, facilitating the testing of PCs before release and therefore seems to be practical for use as a routine screening method.

P11.5

Does Donor Screening with Anti-HBc improve Safety of Blood Products?

E.-M. Zayc-Schmidt, L. Pichl, V. Schottstedt, A. Hoburg
DRK Blutspendedienst West, Hagen, D

Purpose: Routine-screening of donations with Anti-HBc is recommended and ruled by Votum 31 of the Arbeitskreis Blut, a committee composed of members of the Health Authorities, Plasma industry and the Blood Transfusion Services in Germany. Reports of healthy HBsAg negative HBV low level carriers with DNA amounts below the current sensitivity of HBV NAT pool testing led to these recommendations. **Methods:** All blood donations of the Red Cross Blood Transfusion Service West (approx. 1 million/year) are screened since 02/01/06 for Anti-HBc with the Monolisa Anti-HBc Plus (BioRad). Positive donations are retested twice with the Core AxSYM (Abbott), with AUSAB (Anti-HBs, Abbott) and a sensitive (12 IU/ml) single donor PCR for HBV (Roche Diagnostics, CAP/CTM). All donors with Anti-HBs <100 IU/l are deferred permanently. Reactive samples in HBV single donor PCR are reanalyzed in the Fresh Frozen Plasma of the donation to exclude contaminations in the initial sample tube. If HBV DNA is detected in the FFP, a report is sent to the Head of Drug Safety to decide whether former donations have to be checked in a look back performance. **Results:** 270,000 donations have been currently screened. 8070 Anti-HBc positive donors were identified in the Monolisa test and 5554 had also positive results in the Core AxSYM. For 1502 donors with Anti-HBs levels <100 IU/l these results led to permanent deferral. 20 of the 5554 donors with reproducible reactive Anti-HBc results and low Anti-HBs levels revealed initially positive single donor

HBV NAT. 6 of them (Anti-HBs from 0 to 13 IU/l) were confirmed by positive FFP testing. The look back performances are ongoing. **Conclusion:** We found 20 Anti-HBc positive donors who were HBsAg and HBV pool PCR (n = 96 donations) negative in routine testing but reactive in single donor HBV NAT. 6 of them had low amounts of HBV DNA (mostly <1.2 E + 1 IU/ml plasma) in the corresponding FFP. Whether these 6 donors were able to infect recipients in the past or had detectable amounts of HBV DNA in former donations can only be proved by thorough look back currently under investigation.

P11.6

Contamination of Platelet Concentrates with Klebsiella pneumoniae – Still at Risk?

M. Schmidt[1], S.-B. Nicol[2], K. Hourfar[1], W. Sireis[1], W. Weichert[1], E. Seifried[1], T. Montag[2]

[1]DRK Institut Frankfurt, Frankfurt, D; [2]Paul Ehrlich Institut, Langen, D

Background and Objectives: Platelet concentrates (PCs) are the most common source of transfusion-related sepsis. Approximately 1 in 2,000 to 1 in 3,000 units of PCs are contaminated with bacteria originating from the donor's skin or bloodstream. The risk of acquiring a bacterial infection through transfusion is currently 100 to 1,000 times higher than that of transfusion-associated viral infections. **Study Design and Methods:** A 58-year-old patient was transfused with an apheresis platelet concentrate (APC) after bone marrow transplantation. Only five minutes into transfusion, the patient was seized with shivering fits. His temperature rose to 39.8°C and blood pressure fell to 60/40 mmHg. The patient went into septic shock, was intubated and treated in an emergency care unit. He eventually died of multiple organ failure 24 days after infection. Bacterial cultures were taken from the recipient's blood samples and also from samples of the original platelet bags. **Results:** Klebsiella pneumoniae subspecies pneumoniae were detected in blood samples, as well as in the original PCs. DNA fingerprints authenticated the identity. Capsule type was determined as K62. The bacterial number exceeded 108 CFU/ml 24 hours after spiking with an inoculum of 1–10 CFU/ml, which demonstrated very rapid growth kinetics. LPS concentration also increased to 1 µg/mL. The bacterial strain was neither resistant to common antibiotics nor 70% isopropyl alcohol. **Conclusion:** Bacterial infection remains a risk in transfusion medicine. Screening methods or pathogen inactivation methods should add significantly to blood safety.

P11.7

Should Anti-HBc be Introduced in the Screening of Blood Donations?

C. Drexler[1], M. Bayer[1], M. Riegelnegg[1], M.Schmidt[2], S. Sipurzynski[1], M. Vadon[1], G.Lanzer[1]

[1]Medizinische Universität Graz – Uniklinik für Blutgruppenserologie und Transfusionsmedizin, Graz, A; [2]DRK Hessen, Frankfurt/Main, D

Purpose: In Austria a screening of blood donations is mandatory for HBV, HCV and HIV and is performed by serological and molecular diagnostic methods. For HBV the Nucleic acid amplification testing (NAT) is done voluntarily. **Methods:** Screening methods include a serological search for HCV antibodies (Ortho HCV 3.0), HIV antibodies (Enzygnost Anti-HIV1/2 Plus) and HBs antigen (Enzygnost HBsAg 5.0). Negative samples are tested by real time PCR in a maximum pool size of 96 (DRK Hessen). 20368 blood units were additionally tested by anti-HBc (Enzygnost Anti-HBc monoclonal). **Results:** Since the introduction of NAT testing in April 1999 until December 2005, we have screened 421,465 blood donations. 576 (0.14%) samples were found to be repeatedly positive in serological testings for anti-HCV, 319 for anti-HIV (0.08%), and 576 for HBs antigen (0.14%). Within the ELISA-negative donations, no HCV- or HIV-RNA was detected. One HBsAg- and anti-HBs-nonreactive anti-HBc-reactive blood donor was discovered by NAT as being a low level carrier. HBV was quantified with 50 IU/mL, genotype was D. This led to the question whether a general screening for anti-HBc should be adopted. Therefore, 20,368 blood units were additionally tested by anti-HBc. 713 (3.5%) samples were found positive and were retested with a second ELISA (Axsym Core) of which 296 (1.5%) were still positive. 39 donations were positive for HBsAg and another 5 showed positive results for both, anti-HBc and HBsAg. None was confirmed positive neither by neutralization assay nor by single-sample PCR. On all HBsAg negative samples a pool PCR was performed, however, no HBV-DNA was detected. **Conclusions:** The purpose of PCR implementation was a reduction of viral transmission by transfusion of blood components. This summary of our screening results shows that an introduction of routine anti-HBc testing would lead to a maximal loss of further 1.5% of blood donations. Since the only HBV positive donation was detected by pool PCR, the implementation of anti-HBc testing does not seem to be essential in terms of safety in blood products.

P11.8

Results of Eight Years Screening for HBV with Highly Sensitive Pool-NAT in German Red Cross Blood Donor Services Saxony, Berlin and Brandenburg

K. Gubbe[1], K. Frank[1], M. Loehr[2], A. Karl[1]

[1]DRK-Blutspendedienst Sachsen, Plauen, D; [2]DRK Blutspendedienst Berlin und Brandenburg gGmbH, Cottbus, D

Purpose: Our PCR-Lab started in 1998 with routine NAT-screening for HCV, HIV and HBV. Although HBV-NAT screening is on a voluntary basis, HBV NAT has become a standard in blood donor screening in Germany. To detect low viremic donors in the window period highly sensitive pool-NAT is needed. Up to now no commercial test for plasma pools of 96 donations is available with a sensitivity around 100 IU HBV/ml in the single donation. **Method:** We adapted Baxter's IQ-PCR by changing the pool-size (96 donations), the parameters for enrichment of viruses by ultracentrifugation and the extraction method. The 95% detection limit was determined by probit analysis. The analytical sensitivity is 11.1 IU HBV per ml and 107 IU HBV per ml in the single donation. HBV genotypes A-G are detected with comparable sensitivity. Assay specificity was high (99.97%), 1.35% of all tests were invalid. **Results:** Since 1998 3,729,537 donations were screened. Six HBV-PCR-only-positive donations were detected. One of these donations was also found anti-HBc-positive in the confirmation testing. Five window phase donations with titers from 7.6 to 229 IU/ml were identified. The detection rate of window-period units was calculated to be one in 621,589 donations. All these donation were serologically screened for HBsAg with Abbott Prism. By using an alternative experimental PCR-System with a modified Qiagen extraction for pools of 96 donations enhanced analytical sensitivity of about 60 IU/ml in the single donation can be reached. **Conclusions:** When screening all blood donations for HBsAg with Abbott Prism an additional benefit can only be reached with a highly sensitive HBV-pool-PCR. The yield of HBV-Pool-NAT was higher than that of HIV- and HCV-Pool-NAT in the mentioned period. We could show that our HBV-pool-NAT efficiently detects window phase donations and is a useful tool to increment the safety of blood products.

P11.9

Single-Run Parallel Detection of Bacteria in Platelet Concentrates by PCR

H. Kojzar[1], M. Bayer[2], M. Prischl[1], M. Vadon[2], G. Lanzer[2], F. Turnowsky[1]

[1]Karl-Franzens-Universität Graz – Institut für Molekulare Biowissenschaften, Graz, A; [2]Universitätsklinik für Blutgruppenserologie und Transfusionsmedizin, Graz, A

Purpose: Bacterial transmission remains a significant problem in transfusion medicine, and platelet concentrates (PC) are responsible for the majority of bacterial transmissions due to the required storage of the product at 22°C. The risk of bacterial platelet contamination is approximately 1 in 2000 cases. The present standard for detection of bacterial contaminations in PC is an automated bacterial blood culturing system which is very sensitive, but requires some time of cultivation. Therefore, the development of sensitive, but faster methods – such as molecular diagnostic methods – is required. **Methods:** The PCR-assay was optimized with cultures of Bacillus cereus, Escherichia coli, Staphylococcus aureus and Klebsiella pneumoniae. DNA was extracted using the NucleoSpin® Tissue Kit (Macherey-Nagel). Universal 16S rRNA gene primers were used for all tested bacterial strains combined with standard Taq DNA polymerase (Fermentas Life Sciences). In order to test the efficiency of each specific PCR reaction, an internal standard using a yeast gene was established. After optimizing the assay, also spiked PCs were tested and the detection limit for bacterial contaminations was determined. **Results:** Using bacterial cultures, our method showed high sensitivity and detected 10–25 cfu per ml. Under optimized conditions no cross reactions of bacterial DNA with human DNA was observed and no false positive results were caused by reagent contaminations. In spiked PCs bacterial concentrations of less than 100 cfu per ml could be detected by this PCR method. **Conclusions:** We have designed a molecular assay based on a single run polymerase chain reaction (PCR) for detection of bacteria in PC. Until now our work is not completely finished, but our assay allows a cheap and easy way for detecting bacterial contaminations in PC. It is planned to modify the assay in order to detect other pathogens, like Candida albicans, as well.

P11.10

Evaluation of the Greiner EDTA-Gel-Vacuette System for Prolonged Storage of Plasma

K. Gubbe, A. Karl
DRK-Blutspendedienst Sachsen, Plauen, D

Purpose: Preanalytical factors are cruisal for sensitive virus screening by PCR. Plasma sample tubes with gel barrier are standard for such applications. Manufacturers recommend for an optimal stability of viruses a maximum storage time of six hours from sampling to centrifugation. Due to logistical problems in blood donor services a longer storage time than recommended would be of great value. Our goal was to show virus stability in Greiner EDTA-Gel-Vacuette tubes for a time of up to 24 hours from sampling. **Methods:** Fifteen tubes from every three donors were collected. HBV, HCV, HIV, HAV and Parvovirus-B19 were spiked into the 5 ml tubes with a titer of three times of the 95% cut off of the respective NAT. At 6, 15 and 24 hours storage at room temperature five tubes were centrifuged, frozen at –30°C and then unfreezed. 1 ml plasma from each sample was immediately tested for HBV, HCV, HIV, HAV and Parvovirus-B19. NAT testing was done with an adapted Baxter IQ PCR-system. **Results:** Virus was detected in all samples at the time six and fifteen hours after sampling. 24 hours after sampling HCV, HIV, HBV and Parvovirus-B19 could be found in five from five samples from the three donors. Only four samples from donor three were HAV-PCR-positive at 24 hours after sampling. No haemolysis could be noticed. The gel barriere reliably separated the cells from plasma not only at 6 hours after sampling but also at 24 hours. **Conclusion:** The stability of HBV, HCV, HIV, HAV and Parvovirus-B19 in blood samples is guaranteed in Greiner EDTA-Gel-Vacuette-tubes not only at six hours after sampling as recommended from the manufacturer but also up to 24 hours when stored at room temperature. One falsely HAV-negative result at 24 hours corresponds to the statistical probability as in total 225 tests were done. Only 99 from 100 tests become correctly positive at a virus titer of three times of the 95% cut off of the PCR. The complete separation of the cells from the plasma by the gel barrier is guaranteed after 24 hours storage.

P11.11

Transmission of Hepatitis B Virus by a HBsAg-Negative Early Window-Phase Donation

D. Deuble, A. Ender, U. Sugg
Zentralinstitut für Transfusionsmedizin und Blutspendedienst, Stuttgart, D

Purpose: Continuous improvements of blood donor selection and testing protocols have nearly eliminated the risk of HIV or HCV transmission by blood donations. Meanwhile, the focus of interest is put back to posttransfusion hepatitis B. The main reasons for residual risk of HBV transmission include blood collected within the HBsAg-negative window-period of early infection and the existence of chronic carriers with either very low levels of HBsAg or mutant forms of HBV, both escaping detection by current available HBsAg assays. **Case Report:** We report on a multiple-time donor with an asymptomatic acute hepatitis B virus infection who was tested negative by PRISM HBsAg assay in all consecutive donations at the blood bank Stuttgart. **Results:** One donation during the early window-phase of HBV infection contained 725 viral genome copies/ml which was recognized by retrospective pool HBV NAT testing. The recipient of the red blood-cell concentrate remained asymptomatic but showed positive results for anti-HBc and anti-HBs by follow-up testing. Another donation given four months later was retrospectively tested positive for anti-HBc but negative for the presence of HBV-DNA and the recipient of the erythrocyte concentrate showed no evidence for HBV infection. **Conclusion:** This case report demonstrates that HBV transmission of an early window-phase donation could have been prevented by sensitive pool HBV NAT testing but not by anti-HBc testing. The transmission of approximately 1.5×104 viral genome copies to the recipient did not cause any severe health damage and presumably induced immunity.

P11.12

Storage Stability of Theraflex MB-Plasma after 15 Month and Blueflex Filtration Efficiency

S. Reichenberg
Maco Pharma International, Langen, D

Purpose: Virus transmission due to blood products has decreased during the last decades thanks to the introduction of sophisticated testing procedures. Nevertheless, a residual risk still exists. Additionally, the possible appearance of newly emerging viruses in the transfusion chain cannot be neglected. In order to further improve the viral safety of plasma MacoPharma developed the Theraflex MB-Plasma system. It consists of a bag system with a plasma filter (Plasmaflex), Methylene Blue (MB) pill, an illumination bag, a MB retention filter (Blueflex), and a storage bag and includes illumination at 180 J/cm^2 at 590 nm using a Macotronic illumination device. It is of critical importance that a virus inactivation system does not impair the plasma quality. Therefore, the plasma quality after 15-month storage and the efficiency of the methylene blue and photoproduct reduction was tested. **Methods:** 18 plasmas from whole blood were treated within 6 h after donation at three different days. At different steps of the Theraflex MB-Plasma procedure the MB and photoproduct content was measured by HPLC, which was described previously. At each day plasma was pooled and divided into several storage bags. At different time following plasma factors were measured.

1. Global tests (Quick, INR, aPTT, thrombin time)
2. Coagulation factors (Fibrinogen, F II, F V, F VII, F VIII:c, F IX, F X, F XI, F XII, FXIII, vWF Ristocetin Co-Factor)
3. Inhibitors (AT III, Protein C, Protein S)
4. Fibrinolysis (Plasmin inhibitor, alpha-1-Antitrypsin, Plasminogen)
5. Complement (CH50, C3a)
6. Activation (TAT, F XIIa, D-Dimer)

Results: Illumination of MB-containing plasma with visible light using the Macotronic illumination device resulted in the generation of photoproducts. Mean reduction of the total phenothiazine content was 94.5%. Every single filtration yielded in a filtration efficiency of minimum 91%. The mean reduction capacity for MB was above 99.9%. There was no significant change in the plasma factor content after treatment during the whole 15-month storage period. The only difference between the plasma parameters resulted from the treatment itself. Here, an increase in the INR and aPTT (+14.3%; +18.2%), decrease of fibrinogen (−19.3), factor V (−25.3%), factor VIII (−21.8%), factor IX (−25.6%), factor X (−23.4%), and factor XI (−16.8%) was observed. Despite this variations the values were within the ranges found in non-treated plasma. **Conclusions:** Even after 15-month storage the Theraflex MB plasma had a satisfactory quality regarding the activity and composition of plasma factors. MB and photoproducts are depleted by at least 1 log10 step due to the Blueflex filtration step.

P11.13

Implementation of Anti-HBc Blood Donor Screening – Outcome with Regard to HbsAg Negative, HBV NAT Negative, Anti-HBc Positive Blood Donors

W. Sireis[1], E. Schellenberg[1], S. Findhammer[1], K. Frank[2], A. Karl[2], G. Geusendam[3], T. Dengler[1], M. Loehr[4], M. Schmidt[1], E. Seifried[1]
[1]DRK Blutspendedienst Baden-Württemberg-Hessen, Frankfurt, D; [2]DRK Blutspendedienst Sachsen, Plauen, D; [3]DRK Blutspendedienst Schleswig-Holstein, Luetjensee, D; [4]DRK Blutspendedienst Berlin und Brandenburg, Cottbus, D

Background and Objectives: Despite availability of sensitive screening assays for hepatitis B virus surface antigen (HBsAg) and mini-pool NAT, occasional cases of HBV-viremic donors still occur. While only few knowledge about the infectivity of such donors exists, there have been reports describing HBV transmissions due to the transfusion of low titer viremic blood components. To further reduce this risk, the Paul-Ehrlich-Institute (Langen, Germany) has forced the implementation of anti-HBc testing as additional screening marker. Here we describe the outcome of anti-HBc testing after implementation in the German Red Cross Blood Donor Service Baden-Wuerttemberg-Hessen in February 2006. **Study Design and Methods:** Laboratory testing of 345,025 blood donations was evaluated for the presence of anti-HBc. Repeat reactive samples were then further analysed for their anti-HBs titre and for the presence of HBV-DNA. First time donors with repeat reactive Anti-HBc results and repeat donors with additional Anti-HBs titres <100 IU/L and/or DNA positivity were rejected from further blood donations. A "Look Back" procedure was initiated for NAT-positive repeat donors or donors that presented with seroconversion. **Results:** Among 345,025 blood donations 1.34% were repeat reactive for Anti-HBc when negative for HBsAg (1.21% repeat donors and 0.13% first time donors). Among these the anti-HBs-titre was >100 IU/L in 71.8% repeat donors and 65% first time donors. In total 8/185,000 donors were HBV ID-NAT positive (Anti-HBs < 100 IU/L), of which 6 were repeat donors and 2 first time donors. All 8 samples were HBsAg as well as mini-Pool-NAT negative. Look back in 6 Anti-HBc-positive repeat donors is still ongoing. **Conclusion:** Our data show that some blood donors and donations have a history of hepatitis B, which was not identified by HBsAg and mini-Pool-NAT only. From the current data we can not conclude if these donations reflect recent or older infections, respectively. Therefore, the infectious status of such donations is still uncertain and it will need further look back investigations to comment on this important issue. However, the exclusion of Anit-HBc positive donors with Anti-HBs titres <100 IU/L is an important measure to improve the safety of blood components.

P11.14

Introduction of Anti-HBc Testing in Routine Donor Typing

F.F. Wagner, C. Jork, U. Bauerfeind
DRK Blutspendedienst NSTOB, Springe, D

Purpose: Anti-HBc testing was adviced to detect low level carriers of HBV. We started routine Anti-HBc testing in our blood service in February 2006. **Methods:** All donations (including laboratory tests of first time donors not allowed to donate) were tested using Enzygnost Anti-HBc monoclonal (Behring). Reactive donations were checked using AxSym Anti-HBs (Abbott) and COBAS AmpliPrep/COBAS TaqMan HBV Test (95% detection limit: 12 IU/ml). Donations with less than 10 mIU/ml anti-HBs were further evaluated for Anti-HBc, Anti-HBc IgM, Anti-HBe and HBeAg using AxSym tests. The incidence of Anti-HBc reactive donations were checked for eight weeks (minimal redonation interval for whole blood donation) after start of anti-HBc testing. Furthermore, anti-HBe results were checked during the initial 4 weeks. **Results:** Within eight weeks, we tested 14008 first time donations (FTD) and 109556 repeat donations (RD). The following constellations were detected: Anti-HBc reactive, Anti-HBs >100 mIU/ml: FTD 1.14%, RD 1.18%. Anti-HBc reactive, Anti-HBs between 10 and 100 mIU/ml: FTD 0.49%; RD 0.30%. Anti-HBc reactive (Behring and Abbott), Anti-HBs <10 mIU/ml: FTD 0.72%, RD 0.36%. Anti-HBc reactive (Behring only), Anti-HBs <10 mIU/ml: FTD 0.25%, RD 0.21%. Among 216 donations with Anti-HBs <10 checked for anti-HBe, 38 were reactive. All but two of these were reactive in both the Behring and Abbott Anti-HBc tests. In contrast, only 74 of 187 Anti-HBe negative samples were reactive in both Anti-HBc tests. To check the HBc reactive samples of RD 2245 single PCRs for HBV-DNA have been performed. Of these 0.7% (16) were initially reactive but only 0.09% (2) were repeatedly (twice) reactive by PCR. **Conclusion:** The introduction of Anti-HBc testing according to Votum 31 and the PEI Stufenplan strategy leads to the loss of 0.89% or repeat donors. Using a HBV PCR with a sensitivity of 12 IU/ml, the rate of PCR positive, occult HBV infected donors is lower than anticipated. Anti-HBe may be a useful parameter to proof contact with HBV virus and to exclude non-specific Anti-HBc reactivity.

P11.15

Single Sample Testing of Anti-HBc Positive, HBsAg Negative Blood Donations

M. Weber-Schehl[1], D. Hedges[1], F. Weinauer[2]
[1]Blutspendedienst des BRK, Wiesentheid, D; [2]Blutspendedienst des BRK, München, D

Purpose: To investigate the rate of anti-HBc positive donations with detectable HBV DNA, a sensitive single sample PCR of anti-HBc positive, HBsAg negative blood donations was performed. **Methods:** All blood donations collected at the Bavarian Red Cross were screened for Hepatitis B surface antigen (HBsAg) and antibodies to Hepatitis B Core antigen (anti-HBc) by chemiluminescent assay (ChLIA, ABBOTT). In addition to german guidelines all blood donations were routinely screened for Hepatitis B virus DNA by inhouse-PCR in minipools with a sensitivity of 930 IU/ml (95% hit rate). From all anti-HBc repeat reactive donations anti-HBs was determined (AUSAB, ABBOTT). PCR testing of anti-HBc repeat reactive donations was performed in a single sample PCR with a sensitivity of 13 IU/ml (95% hit rate). **Results:** Since september 2001 3,643 anti-HBc repeat reactive, HBsAg negative blood donations were tested in a single sample PCR for HBV DNA. Out of these, three donations were identified with detectable HBV DNA (0.08%). Virus particle concentrations were far below detection limit of routine screening, therefore they could not be identified in routine screening. Only one of the three identified donations showed detectable levels of anti-HBs. **Conclusions:** Low level of HBV DNA could be detected in anti-HBc positive, HBsAg negative blood donations. Screening for antibodies to Hepatitis B Core antigen could identify potentially infectious blood donations from HBsAg negative carriers.

P12: Viral Diseases

P12.1

Progression of HIV/AIDS and Association to the HLA Allelic Diversity in the Sudanese Population

N. Elamin[1], P.A. Horn[1], M. Elbashir[2], I.M. Elkhidir[2], G. Elghazali[2], R. Blasczyk[1]
[1]Medizinische Hochschule Hannover, D; [2]University of Khartoum, SD

Purpose: So far 12,369 cases of HIV/AIDS have been officially reported to the Sudanese National AIDS Control Program, since the 1st case was described in 1986. However, the true frequency of HIV/AIDS cases in Sudan is not known. There are several described associations between HLA types and pathogenic features of HIV-I infections and progression to AIDS. This applies not only to single alleles, such as B35, which is considered a major risk factor for the development of AIDS and for more rapid progression to AIDS in subjects with hemophilia. Also certain haplotypes, for example HLA-A1-B8-DR3 have been reported to be associated with rapid AIDS progression and with a rapid loss of CD4+ lymphocytes. However, there is evidence that HLA associations of disease progression significantly differs in different ethnic groups. It was therefore the objective of the current study to analyse the relationship between HLA typing and the progression to AIDS in the Sudanese population. **Methods:** The three ethnic groups representing the majority of the Sudanese population were studied: Nilo-Saharan, Niger-Congo and Afro-Asiatic. A total of 120 patients and 200 controls were sequenced for HLA-A, -B, -C, -DRB1 and DQB1 to get allele level typing. **Results and Conclusions:** In the course of our study we identified novel HLA alleles in 1.25% of our study subjects, hinting at the yet insufficiently explored HLA diversity in this population. For HLA class I alleles so far no statistical significant correlation with HIV/AIDS progression could be identified. However, for HLA class II alleles we found a positive correlation between HLA-DRB1*0804-DQB1*0201, DRB1*1302-DQB1*0501 and a rapid progression from HIV infection to AIDS, whereas DRB1*1101-DQB1*0301 correlated with a slow progression.

P13: Blood Component Production

P13.1

In-vitro Quality of RBCs Collected by Multicomponent Apheresis Compared to Manually Collected RBCs during 49 Days of Storage

S.M. Picker, S. Radojska, B. Gathof
Klinikum der Universität zu Köln, D

Background: New technological developments enable the automated collection and preparation of RBCs. The purpose of this study was to evaluate quality of apheresis-derived RBCs (ARBCs) collected as double (2-RBCs) or as single units (along with PLTs, RBCP), using four different apheresis systems. **Design:** 66 donors, well matched for pre-procedure baseline parameters, underwent RBC apheresis collection with the BAXTER Amicus (AM, 15 RBCP) and Alyx (AX, 15 2-RBC), the GAMBRO Trima Accel (TA, 9 RBCP, 8 2-RBC), and the HAEMONETICS MCS Plus (MCS+, 9 RBCP, 10 2-RBC). In-vitro properties were analyzed during 49 days of storage and compared to MRBCs (n = 14). **Results:** All units but one AX demonstrated WBCs $<1 \times 10^6$. ARBCs showed lower variability in volume compared to MRBCs. All units met international requirements (European, AABB) for HCT (50–70%), Hb content (>40 g) and RBC mass (≥153 mL). During storage, ARBCs changed from aerobic to anaerobic glycolysis, while MRBCs mainly performed anaerobic glycolysis throughout the entire storage period. Hemolysis (with slight advantages for MRBCs) and pH remained similar without reaching critical limits in any study group. MRBCs were significantly superior in energy maintenance as indicated by better ATP preservation (especially vs. AX) and lower supernatant K+ as surrogate marker for the function of the Na+/K+ pump (especially vs. TA, demonstrating the highest metabolic activity among ARBCs). **Conclusion:** ARBCs were more consistent than MRBCs and demonstrated sufficient in-vitro quality throughout storage, even though lower ATP preservation was observed compared to MRBCs probably due to differences in glucose metabolism.

P13.2

Visual Monitoring of Platelet Concentrates in Routine: Obligatory for Prevention of Transfusion-Transmitted Bacterial Infections

W. Madla[1], V. Schmidt[1], C. Jiménez-Klingberg[2], A. Markovic[1]
[1]DRK Blutspendedienst West Institut Bad Kreuznach gGmbH, Bad Kreuznach, D; [2]DRK Blutspendedienst West, Hagen, D

Purpose: In our blood transfusion service up to 50 platelet concentrates (PC) a day are produced via apheresis or buffy coat pooling technique. In spite of aseptic techniques and accurate preparation PC deserve alertness, as they might be bacterially contaminated. **Methods:** According to EC-GMP and German guidelines for hemotherapy the PC are submitted to inprocess control procedures during single steps of production as well as to visual inspections in areas of inventory. **Results:** Large white aggregates have been identified in routine visual monitoring of both parts of an apheresis platelet concentrate (double product) 72 hours after preparation via single needle technique. 36 hours before there has been no deviation in the scope of controlling the products for release. Testing for sterility and bacterial differentiation revealed high contamination with Serratia marcescens (S.m.). Collection sets and solutions of ACD-A with the lot numbers concerned could be eliminated as possible origin. These as well as additional in-date platelet units, prepared by using the incriminated equipment, were negative in BacT/ALERT cultures. Blood and urine samples provided by the donor were also negative for the presence of S.m. The donor confirmed that he had not any signs of infection before and after donation. Random checks of skin disinfection performance by taking product samples could proof safety and stability of the procedure. Despite extensive investigations the source of the bacterial contamination could not be identified. **Conclusions:** Published hemovigilance data demonstrate that bacteria-contaminated blood products often have been the cause of fatal transfusion reactions. In respect to bacterial contamination of PC an incidence of 0.08 to 0.7% has been reported. These facts, confirmed by the incident described, underline the importance for critical visual inspection of blood products in the course of production, storage and before issue. The same has to be mandatory for users especially before applying PC. Visual monitoring in routine contributes to quality and safety of products for hemotherapy.

P13.3

Vergleich verschiedener Vollblutseparatoren

A. Rabe, C. Krüger, S. Jost, K.-P. Krause
Haema AG, Leipzig, D

Mit automatischen Separationsgeräten kann die Produktivität der Verarbeitung von Vollblutspenden erhöht und die Verarbeitungsqualität stabilisiert werden. Vor der Entscheidung für einen neuen Separator für die Vollblutverarbeitung wurden 5 verschiedene Separationssysteme in einem Feldversuch getestet und einer Bewertung unterzogen (Macopress, Fa. Macopharma; Compomat, Fa. Fresenius; T-ACE II, Fa. Terumo; Optipress, Fa. Baxter; Pressomat, Fa. Hettich). Es wurden nur Separatoren getestet, die für Top-Top-Beutelsysteme geeignet sind.
Kriterien zur Bewertung waren:

1. Leistungsdaten (Verarbeitungskapazität, Plasmaausbeute, Fehlproduktion)
2. Qualitätskontrolldaten der Produkte (HB-Gehalt, Volumina, Reinheit)
3. technische Parameter
4. die EDV-technische Anbindung (Stabilität des Datentransfers, Parameterisierbarkeit)
5. der Firmenservice (während Testung, in Routine)
6. die Bedienerfreundlichkeit (Handbuch, Lautstärke, Anzahl Handgriffe, Fehlererkennung).

Mittels eines Bewertungsscores wurden drei der fünf Systeme bewertet, die prinzipiell geeignet erschienen. Nicht in die Bewertung aufgenommen wurden die Systeme, deren Eignung für den ausschließlichen Einsatz bzw. wegen schwieriger Bearbeitung von TT-Beutelsystemen oder wegen technischer Probleme im Verarbeitungsprozess nicht in Frage kamen. Durch die Komplexität der Bewertungskriterien war es möglich, die Geräte umfassend einzuschätzen. Dabei ergab sich ein deutlicher Vorteil für ein Separationssystem.

P13.4

Donor Variables in Double-Unit PLT Concentrates Compared to Triple-Unit PLT Concentrates

G. Jaster[1], B. Baumann-Baretti[1], K.-P. Krause[2]
[1]Haema AG, Berlin, D; [2]Haema AG, Leipzig; D

Purpose: No comparable data regarding donor- and preprocedure PLT characteristics, the extent and duration of decrease and recovery in PLT count of the donor after plateletapheresis of double-unit PLT concentrates (DU-PC) and triple-unit PLT concentrates (TU-PC) do exist. We compared mean donor and PLT pre- and postprocedure characteristics. **Methods:** We analysed retrospectively data of 236 donors in 355 DU-PC- and 123 TU-PC-apheresis procedures between 09/2005 until 03/2006. For plateletpheresis minimum hemoglobin in female and male donors 12.5 g/dl and 13.5 g/dl and minimum donor platelet count 250 × 10e9/l had to be met. Apheresis PLT concentrates were collected with Trima Accel Version 5, Gambro. Target yields of 6.3 × 10e11 in DU-PC and 9.3 × 10e11 in TU-PC were used. **Results:** The recovery in PLT count after 15 days post donation ranged between 95% of the initial value in male DU-PCD and 92.1% in TU-PCD; whereas in female DU-PCD the recovery was 94.7% of the initial PLT count after 12 days and in TU-PCD after 15 day 95.4%. **Conclusion:** The PLT yield relating to the single platelet concentrate after splitting showed no differencies if collected as DU-PC or TU-PC. There is no significant difference in postprocedure platelet count between donors of DU-PC and TU-PC. The platelet count of female and male donors recovered to almost initial values after 12 to 15 days independent if DU-PC or TU-PC were produced. Donors of TU-PC demonstrate an elevated BMI; female donors of TU-PC groups are rare but with elevated BMI qualified for TU-PC-donation.

Donor and PLT characteristics	DU-PC donor		TU-PC donor	
Variable	male	female	male	female
Preprocedure PLT count ($\times 10^{11}$/L)	302 ± 34	324 ± 46	323 ± 56	335 ± 48
Postprocedure PLT count ($\times 10^{11}$/L)	217 ± 40	215 ± 41	209 ± 48	211 ± 55
Mean PLT decrease ($\times 10^{11}$/L)	123 ± 18.7	142 ± 70.3	157 ± 35	163 ± 33
Body mass index (BMI)	24.4 ± 3.2	26 ± 3.9	26.6 ± 3.6	31.3 ± 5.6
whole blood processed (ml)	5136 ± 645	3872 ± 658	5699 ± 640	4256 ± 658
Concentration ($\times 10^{9}$/L)	1367 ± 170	1339 ± 193	1363 ± 161	1361 ± 259

P13.5

Comparison of Double-Unit PLT Concentrates versus Triple-Unit PLT Concentrates Collected with Gambro Trima Accel Single-Needle Plateletpheresis

B. Baumann-Baretti[1], G. Jaster[1], B. Brys[2], T. Drahs[2], K.-P. Krause[2]
[1]Haema AG, Berlin, D; [2]Haema AG, Leipzig, D

Background: High safety and efficacy of plateletapheresis with the Trima Accel Version 5.1 has been described. Focusing on productivity, donor variables and quality control we compared double-unit PLT concentrates (DU-PC) with triple-unit PLT concentrates (TU-PC). **Methods:** We analysed retrospecitively data of 106 DU-PC and 23 TU-PC apheresis procedures. PLT concentrates were produced by an automatic continuous flow separator (Trima Accel Version 5.1, Gambro). Target yields of 6.3 × 10e11 in DU-PC and 9.3 × 10e11 in TU-PC respectively were used. **Results:** There is no significant difference in postprocedure PLT counts between DU-PC- and TU-PC-donors. In 10 to 15 days after donation 100% of the initial preprocedure PLT count in DU-PC- and TU-PC-donors was obtained. The postprocedure PLT count never dropped under 150 × 10e9/L. PLT concentrations per unit after splitting ranged in 33% between 2.2 to 2.9 × 10e11/unit and in 67% higher than 3 × 10e11/unit. **Conclusion:** Plateletpheresis with target yields of 6.3 × 10e11 and 9.3 × 10e11 meets the German regulations for donor's postprocedure PLT count. All collections passed the minimum PLT yield stated in the German standards. Still in accordance wih the German guidelines a part of the products contains an elevated number of residual WBCs; therefore the control of the residual WBC count after plateletpheresis with the Trima Accel Version 5.1 might be useful.

Residual white blood cells	>1 × 10^6 WBCs (%)	>5 × 10^6 WBCs (%)
DU-PC donation (n = 106)	1.8	1.8
TU-PC donation (n = 23)	8.7	0
Total	3.1	1.8

Mean PLT characteristics

	Volume (ml)	Concentration ($\times 10^9$/L)	PLT ($\times 10^{11}$/ volume)	PLTs ($\times 10^{11}$/ unit splitting)
DU-PC donor	447 ± 40	1456 ± 154	6.5 ± 0.8	3.0 ± 0.4
TU-PC donor	675 ± 39	1455 ± 160	9.9 ± 1.3	3.22 ± 0.3

P13.6

Rotated Overnight Hemolysis as a Parameter for Red Blood Cell Storage Quality

T. Schulzki
Regionaler Blutspendedienst SRK Graubünden, Chur, CH

Purpose: Quality control of erythrocyte products at the end of storage consists in measuring the rate of hemolysis. This parameter has little to do with invivo survival. Furthermore, some problems arise because this parameter depends a lot on preanalytical items leading to differences in the results. We used an overnight, rotated sample to establish a new parameter. **Methods:** We used outdated products (red cells, leukocyte depleted, in SAGM, PALL®) and products for the evaluation of another additive solution (PAGGS-M, from Fresenius® and PALL®). There are four experiments: 1. Checking the effect of volume in the sample tubes (native samples 1.5 ml vs. 4.5 ml over-head; 1.5 ml rolling). 2. Evaluation of free hemoglobin during an 24 h time in different ways (overhead, rolling, samples in nativ tubes and with EDTA and two kinds of clot activator); 3. 24 h-measurement in routine quality control with native samples; 4. 24 h-measurement with the evaluation of PAGGS-M with native samples. To check for the meaning of results we looked for differences in production (short production vs. overnight production). We also measured total hemoglobin, MCV, erythrocyte count, hematocrit and micro hematocrit. **Results:** It could be shown that more volume in the tube resulted in a higher hemolysis. The kinetics of the hemolysis turned out to be exponential with an endpoint with all kinds of handling, usualy reaching the endpoint after about 8 hours. The biggest amount of hemolysis is achieved with the silica tubes due to well known interaction of silica with erythrocyte membrane. The rapid rise of free hemoglobin after starting the rotation is an important result. In preliminary experiments, we saw a difference between products with short and long preparation time, which not could be seen using standard parameters, but is has to be done with a bigger number. Evaluating PAGGS-M we could see rising overnight rotation hemolysis during storage but no difference between the time of preparation. Calculating micro hematocrit and cellcount showed that free hemoglobin consists of destroyed erythrocytes and some release. **Conclusions:** We showed some relevant points to establish a new test for quality control of red cell storage. It is possible to use an overnight hemolysis. There may be differences in production lines (at least for red cells in SAGM), but the relevance for in-vivo-viabilty of red cells remains to be shown. Further, the data shows the relevance of preanalytical items for measuring hemolysis.

P13.7

Remaining Red Blood Cell Allo-Antibodies in Blood Products Donated by Allo-Sensitized Blood Donors. A Comparative Titration Study

E. Matheis, A.E. Böhlen-Bodmer, B. Grossrieder, K. Hardegger, A. Schille, B.M. Frey
Zürcher Blutspendedienst SRK, Zürich, CH

Background: Allocation of transfusion compatible red blood cell concentrates (RBCC) in patients carrying warm-reactive autoantibodies (WRA) is often hampered by the WRA interfering with cross-match procedure. Therefore, simultaneously present alloreactive antibodies (ARA) may escape detection and therefore may cause potentially life-threatening transfusion reactions upon transfusion. Various strategies to uncover coexistent ARA or to overcome interfering WRA are in use, e.g. autologous and homologous serum adsorption of WRA (ASA and HAS resp), dilution strategies of patient's serum and modification of cross-match milieu. However, these serology based strategies are prone to detection deficits and many of them are technically demanding. In addition, they have to be repeated frequently during transfusion episodes. Molecular genotyping (MGT) of red cell antigens predicting RBC phenotype offers a new approach to allocate phenotype compatible RBCCs, which will be transfused irrespective of cross-match results. Retrospectively, we compared the performance of HAS versus MGT based allocation of RBCC in patients with WRA. **Methods:** From 1.5.2003 to 30.3.2006 we assessed 67 patients. Until 10/2003, RBCC allocation was exclusively HAS based. Starting in 11/2003, MGT techniques using commercially available SNP based assays as well as in house designed SNP and RFLP based assays were applied progressively. The main study focus of the study were put on frequency and specificity of ARA detected by HAS, number of allocation procedures needed, new ARA formation following transfusion and cost effectiveness. **Results:** 30/67 (44.8%) patients were examined by HAS as first line examination and 37/67 (55.2%) patients were managed by MGT. Table 1 summarizes the overall outcome of the two strategies.

Table 1. Outcome of RBCC Allocation Strategies in the Presence of WRA

Number/Endpoint	HAS	MGT
Patients	30	37
Investigations	38	37
Repeated investigations	8	0
Allocated RBCCs	196	762
Work-up time/procedure (total, in h)	8 (296)	6 (222)
Preexisting ARA	13	45
Newly discovered ARA following Tx	3	0

Data on ARA specificities as well as genotype pecularities will be provided.

Conclusions:

1. MGT based allocation strategies of RBCCs in patients with WAR are safe, efficient and economic.
2. Commercial available genotyping kits need to be completed by in house adapted procedures to cover all clinical relevant genotypes
3. In any case of transfusion of cross-match positive RBCCs in the presence of WRA, we recommend to search for newly induced ARA after disappearance of WRA and awaiting an appropriate time gap following transfusion

P13.8

Leucodepleted Whole Blood – an Interesting Option to Facilitate Blood Supply?

U. Seyfert, J. Leopoldseder, A. Vogt, P. Hellstern
Klinikum – IHT, Ludwigshafen, D

Leucodepleted whole blood (LWB) is used for autologous donations. We have no certain evidence if it will be appropriate for certain instances of homologous use. **Material and Methods:** 34 units of whole blood (CPDA-1; Fresenius, FRG) donated according to the German guidelines were leucofiltered prestorage and stored upt to 45 days. Leucodepleted red blood cells in SAG-M (N = 30, RCC; Baxter, Fresenius) served as controls. Haematological, biochemical (pH, ATP, 2,3 DPG, potassium, free haemoglobin, C3a, C5a) and coagulation parameters (all plasmatic coagulation factors, protein C, protein S, VWF, RCoF, CBA, plasminogen, F1 + 2 prothrombin fragments) were determined at designed timepoints during storage life using commercially available kits. **Results:** Apart from significant ($p < 0.05$) differences in hematocrit, ATP (27 ± 6.3 umol/dl), potassium (30 ± 3.7 mmol/l) with higher levels detected in RCC no remarkable differences were observed. The filters resulted in C3a and C5a removal. At the end of storage life of LWB there was a significant ($p < 0.001$) decrease in FV- (71 ± 11%), FVII- (59 ± 18.5%), FVIII:C- (59 ± 18.5%), RCoF- (40 ± 28.3%) and CBA (57 ± 35.5 umol/dl) levels. **Conclusions:** Our data indicate that the quality of LWB is comparable to that of RCC and leucodepleted plasma. LWB maintains a satisfactory level of coagulation factors even after the storage life. There is no activation of coagulation or of the complement system. Safety and long term quality, however, remains to be confirmed by clinical trials.

P13.9

The Quality of Fresh-Frozen Plasma in the Period after Thawing Stored at 4°C and Room Temperature

S. Runkel, W.E. Hitzler
Klinikum der Johannes Gutenberg Universität, Mainz, D

Purpose: Fresh frozen plasma (FFP) is clinically indicated for a varieaty of coagulation complications. Mainly acute disseminated intravascular coagulation, plasma exchange, massive transfusion and in some cases coagulation deficiencies are to be mentioned as indications. Once fresh frozen plasma is thawed, the following storage time is limited due to the low stability of coagulation factors. Therefore transfusion should be carried out without delay. Few data is available about stability of the most important cagulation factors in thawed fresh frozen plasma. The aim of this study is to monitor the decrease of activity of coagulation factors 48 hours after thawing and to define an adequate storage time. **Material and Methods:** 42 FFP were thawed at 37°C. 2 bags were each sterilely connected and the plasma was pooled, mixed thoroughly and subsequently dispersed in the original bags. The connected bags were separated and an aliquot was tested immidiately after this manipulation. One bag was stored at 4°C and the other at 22°C for 48 hours. An Aliquot for analysis was taken 1, 2, 3, 4, 5, 6, 10, 24 and 48 hours after thawing. Factor V, Factor VIII, Factor XI were assayed by clotting assay with deficient plasma. Protein S was determined by extension of coagulation time in presence of Protein C and FVa. The Protein C assay is based on a chromogenic reaction. Fibrinogen is determined in the presence of thrombin. Prothrombin time (PT) and activated partial thromboplastin time (aPTT) were also determined. **Results:** Over the whole period of 48 hours PT, aPTT, Factor V, Protein C, Fibrinogen and Factor XI showed no decrease in activity or concentration at 4°C or 22°C. Activity of Protein S showed no loss of activity after 10 hours of storage at 4°C and a slight decrease of 16.3% after 10 hours of storage at 22°C. The decline of activity of Factor VIII after 6 hours of storage at 4°C and 22°C was moderate (9.3%; 13.2%). 10 hours of storage resulted in a loss of activity of 30.5% at 4°C and 38.8% an 22°C. After 24 h of storage at 4°C only Factor VIII activity was reduced to 60% of the original value **Conclusion:** Fresh frozen plasma once thawed should be transfused without delay. Apart from this storage for 6 hours at room temperature does not lead to a significant inactivation of coagulation factors. Above all storage of 24 h at 4°C only reduces activity of factor VIII significantly.

P13.10

Iron Status in Healthy Whole Blood Donors Monitored by Serum Iron, Serum Ferritin, Transferrin and Soluble Transferrin Receptor

F. Fleschutz, D. Hermsen, S. Hasberg, F. Wenzel, G. Giers
Institut für Hämostaseologie und Transfusionsmedizin, Düsseldorf, D

Introduction: Whole blood donation causes a well defined loss of iron in hemoglobin. Monitoring of the iron status can be helpful to prevent iron deficiency in blood donors [1, 2]. Therefore we evaluated the ability of the available tools serum iron (SI), serum ferritin (SF), transferrin (Tf) and soluble transferrin receptor (sTfR) to differentiate iron loss in three groups of blood donors: first time whole-blood (FTWB) donors, rare whole-blood (WB) donors and frequent whole-blood (WB) donors. **Methods:** 20 healthy FTWB donors (10 women, 10 men) and 40 healthy permanent WB donors (20 women, 20 men) between 20 and 40 years (mean age 31 ± 6 years) were included in the study. Rare WB donors had to donate in the last year 1 to 3 donations (women 1 to 2 times, men 1 to 3 times), and frequent WB donors had to donate in the last year more than three times (women ≥ 3 times, men ≥ 4 times). In predonation blood samples SI and SF were photometrically determined by a Vitros Chemistry System 950 (Ortho-Clinical Diagnostics, Germany) and transferrin Tf and sTfR were measured turbidometrically by a Cobas Integra 400 (Roche Diagnostics, Germany). **Results:** In FTWB donors SI, SF, Tf and sTfR were found to be 112 ± 35 μg/dl, 69 ± 35 ng/ml, 271 ± 41 mg/dl and 1.45 ± 0.26 mg/l, respectively. Women showed a significant reduction of SF to 31 ± 28 ng/ml compared to men (105 ± 52 ng/ml). In rare WB donors (2.25 ± 0.4 donations/year, average iron loss <500 mg/year) no significant changes in the examined parameters could be observed. Frequent WB donors (males: 4.8 ± 0.9 donations/year (average iron loss of 1132 mg/year), females: 3.1 ± 0.3 donations/year (average iron loss of 660 mg/year)) showed a significant reduction in SF (in women to 14 ± 7 ng/ml, and in men to 15 ± 13 ng/ml) and a significant elevation in sTfR (in women to 1.6 ± 0.3 mg/l, and in men to 1.9 ± 0.6 mg/l). **Conclusions:** In whole blood donors with iron loss less than 500 mg per year serum iron, serum ferritin, transferrin and soluble transferrin receptor were not altered. However, in frequent WB donors serum ferritin and soluble transferrin receptor showed significant changes. These parameters may be useful in the early detection of iron deficiency in blood donors.

1 Flesland O et al: Transfus Apher Sci 31:11–16, 2004.
2 Brittenham GM: Dev Biol 120:77–82, 2005.

P13.11

Qualitätsaspekte von Source- und Recovered Plasma mit Hinblick auf Weiterverarbeitung durch den Fraktionierer/Quality Aspects of Source and Recovered Plasma for Fractionation

K. Seidel
ZLB Plasma Services, Marburg, D

Seit Jahrzehnten wird die plasmaverarbeitende Industrie mit Plasma beliefert, das mittels 2 verschiedener Methoden gewonnen wird, nämlich Plasma aus der Vollblutspende und Plasmapherese-Plasma. Diese Produkte unterscheiden sich erheblich durch unterschiedliche Gewinnung, Menge, Verarbeitung, Transport, Lagerung, IgG-Gehalt, vWF und FVIII Gehalt, sowie Verfügbarkeit. Diese Unterschiede werden hier beleuchtet. Beide Plasmaarten ergänzen sich und leisten eine wertvollen Beitrag zur Versorgung der Fraktionierer mit diesem hochwertigen Ausgangsmaterial. For decades the plasma industry has been supplied with plasma collected by 2 different methods, plasma from whole blood and plasma obtained by plasmapheresis. These products differ with regards to collection procedure, quantity, processing, transport, storage, IgG contents, vWF and FVIII contents as well as availability. These differences are discussed here. These 2 types of plasma complement each other and make a significant contribution to the supply of the fractionating industry with this valuable source material.

P13.12

Clinical Efficacy of Platelet Transfusion from Storage Bags with Improved Gaseous Exchange in Frequently Transfused Cancer Patients

H. Rühl, H. Hackstein, K. Heidinger, J. Misterek, G. Bein
Justus Liebig University Giessen, D

Background: Platelets become irreversibly damaged if being stored in an environment with low pH. Their metabolism produces carbon dioxide under aerobic conditions (and lactic acid under anearobic conditions) that leads to pH decline over storage. Platelet storage bags that provide a high rate of gaseous exchange allow carbon dioxide to leave and oxygen to enter the bag, thus slowing down the fall in pH. On the other hand, increased pH levels are often observed in these platelet storage containers. These findings have brought up the question whether such storage conditions interfere with platelet function and clinical effectiveness at the end of the storage time. To examine the clinical efficacy of platelet transfusions from storage bags with a high rate of gaseous exchange we prospectively analysed the transfusion results (corrected count increment [CCI]) in cancer patients. **Methods:** Platelet concentrates (n = 21) with a mean platelet content of 3,187 (2,694–3,656) × 10E11/bag were produced by plateletpheresis using the Gambro TrimaTM device. The transfusion recipients were thrombocytopenic patients (pretransfusion platelet values of 7 [1–22] × 10E9/L) with hematological malignancies. Patients with known immune and non-immune causes of platelet refractoriness were excluded. All transfused platelet concentrates were 3–5 days old. The CCI was determined 1 hour after platelet transfusion. **Results:** Platelet values of the transfusion recipients ranged between 16 and 43 × 10E9/L (mean: 28 × 10E9/L) 1 hour after platelet transfusion. In 20 of 21 cases the CCI was higher than 7.5 (mean: 12.45; range 7.27–18.73). **Conclusions:** Platelet concentrates in storage bags with a high rate of gaseous exchange are clinically efficient in frequently transfused cancer patients.

P13.13

The Quality of Leukocyte-Depleted Whole Blood Using the Automate for Blood Collection System

R. Karger, C. Lukow, V. Kretschmer
Philipps-Universität Marburg, Marburg, D

Background: Measures to reduce the storage lesion of red cell containing blood products are always warranted because several unfavourable effects of transfusion appear to be associated with the decreasing quality of the red cells during storage. **Methods:** In a randomized controlled fashion, 2 × 20 CPDA-1 containing leukocyte-depleted whole blood (LD-WB) units were investigated. In one group, anticoagulant was continuously added to the donated blood via a roller pump thereby preserving the correct red cell to anticoagulant ratio during donation in order to prevent the so called citrate shock, using a new drawing device (MacoPharma ABCÒ, Langen). In the other group, WB units were produced using a conventional drawing device. All WB units were leukocyte-depleted 2 hours post donation using the LST2 filter (MacoPharma). Red cell quality parameters (ATP, 2,3-DPG, free haemoglobin, potassium, glucose, lactate, pH) and parameters of coagulation (factor V, VIII, antithrombin, D-dimer) were determined on days 1, 7, 21, 35, 42, and 49 of storage. **Results:** All 40 LD-WB units had less than 2 × 105/unit residual leukocytes. The ABC and conventional group showed comparable unit volumes with 525 (SD 5.3) mL vs. 524 (SD 10.2) mL and haemoglobin content with 65.9 (SD 5.1) g/unit vs. 67.5 (SD 7.8) g/unit. Volumes exhibited a significantly higher variation after conventional blood drawing (P = 0.006). Variation of haemoglobin content also tended to be higher in the conventional group (P = 0.07). During storage, none of the measured quality parameters was significantly different between the two groups. Mean ATP was 1.69 (0.5) and 1.66 (0.4) μmol/g haemoglobin, and mean haemolysis rate was 0.47 (0.14) and 0.44 (0.13)% in the ABC and conventional group, respectively, after 49 days of storage. **Conclusion:** The ABC device provided a better standardized blood product. Maintaining the correct red cell to anticoagulant ratio during donation did not improve red cell storage parameters in LD-WB. However, the red cell quality parameters in both groups suggest that storage of LD-WB might be extended to 42 or even 49 days.

P14: Blood Substitutes

P14.1

Antiplatelet Therapy Preceding Coronary Artery Surgery: Implications for Bleeding and Transfusion Requirements

S.M. Picker, T. Kaleta, H. Khosro, S. Kampe, B. Gathof
Klinikum der Universität zu Köln, D

Background: Bleeding after heart surgery correlates with morbidity and mortality. The purpose of this study was to determine the influence of antiplatelet therapy (APT) with acetylsalicylic acid and/or clopidogrel/ticlopidine on perioperative blood loss and transfusion demands in coronary artery bypass grafting (CABG). **Design:** A cohort of 80 patients undergoing CABG was reviewed retrospectively. 40 patients who received APT within 7 days prior to surgery were compared with 40 control patients (CONs) without APT for at least 1 week. CONs and APTs underwent CABG at the same day by the same team. Chest tube output was evaluated postoperatively for up to 12 hours. Transfused units were measured intraoperatively and during ICU stay. **Results:** APTs demonstrated lower CK-MB values (5.8 ± 3.1 vs. 8.2 ± 4.1% of total CK, p = 0.004) and infarction rates (0 vs. 3, p = 0.24) compared to CONs, but had significantly more haemorrhages (939.9 ± 861.2 ml vs. 411.5 ± 590.1 ml; p = 0.002) and transfusion requirements (RBC: 4.5 ± 4.9 vs. 1.5 ± 2.3; FFP: 4.9 ± 6.4 vs. 1.3 ± 2.5; PLTs: 1.5 ± 1.3 vs. 0.1 ± 0.2, all p ≤ 0.001), particularly for only short APT free intervals (* significant to CON). There was no difference between single or combined APT.

APT free; CK-MB (%); Blood loss (ml); RBCs; FFP; Platelets
≤2 days; 5.6 ± 3.3*; 1224.4 ± 1064.6*; 6.0 ± 5.5*; 6.2 ± 7.9*; 1.8 ± 1.1*
3–5 days; 6.2 ± 2.7; 681.2 ± 601.1; 3.3 ± 4.4; 3.7 ± 4.0; 1.5 ± 1.6*
6–7 days; 5.7 ± 3.7; 744.4 ± 575.6; 3.3 ± 4.1; 4.2 ± 6.0; 0.1 ± 0.2

Conclusion: Elevated blood loss and transfusion requirements have to be expected, if APT is not discontinued for at least 2 days before elective CABG. Whesther the beneficial effect of APT for perioperative infarction rates is still observed with discontinuous treatment, remains subject of further investigations.

P14.2

Transfusion Requirements in Relation to Chemotherapeutic Interventions

S. Picker, B. Assefa, C. Scheid, B. Gathof
Klinikum der Universität zu Köln, D

Background: The aim of this study was to evaluate transfusion requirements during treatment with different chemotherapeutic regimens (CTRs) for acute myeloid and lymphatic leukaemia. Design: 100 cytostatic cycles (34 HAM, 35 TAD, 8 S-HAI, 11 IND 1, 12 IND 2) in patients, comparable for age, body mass index and body surface were retrospectively reviewed. Pre-transfusion WBC counts, CRPs, temperatures, aPTT and Quick values as well as Hb and PLT takes were recorded for each RBC and PLT transfusion during 28 days after cytostatic induction (day 0). Blood cell take was related to storage age (RBCs: #/. 10 days; PLTs: #/. 3 days) and PLT dose (#/. 2.5 3 1011/unit). Transfusion triggers were 80g Hb/L and 10,000 3 109PLTs/L. Results: Probably due to significantly lower pre-transfusion WBC counts and higher CRPs, S-HAI demonstrated the highest demands for RBCs (11.5 6 6.8 vs. 9.8 6 6.2 in TAD and 9.0 6 4.1 in HAM) and PLTs (10.4 6 6.6 vs. 9.9 6 7.0 in TAD and 8.5 6 4.6 in HAM), while IND 1 (RBCs: 3.1 6 2.4; PLTs: 1.3 6 2.0) and IND 2 (RBCs: 5.8 6 4.1; PLTs: 2.2 6 3.1) were the significantly lowest. In HAM and IND 1, transfusion peaks for RBCs (2.91 6 2.63; 1.36 6 1.29) and PLTs (3.24 6 1.92; 0.55 6 0.69) were observed already in week 1/2, whereas TAD, S-HAI, and IND 2 had peaks for RBCs (2.97 6 2.67; 3.50 6 0.93; 2.00 6 1.48) and PLTs (3.11 6 2.69; 3.75 6 3.45; 0.75 6 1.22) in week 3/4. As expected from the lower transfusion demand, Hb (g/dL/unit) and PLT take (3109/L/unit) was higher with IND 1 (Hb: 0.77 6 0.41; PLTs: 11.93 6 13.18) and IND 2 (Hb: 0.87 6 0.41; PLTs: 15.39 6 16.10) compared to the other groups (Hb take: 0.63 to 0.69; PLT take: 8.11 to 11.40), particularly for short-stored RBCs (IND 2). Except for IND 1 and IND 2, PLT take was higher for short-stored units (9.06–13.16 vs. 7.10–9.98) and ranged from 6.52–13.11 and 8.67–16.47 for low and high dose PLTs, respectively. Conclusion: Transfusion requirements differed between different CTRs with TAD and S-HAI the highest, and IND 1 and IND 2 the lowest. The results of our study could help to optimize blood supply, particularly PLTs, for hematological malignancies.

P15: Health Economic Impacts

P15.1

Is European Source Plasma Different from Plasma from the US?

K.-P. Krause
Haema AG, Leipzig, D

Introduction: If one read different publications it has to be recognized that the price for European plasma is up to 10% less than the price of plasma from the US. Additionally plasma collectors face different difficulties if they want to contract there plasma with different fractionators. The question arises, what are the reasons for these differences. **Material and Methods:** Quality characteristics of US and European plasma and regulatory background of plasma production in the US and Europe were lighted. **Results:** Hellstern et al showed differences in total protein, albumin and IgG levels whereas for these parameter higher data where found in plasma from Europe. The content of FI, FV and FVIII was less in US plasma. Different regulations apply for European and US plasma. While the EU directive 2002/98/EC, PIC Guide, Drug & Transfusion Law and the Recommendations of the German Physician Association regulate European and German plasma collection in the US 21 CFR 640 is mandatory. The different applying guidelines lead to differences in the plasma production. Main differences are: NDDR, rejection of donors stood a certain time in Europe because of CJD, interviewed questionnaire, testing for West Nile, use of medical substitutes, urine analysis, serum protein electrophoresis, softgoods 510k, serology tests (2nd generation tests) FDA-approved in the US; use of self administered questionnaire, serum total protein, IgG-measurement, presence of physician at every donation, use of 3rd generation CE-marked serology tests in the EU. If one compares the usability of products got from US or European plasma it can be seen, that products from US-plasma are accepted world wide, while products from European plasma are excluded from the US market and some other countries. **Conclusion:** Yes, there is a difference between European and US plasma but comparing different aspects leads to the conclusion that European has at least the same quality compared to US plasma. Excluding European plasma and products from European plasma from the US market is not justified and dangerous in cases of occurrence of new pathogens in the US.

1 Hellstern et al: The impact of the intensity of serial automated plasmapheresis and the speed of deep-freezing on the quality of plasma. Transfusion 2001; 41:1601–1605.

P15.2

Rejection of Blood Donors in the Greifswald Blood Donation Centre: A Retrospective Study

F. Hartung, U. Alpen, A. Wessel, N. Lubenow, A. Greinacher
Ernst-Moritz-Arndt-University Greifswald, D

Purpose: Demographic changes will lead to an older population with consecutively increasing need for blood transfusions due to an increase of malignant disease and major surgery. A significant fraction of donors presenting for blood donation is currently rejected. We analyzed the frequency and the reasons for rejection to identify strategies to reduce the number of rejected donors. **Methods:** Reasons for rejection of blood donors in the blood donation center of the University Hospital Greifswald between 01/01/2005 and 31/12/2005 were retrieved from the donor records and related to donor age and gender. **Results:** Of 24816 donors presenting for donation, 4037 (16.3%) were rejected, while whole blood 20779 donations were obtained during the same time period. 2602 (64%) rejected donors were female and 1435 (36%) were male. Reasons for rejection were low haemoglobin (Hb) n = 2088 (52%), followed by infections/visit to the dentist n = 512 (13%), surgical intervention/tattoo/piercing n = 438 (11%) and others, e.g. high blood pressure, body weight <50 kg or medication n = 999 (25%). Low Hb occurred significantly more often in female (n = 1602; 77%) than in male (n = 487; 23%; $P < 0.0001$) donors. The majority of donors rejected because of low haemoglobin were in the age group of 18–29 years and were regular donors (n = 1441 vs. n = 185 first time donors). **Conclusions:** About 50% of rejected blood donors showed a low haemoglobin, most likely induced by previous blood donations. Prevention of iron depletion in regular donors, especially women, could result in a substantial reduction of rejected donors.

P15.3

The Cost-Effectiveness of Autologous Haemotherapy in 2006

R. Karger, V. Kretschmer
Philipps-Universität Marburg, D

Background: During the last 15 years numerous economic evaluations of autologous haemotherapy methods (AHM) have been published. There is still an ongoing debate whether these measures are cost-effective when compared to each other or to other medical interventions. **Methods:** A search in MEDLINE and the British National Health Service Economic Evaluation Database (NHS EED) was conducted in order to retrieve cost-effectiveness analyses of AHM focusing on preoperative autologous blood donation (PABD), acute normovolaemic haemodilution (ANH), or perioperative cell salvage (PCS) methods. The search encompassed the years from 1991 to 2006. The quality of retrieved papers was assessed using published criteria for the evaluation of economic analyses of health care measures. Articles were included in the systematic review if they provided a full economic evaluation; i.e. either a cost-minimization- (CMA), cost-effectiveness- (CEA), or cost-utility analysis (CUA). **Results:** 26 studies were identified: 10 for PABD, 4 for ANH, 7 for PCS. 5 studies evaluated strategies combining different AHM. 9 studies were considered a CUA, 17 studies were a CEA, 4 of which reduced to a CMA, because effectiveness was regarded as identical in the compared study groups. 19 (73%) studies were conducted in the USA, including all PABD studies. Only one study included indirect costs in its cost estimates. The majority of analyses were based on suboptimal study designs. Only 6 studies employed randomized controlled trials (RCTs). In most of these studies, avoidance of allogeneic transfusion was chosen as effectiveness parameter. 8 studies used decision-analysis-models for the estimation of the outcome (effectiveness) data, and calculated cost-effectiveness ratios based on quality-adjusted life years in a CUA. These included 8 PABD studies and 2 PCS studies. However, the assumptions needed for the models were often either outdated or were derived from unsystematic reviews of the pertinent literature, leaving much space for a critical discussion of the appropriateness or justification of these assumptions. **Conclusions:** Economic analyses of AHM are heterogeneous with respect to several aspects of study design, including analysis method, cost estimation, perspective, outcome conceptualization, conduction of sensitivity analyses, etc. The currently available scientific evidence is of limited quality owing to considerable uncertainties in estimates of several of key variables supposed to substantially affect the results of the economic analyses. A concerted effort of health economists, clinical epidemiologists and clinicians is needed in order to define the best approach for determining the cost-effectiveness of AHM.

P16: Other Subjects

P16.1

Allergic Reactions to Aprotinin Administration? Prospective Analysis in 1,307 Major Orthopedic Surgery Patients

G. Singbartl[1], L. Schwarz[1], C. Hoenemann[2]
[1]ENDO-Klinik Hamburg GmbH, Hamburg, D; [2]St. Marien-Hospital, Vechta

Introduction: Aprotinin (APR) is known to reduce periop. blood-loss. Since it is made of bovine tissue, it bears the risk of allergic reactions (AR). Very few prospective studies analysed frequency/severity of AR to APR; whether w/ or w/o antihistaminic H1-/H2 drugs remains mostly unclear; w/or w/o known pre-existing allergic diseases is even lacking. **Methods:** Prospect. study in 1,307 continuous orthopedic surgery pts. Administering H1-/H2-blocking drugs; i.v. test-dose of 1 ml of APR; ten min. later bolus infusion of 2 mio KIU of APR, followed by 0.5 million KIU p. hour. AR were assessed to Ring and Messmer. Statistics by multiple linear regression analysis, Chi?-test referring to frequency/severity of AR w/ considering degree of freedom (df); $p < 0.05$. **Results:** Total AR-rate was 1.3% (17/1,307 pts); w/'first-time APR' it was 0.74% (9/1,209 pts), and w/'repeat APR' it was 8.16% (8/98 pts). 6 of these 8 AR w/ ?repeat APR? happened within 3 months after previous APR. AR was more severe in 'repeat APR' than in ?first-time APR?. Table 1 summarizes results.

	Frequency of AR			Severity of AR		
variable	Chi^2	df	p	Chi^2	df	p
age	0.004	1	0.9527	2.32	4	0.6780
gender	0.02	1	0.8815	5.71	4	0.2219
known pre-existing allergic dis.	1.86	1	0.1724	3.73	4	0.4437
time H1-/H2-blocking-APR	2.35	2	0.3082	10.98	8	0.2026
intra-/postoperative APR	2.35	2	0.3094	12.07	8	0.1480
type of anesthesia	4.26	2	0.1187	19.45	8	0.0126
time previous-actual APR	8.59	1	0.0034	9.21	2	0.0100
first-time vs. repeat APR a	19.86	1	<0.0001	32.34	4	<0.0001

Discussion: 'Repeat APR' and 'time-interval from previous to actual APR of <3 months' has been demonstrated of impact on frequency and severity of AR to APR. Known pre-existing allergic diseases have not been shown of relevance on AR to APR.

P16.2

Preoperative Autologous Deposit or Perioperative Blood Salvage: Mathematical Analysis and Comparison on Preoperative Autologous Deposit Data from the Literature

G. Singbartl
ENDO-Klinik Hamburg GmbH, Hamburg, D

Background: Previous data have demonstrated perioperative blood salvage (PBS) more efficacious (i.e. increase in total RBC-mass [+RBC]) and effective (maximal allowable blood-loss [MABL] compensated w/ +RBC) than preoperative autologous deposit (PAD). Since this result might have been due to a not-optimal PAD-concept, we decided to mathematically analyse PAD-data from the literature, to either confirm or reject these previous data. **Methods:** Review of the literature on PAD to find papers with complete data-sets necessary for this mathematical analysis by mean-/median-data reported. RBC-recovery-rate to PBS was set w/30%, hct min for re-transfusion w/ 24 and 21. Re-transfusion of +RBC together w/ additional colloid to maintain hct min and normovolemia despite ongoing blood-loss; thereby, resulting in MABL (ltr.) compensated by +RBC (ml) to either PAD or PBS. **Results:** Few papers were found w/ data-sets appropriate for this mathematical comparison. Table 1 summarizes the results. As in PAD preop. hct is lower than initial hct, retransfusion of +RBC will start earlier, and, thus, compensate for a lesser MABL than PBS30; even w/ a smaller +RBC to PBS30. **Discussion:** When intra-indivudually mathematically compared to PBS w/o preceding PAD, data from the literature demonstrated PAD inferior to PBS. Thus, only with an excellent schedule can PAD be superior to PBS, and, thus, be a reasonable alternative.

P16.3

Results of a Pre-Test in Preparation of an Improved Measurement of Customer Satisfaction

J. Hettinger
DRK-Blutspendedienst West Institut Bad Kreuznach gGmbH, Bad Kreuznach, D

Background: The DRK-Blutspendedienst West gGmbH is an association of the red cross blood donation services in the German states of Nordrhein-Westfalen, Rheinland-Pfalz and Saarland. The institute of Bad Kreuznach which is certified by ISO 9001:2000 since 2003, performs approximately 250,000 blood donations p.a. in 2,250 events with 12 mobile and 1 stationary team. The first wide-ranging measurements of customer satisfaction were done in November 2004 at 10 blood donation events by questionnaires. The contents that should be evaluated were categorized by the institute. The survey reached high acceptances by the blood donors. **Purpose:** To find out which critical points are of specific importance to the blood donors, we started a pre-test based on interviews of our blood donors by telephone in order to prepare an improved questionnaire to measure customers satisfaction. **Methods:** Blood donors were interviewed, categorized by sex, age and donor status (multiple vs. primary donor). 200 donors received ex ante written informations. Finally 120 interviews by telephone could be evaluated. **Results:** Nearly 30 points could be identified which were of particular importance for the blood donors. Based on broad common aspects, under the "top three" there could be found interesting differences between the donor categories. **Conclusions:** This pre-test showed, that individual recognition, short waiting time and a good atmosphere were the most important things during an event to our blood donors. A completely improved measurement of customer satisfaction will be developed from the results of this pre-test.

P16.4

A Two Center Analysis of Donor Recovery Rate in 2005 and 2006 Based on Data of Donations and Deferrals in 2003 and 2004

J. Rivero[1], E. Ulrich[1], K. Krause[2]
[1]Haema AG, Dresden; [2]Haema AG, Leipzig, D

Based on the total donation data and total donor deferral data in 2003 and 2004 presented in a study last year, we tracked the donor return rate after 2 and 3 years. We analyzed the donor return rate using the blood bank software PC Blut. Our aim was the determination of a possibly increase of donor recovery rate after 2 or 3 years.

Results:

Parameter	2003 total donations: 217,026	2004 total donations: 153,019
Total Deferrals	N = 14,346 (6.61%)	N = 12,117 (7.91%)
Gender	Male: 45% Female: 55%	Male: 47% Female: 53%
Return rate of donors Survey of 2005	N = 8,557 (59.6%)	N = 7,111 (58.68%)
Return rate of donors Survey of 2006	N = 10,351 (72.1%)	N = 7,959 (65.68%)
Increase of return rate	N = 1,794 (12.5%)	N = 848 (7%)

After determination of the donor return rate of deferred donors in 2003 and 2004 extracted from our research in 2005 we found a loss of donors of 40.4% in 2003 and 41.32% in 2004. We have determined the donor return rate from the year 2003 and 2004 again in 2006 and have found an increase. The donor return rate increased by 12.5% (deferral group 2003) and by 7% (deferral group 2004). So the loss of donors could be reduced to 27.9% in the group of donors deferred in 2003 and to 34.32% in the 2004 group respectively. **Conclusions:** The donor recovery rate of deferred donors is increasing constantly also after 3 years. This knowledge of donor behaviour is important and should be used for promotion and motivation of donors.

1 Whyte G: Quantitating donor behaviour to model the effect of changes in donor management on sufficiency in the blood service. Vox Sang 1999; 76:209–15.

Table 1 for Abstract P16.2

	PAD	+RBC (ml)	MABL (L)		PBS30	+RBC (ml)		MABL (L)	
Hct. min calculated	Data from literature		24%	21%	(Calculated) PAD from original data on the left	24%	21%	24%	21%
Kasper 1997 (osteoarthritis)		386	4.0	4.9		298	342	4.2	5.3
Kasper 1997 (osteoarthritis)		239	2.8	3.5		214	254	3.2	4.1
Kasper 1998 (osteoarthritis)		220	2.6	3.6		290	334	4.1	5.2
Monk 1999 (urology)		105	2.3	3.1		294	343	4.3	5.4
Singbartl 2000 (rheum.arthr.)		51	1.3	1.9		124	163	2.0	2.8

P16.5

Look-Back Investigation of Anti-HLA Antibody Positive Tested Plateletpheresis Donors

M. Mosebach, K. Schliwka, M.U. Heim
Otto-von-Guericke University Magdeburg, D

Background: Transfusion-related acute lung injury (TRALI) is one of the most important severe complication after transfusion of plasma-rich blood components. TRALI expresses clinical pictures like noncardiogenic pulmonary edema, dyspnoea, hypotension, chills and fever. Typically TRALI evolves within 1–2 hours after transfusion. Transfused donor anti-leukocyte antibodies seem to be the main risk factor for the development of TRALI. **Materials and Methods:** Serum samples from 210 plateletpheresis donors were screened by ELISA for the presence of anti-HLA class I and/or class II antibodies (AbScreen, Biotest, Germany) and subsequently confirmed by an ELISA panel (AbIdent, Biotest, Germany). According to anti-HLA-antibody positive tested donors, 6 year look-back investigation for transfusion-related complications for all transfused platelet donations were done. **Results:** Six plateletpheresis donors were screened positive for anti-HLA-class I antibodies and nine were screened positive for HLA-class II antibodies. Hereof only three anti-HLA class I antibodies positive results could be confirmed by ELISA determination. Concerning anti-HLA class II antibodies five sera were screened false positive. Only seven donors have tested positive for specific anti-HLA class or class II antibodies. These seven donors all together donated 244 apheresis platelets. Look-back investigations in our blood-bank records for documented transfusion reactions identified only one patient with announced transfusion reactions (fever and strong chill) among all recipients of the platelets-products, from the donors with anti-HLA antibodies. In the listed case the determined antibodies of the donor (anti-HLA-DR15, anti-HLA-B7) were specific against the patients HLA-antigens. Thus we assumed a mild form of TRALI. **Discussion:** Positive results found during ELISA screening for anti-HLA antibodies have to be confirmed by panel-ELISA differentiation. Otherwise a high number of false positive results (in our case 53%) could be found. Due to the fact, that only one mild form of TRALI was announced after the application of 244 apheresis platelets, which hypothetically contain anti-HLA-antibodies, our look-back study suggests that even in the setting of donor anti-HLA-antibodies, TRALI does not occur in the recipients or remains undetected.

P16.6

Validation of a Cell-Based Assay Following the ICH-Guidelines: Quantification of EBV-Specific Cytotoxic T Cells Using the ELISpot Assay

S. Tippmer[1], A. Moosmann[2], H. Lindena[1], J. Urlacher[1], H.-J. Kolb[3], D.J. Schendel[4], I. Bigalke[1]
[1]GSF – National Research Center for Environment and Health, Martinsried, D; [2]Clinical Cooperative Group Molecular Oncology, Munich, D; [3]III. Medical Clinic Großhadern, LMU, Munich, D; [4]GSF, Institute of Molecular Immunology, Munich, D

Recently cellular therapeutics have come into focus to overcome immunological barriers in order to treat malignancies or viral infections resistant to classical therapies. Although these therapeutics are novelties, their preparation must follow general guidelines regulating production and quality control as summarized in the ICH-guidelines. In the generation of EBV-specific T cell populations the enumeration of reactive cells is part of quality control which can be achieved by determination of IFN-gamma-producing T cells. We have chosen an IFN-gamma-specific ELISpot assay which we validated according to the ICH-guidelines. The assay was performed using the IFN-gamma-specific ELISpot kit from Mabtech together with 96 well filter membrane plates from Millipore. T cells were activated by co-incubation with EBV-transformed LCL, either HLA-matched or -mismatched. The assay was done according to the manufacturer's instructions. Spots were quantified using a Zeiss ELISpot reader. Validation was done by determining the following parameters: intra- and inter-assay precision, linearity, specificity, range, and robustness. Within a donor-specific range the number of T cells and spots showed a linear proportion. The intra-assay variation was very high with CV of ~ 25%, but the results were reproducible leading to a sufficient inter-assay precision. The ELISpot assay proved to be highly specific for HLA-matched EBV-transformed LCL. Cell numbers as low as 100 T cells/well led to satisfactory results. Since the parameter "trueness" could not be analysed we tried to strengthen our ELISpot results by analysis with an alternative technique, the determination of intra-cellular IFN-gamma by FACS. Furthermore the percentage of reactive T cells was correlated to the cytotoxic potential of the populations determined with the Europium assay. Our results show that the ELISpot assay can be validated following ICH guidelines in order to be used as a method for GMP-conform quality control of cellular therapeutics.

P16.7

A Two Center Analysis of the Donor Population Under Demographical Aspects Based on Data of Donations in 2004 and 2005

J. Rivero[1], K. Krause[2], E. Ulrich[1]
[1]Haema AG, Dresden, D; Haema AG,Leipzig, D

The availibity of donors is limited by stringent exclusion criteria of the german national guidelines and the recommendations of the council of Europe and generally shrinking and aging populations [1]. With this background we were especially interested in the demographic distribution of our donor population. A two year analysis (2004 and 2005) was performed using the blood bank software PC Blut. **Main Results:** Differences we found in the group of first time and requalified donors with 5% more female donors and a dominance of female donors in the age group >34–<54 years in all categories in 2004 and 2005. A higher rate of employment of male donors could be an explanation for the findings. Additionally we found a loss of 36% of first time donors between 2004 and 2005, 59% of our first time donors are younger than 25 years. This loss is comparable with the shrinking birth rate in the years from 1985 to 2000 in Germany [1].

1 Birg H: Ursachen und Folgen des Fertilitätsrückgangs in Deutschland und Europa. Zentralbl. Gynäkolog 2004;126:101–111.

Table for Abstract P16.7

Parameter	First time donors 2004 vs. 2005	Qualified blood donors* 2004 vs. 2005	Qualified plasma donors** 2004 vs. 2005	Requalified blood donors 2004 vs. 2005
Gender [Male = m Female = f]	5964 m (45%)/7242 f (55%) vs. 3786 m (45%)/4607 f (55%)	7511 m (53%)/6575 f (47%) vs. 6891 m (50%)/ 6710 f (50%)	7948 m (56%)/6127 f (44%) vs. 7930 m (56%)/6254 f (44%)	853 m (46%)/1005 f (54%) vs. 2485 m (45%) /3034 f (55%)
Reduction of donors	13206 /8393 −36%	14086/13601 −4%	14075/14184 +1%	1858/5519 +279%
Age group >34–<54 years Gender	19.7% m/23% f vs. 12.5% m/22.3% f	24.4% m/35.2% f vs. 25% m/36% f	21.8% m/32.8%f vs. 22.5% m/24.5% f	24.4% m/26.9% f vs. 21.8%m/30.9% f
Donation frequency Gender		2.37 m/1.96 f vs. 2.29 m/1.97 f	8.02 m/6.57 f vs. 9.74 m/7.97 f	

*last donation within 6 month; ** last donation >6 until 24 month

P16.8

Perioperative Serum Erythropoietin and Thrombopoietin Levels in Patients after Coronary Artery Bypass Grafting (CABG)

T. Gettmann[1], M. Kurt[1], N. Zimmermann[2], Klein[1], R. Görlich[3], F. Wenzel[1], G. Giers[1]
[1]Universitätsklinik Düsseldorf, D; [2]Bonn, D; [3]Aachen, D

Introduction: Erythropoietin (EPO) and thrombopoietin (TPO) are main regulators of erythro- and thrombopoiesis, and serum concentrations of the hormones are inversely correlated to the corresponding cell count. Perioperatively anemic states could be observed in cause of loss of erythrocytes, whereas referring to regulatory mechanisms of thrombopoiesis reactice thrombocytosis is a well known phenomenon. Therefore we evaluated the perioperative behaviour of the hormones. **Material and Methods:** Blood samples from 8 patients (mean age 64 ± 8 years) were obtained before and on days 1, 5 and 10 after CABG. sEPO and sTPO levels were determined by commercially available ELISA-Kits (R&D Systems, Germany). In addition, platelet count (PC) and hemoglobin concentration (Hb) were determined. **Results:** Prior to CABG, sEPO (12.8 ± 7.9 mU/ml), sTPO (188.7 ± 64.9 pg/ml), PC (248.8 ± 124.7/nl) and Hb (8.8 ± 1 mmol/l) were within a normal range. At day 1 after surgery, Hb and PC were significantly decreased to 6.4 ± 0.6 mmol/l and 145.5 ± 90.2/nl. In contrast, sEPO and sTPO were significantly elevated to 36.8 ± 28.4 mU/ml and 333.2 ± 105.1 pg/ml, respectively, in spite of perioperative influences such as hemodilution. Accordingly, at day 5 and 10 after surgery increases in Hb and PC could be observed. In particular sTPO elevation was followed by a significant increase in PC (338.2 ± 162.3/nl) at day 10 after surgery compared to preoperative values. **Conclusions:** Serum erythropoietin and thrombopoietin levels were postoperatively elevated corresponding to mild anemia and decreases in platelet count, respectively. Whereas hemoglobin concentration returned nearly in a normal range at follow up, the alterations of the hormones were especially accompanied by the phenomenon of reactive thrombocytosis.

P16.9

Serum Thrombopoietin Levels in Patients with Chemotherapy-Induced Aplasia in Comparison to Patients with Postoperative Thrombocytopenia

I. Kafka, T. Gettmann, R. Görlich, F. Wenzel, G.Giers
Universitätsklinik Düsseldorf, D

Purpose: With regard to the regulation of serum thrombopoietin (sTPO) concentration thrombopoietin clearance by megakaryocytes and bone marrow is still in discussion. Therefore sTPO levels were determined in patients with marked thrombocytopenic states: patients with chemotherapy-induced aplasia in comparison to patients with postoperative thrombocytopenia but intact bone marrow function. **Methods:** Serum blood samples were obtained from 6 patients before and during chemotherapy-induced aplasia and from 7 patients with postoperative thrombocytopenia. In addition, in in vitro experiments TPO clearance were measured by incubation of thrombocytes and MEG-1 cells (megakaryocytic cell line) with TPO. TPO levels were determined by a commercially available ELISA-Kit (R&D Systems). **Results:** During chemotherapy-induced aplasia PC decreased to 36 ± 16/nl. In contrast, sTPO showed a clear increase from 244 ± 201 pg/ml (before start of the chemotherapy) to 2,977 ± 878 pg/ml ($p < 0.05$). In patients with postoperative thrombocytopenia (PC 61 ± 23/nl) sTPO were found to be 274 ± 215 pg/ml. After a postoperative follow-up for two weeks PC was in a normal range (303 ± 113/nl), and sTPO decreased to 210 ± 176 pg/ml. In the in vitro experiments, thrombocytes reduced TPO concentration of about 50 percent after 5 h incubation, whereas MEG-1 cells caused only a reduction of about 10 percent. **Conclusions:** In patients with chemotherapy-induced aplasia, decrease in platelet count was accompanied by a significant clear increase in serum thrombopoietin levels. In contrast, patients with postoperative thrombocytopenia showed only a tendency to elevated serum thrombopoietin levels instead of thrombocytopenia. In aplasia, increase in serum thrombopoietin concentrations may be due to low binding capacity of peripheral thrombocytes and due to suppressed megakaryocytic thrombopoiesis, whereas in postoperative states compensatory megakaryopoiesis may lead to less pronounced alterations of serum thrombopoietin levels.

P16.10

Erythropoietic Response after Preoperative Autologous Blood Donation: The Predictive Value of the New Hematologic Indices "CHr" and "HYPO" in Non Iron-Deficient Patients

V. Weisbach, K. Schmidt, J. Zingsem, R. Zimmermann, R. Eckstein
Universitätsklinikum Erlangen, D

Purpose: The hematologic indices "reticulocyte haemoglobin content (CHr)" and "proportion of hypochromic red cells (HYPO)", which can be determined by means of the Advia 120 automated haematology analyzer (Bayer Diagnostics) are useful tools to determine deficient red cell hemoglobinization and functional iron deficiency. Thus, these elementary and inexpensive parameters might be useful to predict the power of the erythropoietic response after repeated preoperative autologous blood donation (PABD). **Methods:** Before each donation, we measured standard blood count, reticulocyte count, CHr, HYPO and ferritin in 33 adult, non iron-deficient patients without chronic disease, 19 women and 14 men (mean age, 66 years; range, 42–80 years), having two units of autologous blood collected in a weekly interval. The net preoperative red blood cell production (NET) was calculated. Multiple regression analysis was performed to find predictors for erythropoietic variability. **Results:** NET was 291 ± 123 mL (range, 55–585 mL). The baseline values of HYPO showed a significant correlation to the baseline values of Hb ($R = -0.4$; $p = 0.03$), leukocytes ($R = 0.6$; $p = 0.001$) and platelets ($R = 0.4$; $p = 0.02$). The baseline values of CHr showed a significant correlation to the baseline values of ferritin ($R = 0.6$; $p = 0.001$) and Hb ($R = 0.5$; $p = 0.01$). HYPO showed a significant increase from before the first to before the second donation (from 1.4 ± 2.7% to 2.1 ± 3.7%; $p < 0.0005$) while CHr did not (33.6 ± 1.8 pg, 33.7 ± 2.3 pg; $p = 0.64$). Neither the baseline values of HYPO and CHr nor their changes from before the first to before the second donation nor their values before the second donation showed any correlation to NET in multiple regression analysis, while the positive effect of the duration of the interval between the days of first donation and the day of surgery on NET was confirmed ($R = 0.8$; $p < 0.0005$). **Conclusions:** Deficient red cell hemoglobinization increases during repeated PABD. The hematologic indices "reticulocyte haemoglobin content (CHr)" and "proportion of hypochromic red cells (HYPO)" were not useful in the prediction of the power of the erythropoietic response after repeated PABD.

P16.11

Removal of Brain PrPres in Leukoreduced Human RBC Using the MacoPharma Prion Capture (P-CAPT™) Filter

L. Gregori, B.C. Lambert, R. Rohwer
Veterans Affairs, Maryland Health Care System and University of Maryland, Baltimore, USA

Purpose: Blood-borne TSE infectivity can harbor undetected for years in the blood of an asymptomatic variant Creuzfeld-Jakob diseases (vCJD) patient, who during this period could donate blood and eventually transmit the disease. Pathogen Removal and Diagnostic Technologies Inc. (PRDT) developed a strategy to select resins that best adsorbed the TSE causative agent from blood. One resin able to capture brain PrPres in red blood cell concentrate (RBC), whole blood, and plasma was incorporated into a prion capture filter termed P-CAPT™ by MacoPharma. The purpose of this study was to investigate the performance of the P-CAPT™ filter to capture PrPres from scrapie infected hamster brain homogenate mixed in leukoreduced human RBC as assessed by Western blot analysis. **Methods:** Hamster brain homogenate infected with the 263 K strain of scrapie was added to a unit of leukoreduced human RBC. The unit bag was sterile docked to a kit containing an in-line P-CAPT™ filter and a transfer bag to collect the treated RBC. The spiked RBC was filtered by gravity at ambient temperature according to the manufacturer's instructions. At the end of filtration the filter was extensively washed until most of the red blood cells were removed. The proteins captured by the filter were eluted for Western blot analysis using 3F4 antibody to specifically detect PrP.

Evaluations were also performed with two P-CAPT™ filters in series to investigate the level of PrPres removal provided by the filter. **Results:** Western blot analysis of the filter-bound proteins indicated that the P-CAPT™ filter captured brain PrPres from a unit of human leukoreduced RBC. The binding was reproducible within the experimental variability of the Western blot signal. Filtration time was also reproducible. In the experiments using series of filters, no detectable signal was observed in the following second filter. **Conclusions:** The studies described here demonstrated that the selected resin when incorporated into a filter was still capable of capturing brain PrPres. Furthermore, one P-CAPT™ filter removed all PrP input to the limit of detection of the Western blot.

P16.12

Collection, Manufacture, Consumption, Imports and Exports of Blood Components – Data Pursuant to Article 21 Transfusion Act (TFG) for 2003 and 2004

B. Haschberger, A. Waterkamp, J. Hesse, M. Heiden, R. Seitz
Paul-Ehrlich-Institut, Langen, D

Is Germany self-sufficient in the supply of blood products? How does the supply with blood products in Germany compare in the European context? The data collected by the Paul-Ehrlich-Institut (PEI) pursuant to Section 21 Transfusion Act (TFG) are designed to provide an overview on this issue. Whole blood donations still provide the basis for the supply with blood and blood products. In 2003, 54 whole blood donations were collected per 1,000 inhabitants, and in 2004, this figure was 58. As defined by the European Health Committee which considers 40–60 whole blood donations as sufficient for an optimum supply with blood products, blood supplies in Germany can be regarded as sufficient. The manufacture of erythrocyte concentrates (EC), the most important medicinal product derived from whole blood donations, is at the level of previous years, however, a peak value was reached in 2004 with 4.53 million transfusion units (TU). 4.24 million TU were manufactured in 2003. As in previous years, the consumption of EC reported to the Paul-Ehrlich-Institut was clearly lower with 44 or 43 TU per 1,000 inhabitants, respectively. This compares with an average consumption of EC of 35 units per 1,000 inhabitants for the whole of Europe. The quantity of plasma for fractionation for 2003 reached a peak of 2.4 million L, which is equivalent to an increase of 15% compared with 2002. For 2004, a slight negative trend of –4% can be recognised (2.3 million L plasma for fractionation). The increase in the amount of plasma 2003 compared with 2002 corresponds to figures in apheresis donations: In 2003 the apheresis donations are above 2.3 million and the portion of plasma for fractionation from apheresis was 62% (48% in 2004). The calculated amount of plasma for fractionation, taking into account the data for exports and imports, that would be available for the German market, would be 1.7 million L for 2003 and 2.1 million L for 2004. This means that according to the data available, more plasma for fractionation was manufactured in Germany than was required for further processing. This is also confirmed by the questions contained in the reporting questionnaire introduced in 2004, which refers to the actual amount of fractionated plasma in Germany. The evaluation of these data showed that 734,000 L plasma were processed in Germany, corresponding to roughly 1/3 of the amount that can be calculated from plasma available to the German market.

P16.13

Preoperative Autologous Blood Donation and Immunomodulation in Patients Undergoing Elective Hip Arthroplasty

R. Karger, C. Weber, J. Schmidt, V. Kretschmer
Philipps-Universität Marburg, D

Background: Preoperative autologous blood donation (PABD) has been shown to decrease NK cell function in cancer patients. It is unclear whether PABD leads to other immunomodulatory effects that might affect more short term risks like postoperative infectious complications in surgical patients. **Methods:** Leukocyte (granulocytes, lymphocytes, monocytes) and lymphocyte subsets (CD4 ± T-cells, CD8 ± T-cells, B-cells, NK cells) were determined in 86 consecutive patients donating 2 units of autologous whole blood, 500 mL each, in two successive weeks, two to five weeks prior to elective hip replacement surgery. In addition, in a random subgroup of 58 patients, tumour necrosis factor (TNF) secretion of monocytes upon stimulation with lipopolysaccharide, and interferon gamma (IFN-gamma), interleukin 2 (IL-2), IL-4, and IL-10 secretion of lymphocytes upon stimulation with either phytohaemagglutinin or concanavalin A were determined after 24-hour incubation in a whole blood cell suspension culture. Analyses were performed from samples taken before the first donation and on the day prior to operation. **Results:** The total number of leukocytes did not change between measurement time points: 6.7 (1.8) vs. 6.6 (2.0) G/L. The following changes were statistically significant with a Bonferroni adjusted p-value <0.01 (subset proportions are presented as means, with standard deviation in parentheses, TNF secretions presented as medians, with interquartile range given in parentheses): granulocytes increased from 63.3 (7.3) to 66.2 (7.9)% (+4.6%) during the donation phase; lymphocytes decreased from 29.4 (7.1) to 26.8 (7.6)% (−8.8%), accompanied by a relative increase of CD4 ± T-cells from 44.7 (9.4) to 49.5 (8.5)% (+10.7%) and B-cells from 11.6 (4.6) to 12.8 (4.7)% (+10.3%), and a remarkable fall in NK cells from 18.2 (8.4) to 14.4 (7.4)% (−20.9%); the stimulated TNF secretion of monocytes was suppressed from 9.45 (6.01) to 8.29 (7.27) nanograms per 1 million monocytes (−12.3%). The effect of PABD on cytokine secretion of lymphocytes and the Th1/Th2 balance was variable and was dependent on the antigenic stimulus used in vitro. **Conclusions:** In autologous blood donors, immunological changes occur, only part of which can be explained by psychological stress presumed to develop prior to surgery. Thus, donation of one litre of autologous blood within two weeks appears to modulate several parameters of the immune system of patients undergoing elective hip replacement surgery. Although the net effect and clinical relevance of these changes need further evaluation, this study suggests that PABD might influence the propensity to perioperative infectious complications

P16.14

Meningioma – HLA Phenotyping and Analyzing Potential Disease Associations

M. Tschigrjai
Winterbergkliniken, Saarbrücken, D

Several studies investigated the expression of human leukocyte antigens (HLA) and cytokine levels in tumors as well as meningiomas. Expression of HLA and modulated cytokine levels are important for the immune response against infectious agents and malignant cells and are found to influence the development and recurrence, respectively, of such diseases. However, only little is known about the effect of HLA-phenotype. Association of single HLA antigens or HLA haplotypes with disease has been investigated previously, and positive correlations between HLA and some cancers, such as cervical, nasopharyngeal carcinomas or glioma have been reported. The present investigation was aimed to study such correlations in 81 Caucasian patients with intracranial meningioma, an extracerebral tumor of mesenchymal origin compared with 157 Caucasian blood donors from the states Thuringia and Saxonia-Anhalt. Both standard serologic and PCR techniques for HLA typing were employed for all patients and controls. Our results suggest a positive association between single HLA antigens and presence of symptomatic meningioma. Compared with the control population, patients positive for HLA-A*02 had a 2.5-fold increased risk of meningioma ($p < 0.02$) and patients positive for HLA-DQB1*05 a 1.8-fold risk ($p < 0.05$), whereas HLA-A*01; HLA-B*08 and HLA-DRB1*03 were associated with a 0.4-fold decreased risk of meningioma ($p < 0.008$; $p < 0.05$ for the last two antigens). Occurrence rate of combinations and estimated haplotypes containing those HLA antigens were also different in meningioma patients. In conclusion our data suggest a background effect of HLA system on development of intracranial meningioma.

P16.15

The FCGR2A Gene Polymorphism: No Evidence for an Influence on Mortality in the Elderly

B. Flesch, S. Nikolaus, N.E. El Mokhtari, S. Schreiber, A. Nebel
University Hospital Schleswig-Holstein, Kiel, D

Background: Fc receptors for immunoglobulin G (FcgR) are potent links between the cellular and the humoral immune response. The functional single nucleotide polymorphism (SNP) rs1801274 (His131Arg) in the FCGR2A gene which encodes the FcgRIIa influences the efficiency of hIgG2-binding, the main isotype produced in response to encapsulated bacteria like Streptococcus pneumoniae and Haemophilus influenzae. In contrast to the receptor with the His131 allele, FcgRIIa-Arg131 binds hIgG2 poorly and carriers of this variant have been shown to be much more susceptible to succumb to bacterial pneumonia or meningitis. Since bacteremic pneumonia is one of the leading causes of death in elderly individuals, we hypothesized that the Arg131 variant could be a major mortality factor in the old. **Methods:** We analyzed the FCGR2A-His131Arg polymorphism (rs1801274) with a TaqMan® SNP Genotyping Assay in a group of 408 German centenarians and two samples of younger Germans aged 60–75 and 18–49 years, respectively. **Results:** No statistically significant differences were observed between the three age groups, neither at the allele nor at the genotype level. **Conclusion:** Apparently, the advantage of FcgRIIa-His131in the defense of life threatening infectious diseases like bacteremic pneumonia leaves the ability to attain old age largely unaffected.

P16.16

Successful Treatment of Patients with Autoimmune Thrombocytopenia with Subcutaneous Anti-D Injections

O. Meyer[1], H. Kiesewetter[1], M. Hermsen[2], P. Petriedes[3], M. Rose[4], H. Seibt[3], A. Salama[1]
[1]Charité, Universitätsmedizin Berlin, D; [2]Evangelisches Krankenhaus, Hamm, D; [3]Hämatologisch-onkologische Praxis, München, D; [4]Klinik für Kinder- und Jugendmedizin, Minden, D

Purpose: Intravenous (i.v.) anti-D is still used in the treatment of ITP. This treatment may results in fever, chills, headache, nausea, dizziness, intravascular haemolysis, and disseminated intravascular coagulation. We decided to investigate whether subcutaneous (s.c.) delivery could produce the beneficial effect of i.v. anti-D without these sequelae. **Patients and Methods:** Until now, a total of 24 Rh D-positive patients (three children and 21 adults) have been treated. The patients received 50 µg/kg anti-D (Rhophylac or Rhesogam, ZLB Bioplasma, Bern, Switzerland) within 3–5 min. subcutaneously. **Results:** The platelet count increased in 19 (79%) of the treated patients within one week after s.c. injection of anti-D. Three patients had previously been treated with i.v. anti-D and developed acute adverse reactions. These patients tolerated s.c. anti-D, and the effect was comparable to that observed with i.v. anti-D. The administered volume of anti-D was about 0.33 ml/kg, and was not associated with any local complication, and did not lead to a clinically relevant haemolysis in a single case. In addition, s.c. treatment was repeatedly effective in all patients who required retreatment. **Conclusion:** Although s.c. anti-D may take one or two days longer to reach maximum effect, a clinical effect seemed to take place within the first two days. This was supported by the fact that bleeding in affected patients completely vanished within two days, and by the fact the platelet count also began to increase within two days. Most importantly, patients treated with s.c. anti-D must not be monitored as closely for signs and symptoms of acute adverse reactions as those treated with i.v. anti-D.

P16.17

Induction of Significant Interferon-Alpha Production in Human Monocytes

L. Hansmann, S. Groeger, G. Bein, H. Hackstein
Justus Liebig University Gießen, D

Interferon-alpha (IFN-á) plays a critical role in anti-viral immunity and plasmacytoid DCs (pDCs) have been demonstrated to represent the principal source of this cytokine after Toll-like receptor (TLR) 7 and 9 stimulation. Our data show that human monocytes can be stimulated to produce high amounts of alpha-interferon after stimulation with Poly(I:C) and DOTAP (mediator of cellular uptake). Addition of DOTAP dramatically increased Poly(I:C)-induced IFN-á production of human monocytes (12-fold higher IFN-á production compared to Poly(I:C) alone). Using an array of TLR ligands, we reveal that Poly(I:C) and DOTAP represent the second strongest IFN-á stimulus in total peripheral blood mononuclear cells (PBMC), besides the pDC specific TLR9 ligand CpG-ODN2216 (CpG). This stimulus was able to induce approximately 1100 pg/ml IFN-á ($5*10^6$ PBMC/ml), compared to 4200 pg/ml after pDC specific CpG and 320 pg/ml after TLR7/8-ligand (ssRNA/R848). Therefore, Poly(I:C) and DOTAP are able to induce approximately three times more IFN-á in total PBMC when compared to TLR7 stimulation of pDC. Sorting experiments revealed that untouched monocytes are the main IFN-á producers after Poly(I:C) and DOTAP stimulation. These results were confirmed on a single cell basis by ELISpot analysis after Poly(I:C)/DOTAP stimulation. Additional analysis of the influence of more than 30 different cytokines on Poly(I:C)/DOTAP-induced IFN-á in monocytes indicated only IFN-â1a as a moderate enhancer and TNF-á as a weak suppressor of IFN-á production. To further characterize IFN-á production in PBMC we used ELIspot technique that showed the highest spot number after Poly(I:C)/DOTAP stimulation followed by R848 and CpG. Finally we compared IFN-á production in 40,000 highly purified pDCs and untouched monocytes using IFN-á specific ELISA. PDCs stimulated with CpG produced unsurpassed IFN-á amounts (32,000 pg/ml) followed by R848-stimulated pDCs (957 pg/ml) and Poly(I:C)-DOTAP-stimulated monocytes (200 pg/ml). Although pDCs stimulated with CpG or R848 produce the highest IFN-á amounts per cell, in total PBMC monocytes can be stimulated to produce more IFN-á than R848-stimulated pDC. We suggest that human monocytes represent the second major leukocyte subset producing IFN-á after viral infection.

P16.18

Ferritin Levels of Blood Donors (Whole Blood, Apheresis, Double Red Cells), A 2 Year Observation

C. Stebler, L. Infanti, B. Eiche, M. Santoro, H. Lüscher, M. Rüesch
Blutspendezentrum SRK Beider Basel, Basel, CH

Purpose: Donor safety, especially in regard of iron depletion is becoming a major concern, especially in the double red cell donation. To evaluate the extent of iron depletion in different blood donation types, ferritin data should be compared to the equivalent data in regular whole blood donors (WB). **Methods:** Since Jan. 2004 ferritin (ng/L), haemoglobin (Hb, g/dL) and MCV (fL) levels were measured at each donation, independent from the donation type. This allowed a comparison of iron status in WB donors, double red cell donors (DRC) and apheresis donors for plasma and platelets. Repeat donors and first time donors were analyzed separately, allowing a control of normal values in a random population. A subgroup of female WB donors with haemoglobin count above 12 g/dL and low ferritin levels presenting possible symptoms of iron deficiency was followed up. **Results:** Values as average (±SD) in first time donors:ferritin 83 ng/L (±43), Hb15.7 g/dL (±0.96), MCV 88 fL (±3) in 745 males and ferritin 30 ng/L (±23), Hb 13.7 g/dL (±0.95), MCV 89 fL (±4) in 1003 females.

Repeat donors ferritin/Hb/MCV
1st donation whole blood (n = 2614) 43/15.2/87
2nd donation whole blood (n = 2614) 36/15.2/87, ferritin drop 14.5%
3rd donation whole blood (n = 2126) 31/15.2/88, ferritin drop 14.3%
4th donation whole blood (n = 1704) 29/15.4/88, ferritin drop 6.9%
5th donation whole blood (n = 1307) 28/15.3/89, ferritin drop 4.4%
1st donation DRC (n = 338) 60/15.7/88
2nd donation DRC (n = 308) 53/15.8/89, ferritin drop 11.6%

3rd donation DRC (n = 137) 51/15.9/89, ferritin drop 5.4%
4th donation DRC (n = 22) 44/15.8/89, ferritin drop 13.6%

The ferrtitin drop between the first WB donation and the third was 26%, compared to 11.6% in DRC at the second donation. After 5 WB donations 11%, compared to the equal amount of DRC donation at 5.4%. A subgroup of 34 female regular WB donors with an average haemoglobin count of 13.2 g/dL (±0.72) and average ferritin of 5 ng/L (±1.7) presented symptoms of iron depletion. After oral iron substitution average haemoglobin was 14.2 g/L (±0.8) and ferritin 22 ng/L (±8.5). **Conclusions:** The first time donors have shown surprisingly low average ferritin levels for female and male compared to the given standards of 20–200 ng/L. Haemoglobin and MCV values were still normal. The 34 female WB donors needed 4 months of oral iron substitution to correct their ferritin levels. This shows the advantage of baseline ferritin levels in blood donors in order to prevent iron depletion causing deferral from blood donation. Our data do not confirm the fear of greater iron depletion after DRC donation.

Transfusion Medicine and Hemotherapy

Author Index · Autorenverzeichnis

KARGER
Fax +49 761 4 52 07 14
E-Mail Information@karger.de
www.karger.com

Accessible online at:
www.karger.com/tmh